The Mangled Extremity

Raymond A. Pensy • John V. Ingari

Editors

The Mangled Extremity

Evaluation and Management

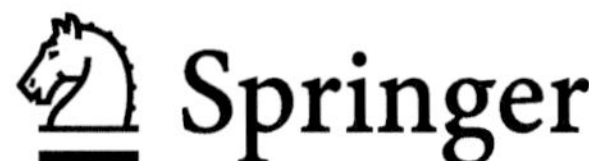

Springer

Editors
Raymond A. Pensy
Department of Orthopaedic Surgery
R Adams Cowley Shock Trauma Center
Baltimore, MD
USA

John V. Ingari
Hand Surgery Division
Department of Orthopaedic Surgery
Sinai Hospital of Baltimore
Baltimore, MD
USA

ISBN 978-3-319-56647-4   ISBN 978-3-319-56648-1   (eBook)
https://doi.org/10.1007/978-3-319-56648-1

This Springer imprint is published by the registered company Springer Nature Switzerland AG
The registered company address is: Gewerbestrasse 11, 6330 Cham, Switzerland

To my wife, Mara, who has made everything I hold dear possible.
– Raymond A. Pensy

*This book could not have happened without the steadfast
support of my wife, Arlene, undeniably my best friend.*
– John (Jack) Ingari, MD

Preface

Alacrity. Detail. Patience.

It is my hope that the reader has heard, annunciated, and professed these words in the operating room prior to handling this text, as these words hold what we the authors believe to be at the core of successful limb salvage efforts and the treatise that follows.

Alacrity: n.1. A cheerful readiness, willingness, or promptitude.

Those charged with the care of the patient with a mangled extremity know this attribute is central to success. A limb, particularly the hand and arm, represents an integral part of human identity. Thus, the physician presented with the mangled upper or lower extremity, rendered to a disorganized collection of torn sinew and shattered bone after massive trauma, reflexively feels the weight of sorrow and depression realizing that their patient has forever lost a portion of their identity and capability. For what possibly amounts to a select few physicians, however, another reflex will similarly occur, one which prompts these individuals to manifest an almost cheerful readiness to put the pieces together, to teach others what they have learned in so doing, and to investigate ways in which to improve the process. Alacrity.

Detail: n. 1. A particular fact or item of information, often noticed only after giving something close attention, or such facts or items considered as a group.

Few would argue that the disciplines of human anatomy, physiology, and psychology represent a seemingly infinite complexity. Students of anatomy recognize that the components of our species, not to mention their physiologic interplay and incorporation with the human psyche, are nearly endless, and complete comprehension of the parts alone for any one individual is virtually impossible. Perhaps it is this challenge, a recognition that improvements in skill and outcome can be achieved with a deeper and more comprehensive understanding of the particular facts that make us "tick," which provides additional motivation to the surgeon who commits to limb salvage. Restoring these pieces of bone, nerve, tendon, and vessel, to provide the most benefit to the patient, requires a watchmaker's attentiveness to individual components. "Operating on a hand without a tourniquet is like trying to fix a watch in an inkwell" – *Sterling Bunnell, MD*. Detail.

Patience: n.1. The capacity to endure what is difficult or disagreeable without complaining.

The ability to persist in the face of difficulty is a common trait among surgeons, so basic and integral for the limb salvage specialist that it goes almost without mention. Understanding the human body's remarkable healing potential and the surgical methods to effect positive change represents a substantial portion of this discipline. The surgeon who faces the mangled limb must also understand *when* to intervene, as there are instances where any given surgical technique may be best suited as the first intervention, or the last intervention, depending on the exact circumstances, as well as the needs and wishes of the patient. Undoubtedly, the mangled limb will require many interventions, and the carefully prescribed timeliness of these operations and therapies is learned only through experience. Patience.

Finally, my suggestion to those who embark on this work is to remember that we, as physicians, treat patients as a whole. Perhaps one of the most challenging aspects of this work is to remember that the technical refinements of skeletal, vascular, and microsurgery, learned through years of training and experience, must go hand in hand with a comprehension of the overall well-being of the patient. The physical, psychological, and social needs must be carefully balanced, as every patient that presents with a limb that could either be salvaged or amputated warrants careful assessment and education, to ensure that the patient and family, to the best of our ability, understand the risks, cost, and duration of our attempts at preserving a limb.

Raymond A. Pensy
Department of Orthopaedic Surgery
R Adams Cowley Shock Trauma Center
Baltimore, MD, USA

Contents

Contributors

Ashley B. Anderson, MD Walter Reed National Military Medical Center, Department of Surgery, Division of Orthopaedics, Bethesda, MD, USA

Uniformed Services University, Bethesda, MD, USA

Michael J. Assayag International Center for Limb Lengthening, Rubin Institute for Advanced Orthopedics, Sinai Hospital of Baltimore, Baltimore, MD, USA

Keith T. Aziz Department of Orthopaedic Surgery, The Johns Hopkins University, Baltimore, MD, USA

Oded Ben-Amotz Department of Orthopaedic Surgery, University of Pennsylvania, Philadelphia, PA, USA

Michael J. Bosse Atrium Health – Carolinas Medical Center, Charlotte, NC, USA

Kevin Carroll Hanger Clinic, New York, NY, USA

Renan C. Castillo Health Policy and Management, Johns Hopkins Bloomberg School of Public Health, Baltimore, MD, USA

Janet D. Conway International Center for Limb Lengthening, Rubin Institute for Advanced Orthopedics, Sinai Hospital of Baltimore, Baltimore, MD, USA

Joseph Dubose Department of Surgery, Uniformed Services University of the Health Sciences, Baltimore, MD, USA

John C. Dun William Beaumont Army Medical Center, El Paso, TX, USA

Uniformed Services University of the Health Sciences, Bethesda, MD, USA

W. Andrew Eglseder Department of Orthopaedics, University of Maryland Medical System, Baltimore, MD, USA

Jonathan A. Forsberg, MD, PhD Walter Reed National Military Medical Center, Department of Surgery, Division of Orthopaedics, Bethesda, MD, USA

Uniformed Services University, Bethesda, MD, USA

Department of Orthopaedic Surgery, Johns Hopkins University, Baltimore, MD, USA

Alexander Hahn Orthopaedics, University of Maryland Medical Center, Baltimore, MD, USA

John E. Herzenberg International Center for Limb Lengthening, Rubin Institute for Advanced Orthopedics, Sinai Hospital of Baltimore, Baltimore, MD, USA

Steven A. Horton Department of Orthopaedics, University of Maryland Medical Center, Baltimore, MD, USA

John V. Ingari Hand Surgery Division, Department of Orthopaedic Surgery, Sinai Hospital of Baltimore, Baltimore, MD, USA

Ryan Katz The Curtis National Hand Center, MedStar Union Memorial Hospital, Baltimore, MD, USA

Lauren E. King Rehabilitation Services, University of Maryland Medical Center, Baltimore, MD, USA

Tyler Klenow Martin Bionics Innovations, Clinical Care, Tampa, FL, USA

Stephen J. Kovach Department of Surgery, Division of Plastic Surgery, University of Pennsylvania, Philadelphia, PA, USA

Erwin A. Kruger Department of Orthopaedic Surgery, University of Pennsylvania, Philadelphia, PA, USA

Chris Langhammer University of Maryland, Department of Orthopaedics, Baltimore, MD, USA

L. Scott Levin Department of Orthopaedic Surgery, University of Pennsylvania, Philadelphia, PA, USA

Department of Surgery, Division of Plastic Surgery, University of Pennsylvania, Philadelphia, PA, USA

Naji Madi Department of Orthopaedic Surgery, Rutgers University, Newark, NJ, USA

Theodore T. Manson Towson Orthopaedic Associates, University of Maryland St. Joseph Medical Center, Department of Orthopaedic Surgeon, Towson, MD, USA

Lucas S. Marchand Department of Orthopaedic Surgery, University of Utah, Salt Lake City, UT, USA

Anna McGinnis Health Policy and Management, Johns Hopkins Bloomberg School of Public Health, Baltimore, MD, USA

Shaun D. Mendenhall Department of Orthopaedic Surgery, University of Pennsylvania, Philadelphia, PA, USA

Manas Nigam Department of Plastic and Reconstructive Surgery, MedStar Georgetown University Hospital, Washington, DC, USA

Ebrahim Paryavi Orthopaedic Surgery, Alaska Native Medical Center, Anchorage, AK, USA

Raymond A. Pensy Department of Orthopaedic Surgery, R Adams Cowley Shock Trauma Center, Baltimore, MD, USA

John Rheinstein Hanger Clinic, New York, NY, USA

Jessica C. Rivera International Center for Limb Lengthening, Rubin Institute for Advanced Orthopedics, Sinai Hospital of Baltimore, Baltimore, MD, USA

Anna Romagnoli R Adams Cowley Shock Trauma Center, University of Maryland Medical System, Baltimore, MD, USA

Thomas Scalea R Adams Cowley Shock Trauma Center, University of Maryland Medical System, Baltimore, MD, USA

Marcus F. Sciadini R Adams Cowley Shock Trauma Center, Department of Orthopaedics, University of Maryland School of Medicine, Baltimore, MD, USA

Jaimie T. Shores Department of Plastic and Reconstructive Surgery, The Johns Hopkins University School of Medicine, Baltimore, MD, USA

Phil Stevens Department of Clinical and Scientific Affiars, Hanger Inc., Salt Lake City, UT, USA

Scott M. Tintle Uniformed Services University of the Health Sciences, Bethesda, MD, USA

Walter Reed National Military Medical Center, Bethesda, MD, USA

Rebuilding the Mangled Extremity: Foundation to Rooftop

Naji Madi and Raymond A. Pensy

Definition

Permitting/Planning Job Site

The human limb, particularly the upper extremity, provides the individual the obvious ability to interact with the environment through endless manners of work, play, communication, and self-care. The extremities provide us with much of our identity, both in the obvious sense of physical attribute, but perhaps much further in regard to how we manifest ourselves in each of the above activities [1, 2]. Loss of part or all of the function of a limb is therefore devastating, both psychologically and physically [3]. The many millions of hours and dollars invested in researching the cause, treatment, and outcomes of these injuries underscore the importance of this work [4, 5].

Several large, multi-center, prospective studies [6, 7] have demonstrated that the decision between limb salvage and amputation is far from straightforward. The interplay of the integral physical components of bone, skin, muscle, etc., cannot be isolated from the psychological and social components when comparing outcomes

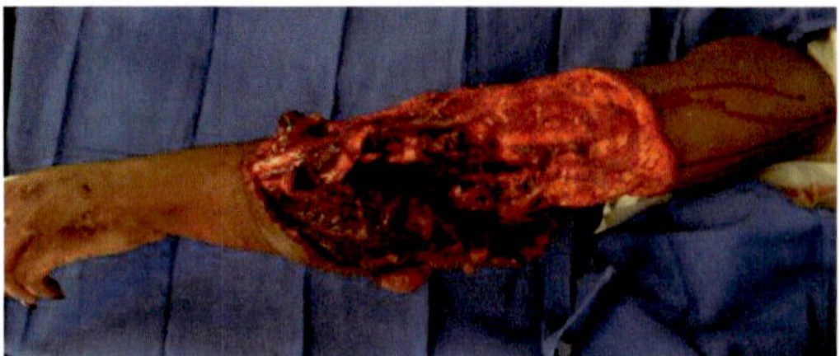

Fig. 1.1 An 18-year-old female with crush injury to her left forearm and typical presentation of mangled extremity with soft tissue, bone, nerve, and vessel injuries

and therefore must also be considered when treating the patient [6, 8]. That being said, the decision to amputate or attempt salvage should begin with a definition, an understanding of how to evaluate to the extremity, and the overall framework of what salvage might entail, so that, at the very least, an educated discussion can be held with the patient on a case-by-case basis and in the hopes of improved future investigations. The bone, soft tissue (muscle, skin, tendon, ligament), vessel, and nerve comprise the key basic components of the limb. It is defined as mangled when three or more of these core four components have been traumatized [9] (Fig. 1.1). The mangled extremity is immediately recognized by the experienced surgeon and the novice alike. The shape and character of the wound are often overwhelming: making sense of the contorted and disfigured limb is often impossible at first. Often covered in blood and debris, torn clothing, sometimes shrapnel, with exposed bone and internal structures,

N. Madi
Department of Orthopaedic Surgery, Rutgers University, Newark, NJ, USA

R. A. Pensy (✉)
Department of Orthopaedic Surgery, R Adams Cowley Shock Trauma Center, Baltimore, MD, USA
e-mail: rpensy@som.umaryland.edu

© Springer Nature Switzerland AG 2021
R. A. Pensy, J. V. Ingari (eds.), *The Mangled Extremity*, https://doi.org/10.1007/978-3-319-56648-1_1

Table 1.1 Comparison of limb salvage phases to construction phases

Phase of construction	Phase of limb salvage
Plans/permitting	Physical exam X-rays, CT, angiogram/consent
Site location	OR set-up: good lighting, right team, radiolucent tables, tourniquet control
Excavation	Debridement
Foundation	Skeletal repair (external, IM, and internal fixation methods)
Plumbing	Arterial reconstruction and hemostasis (suture ligature, vein grafting, shunts, thrombectomy catheters, etc.)
Electrical	Nerve reconstruction (repair, grafting)
Interior finish	Tendon repair/grafting
Exterior finish	Skin (primary closure, temporizing VAC, grafting, flap)

presents even the seasoned clinician a "chaotic" appearance that initially is a struggle at best in discerning salvageable parts, let alone those that can be brought back together as a functional unit.

Thus, a mangled limb can only be effectively deemed salvageable by an experienced surgeon in an environment that permits some "control": an operating room that can provide sufficient lighting, limited external distraction, appropriate tests, and operative inspection. During the above maneuvers, it is mandatory that the surgeon takes inventory of critical structures necessary for salvage and function. This assessment is often only thoroughly achieved when one has completed removal of debris and frankly non-viable tissue. The remaining inventory of viable components will vary enormously based upon the injury mechanism and the degree of contamination. This process of debridement, although the most difficult to study in its effect on successful limb salvage, is widely believed to be the single most important step in the initial treatment of the mangled limb [10].

The planning for reconstruction of the mangled limb is analogous to that required for the construction of a residential home. Although far more complex, the similarities between the functional limb and a quality home construction provide a rationale framework of thinking and an educational tool and provide the outline for the remainder of the text (Table 1.1).

Phases of Limb Salvage

Starting with planning and "permitting," an understanding of the mechanism of injury (crush, sharp or ballistic penetrating, avulsion, etc.) is critical, as well as a thorough physical examination and understanding of the patients traumatized state. As discussed in the next chapter, the patient's physiology will frequently determine the initial course of action and recommendations [9]. Radiographs, Doppler exam, and possible angiogram [11, 12] are frequently useful in providing definitive objective measures of the degree of injury to the bone and artery (Figs. 1.2, 1.3, and 1.4).

This can provide the surgeon the ability to provide at least a preliminary informed consent (permit) to the patient for the initial surgical effort, but the degree of muscle loss, nerve, or tendon injury, can be very difficult to assess from the clinical exam and initial tests alone. Therefore, the consent should be broad and empathetic. These initial steps are paramount [13].

Many authors have suggested scoring systems to aid in the management of mangled extremities including the Predictive Salvage Index (PSI) [14], the Mangled Extremity Severity Score (MESS) [15], the Limb Salvage Index (LSI) [16], and the Nerve injury, Ischemia, Soft tissue contamination, Skeletal injury, Shock, and Age (NISSA) [17]. However, these indices are complex, do not show consistent reproducible results, and lack validation using large cohorts [9, 18]. In some ways, these scoring systems promote the formation of an "inventory"; which is essential to formulating a rational treatment plan, similar to algorithm delineated in Table 1.1.

The operating room (site location) requires an experienced and well-trained team, as well as the necessary equipment. Individuals familiar with skeletal, vascular, and soft tissue surgery, including the anesthesia providers, nurses, radiology

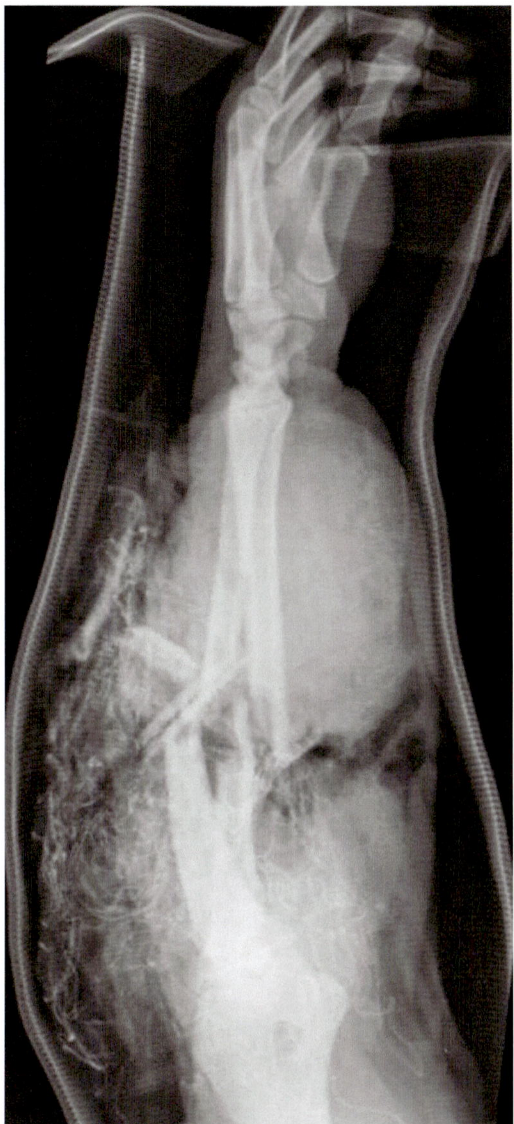

Fig. 1.2 Lateral radiograph of a mangled forearm taken in a sugar tong splint. Comminuted fractures of both bones with ventral and dorsal soft tissue defects

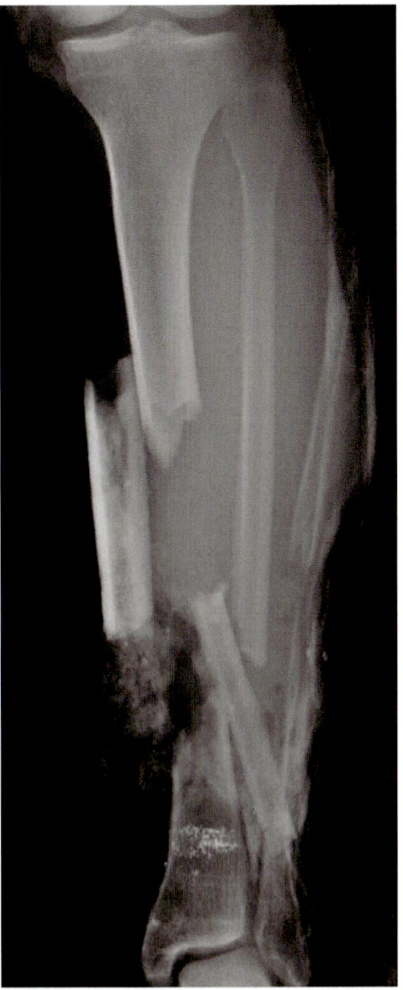

Fig. 1.3 Antero-posterior radiograph of a mangled leg showing segmented, displaced tibial, and fibular shaft fractures with bone loss and soft tissue defects

technicians, and circulators, are key to success, much as would be the right team for any phase of home building. Similarly, the location of these requisite procedures requires forethought—an operating room with sufficient space for fluoroscopy, possible angiography, and available space for instrumentation should be the "job site" for the limb salvage surgeon. Excellent lighting, pneumatic tourniquets, and radiolucent operating tables are essential.

Debridement (Excavation)

The debridement that occurs immediately, or in conjunction with initial revascularization, cannot be over-emphasized [19, 20]. A thorough knowledge of the surgical planes, neurovascular structures, muscular innervation, origins, and insertions is essential to completing a safe, effective, and thorough debridement. The surgical approach to the un-injured limb is far easier than the one contorted and twisted, crushed, or partially avulsed. Nonete-less, "avoiding cutting round structures" is paramount. In order to do so, tourniquet control

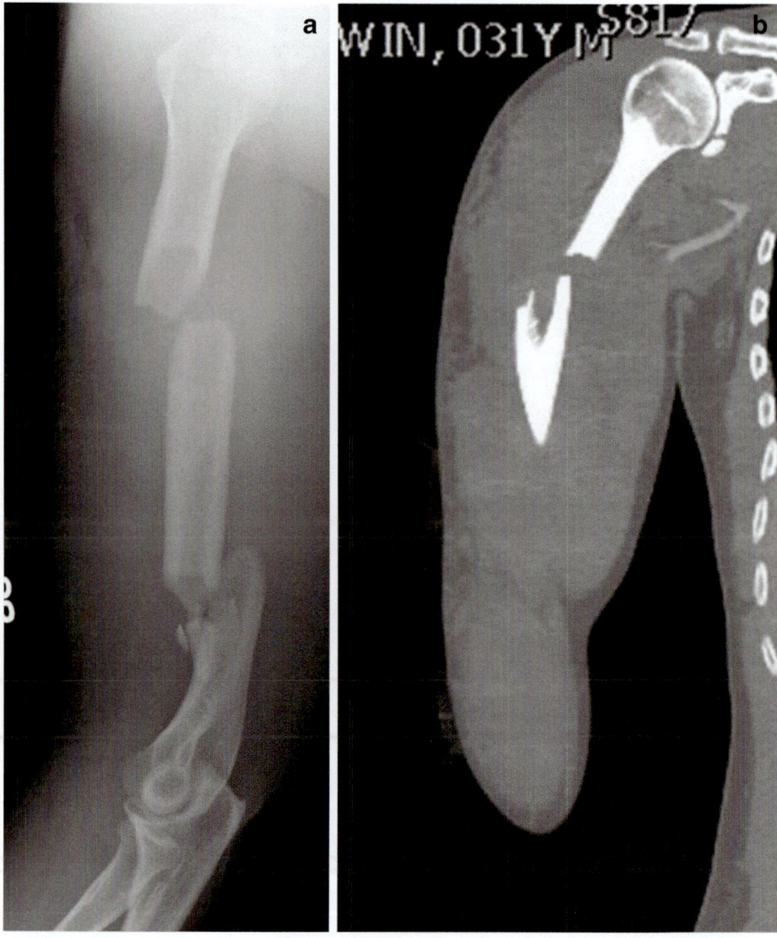

Fig. 1.4 (**a**) Lateral radiograph of the arm showing segmental displaced humeral shaft fracture. (**b**) Coronal reconstruction of a computed tomographic angiogram, showing disruption of the brachial artery and an inferior glenoid fracture

is preferred. In certain instances, particularly those in which ischemia is significant and protracted, re-perfusion via shunting and completing the surgical effort without tourniquet is preferred. In the vast majority of cases, however, it is the author's opinion that tourniquet control affords the surgeon a bloodless field, critical to the identification of critical structures (particularly nerves) and appropriate planes. Once the surgeon has identified those structures within or coursing through the zone of injury, then, and only then, can an effective debridement be completed. A transected nerve results in a permanent and immediate deficit, whereas non-viable muscle or debris left within a wound will invariably result in suppuration, which in turn may render the limb non-salvageable and difficult to justify.

A good debridement must be emphasized. As described above, the use of a tourniquet and thorough knowledge of anatomy will, in most cases, prevent iatrogenic injury to critical neurovascular structures. The author believes that there are generally two types of wounds associated with open fractures: those which will require a marginal excision and those which require radical excision. Those open fractures which represent a simple "inside-out" mechanism with minimal contamination, degloving, periosteal stripping, and devitilization will do well with simply performing a standard approach to the fracture, while removing a minimal amount of the skin, subcutaneous tissue, muscle, and bone, without necessarily beginning the plane of dissection through completely normal tissue. Other injuries, as the result of blast, shot gun, crush via roll-over, fork lift, entrapment, high velocity gun shot, and particularly those with significant ground in foreign debris, will require a radical excision. This dissection must occur as if the surgeon is resecting a cancer, and the surgeon should assume that any remaining cancer will *only* result in positive margins, requiring re-resection at best, and at worst, end in amputation or possibly fatality.

For the marginal excision, the author prefers to use a scalpel to sharply debride skin until there is demonstrable bleeding. Anything less will eventually result in necrosis, with the devastating effects of exposed hardware, tendon, or bone. These tissues will quickly dissecate and rendered functionally useless. Similarly, the muscle is debrided until there is obvious bleeding. The muscle must be contractile and bleeding, or it is removed. Anything less will at best result in suppuration, fever, and pain and, at worst, result in metabolic instability, sepsis, and possibly death. Regarding muscle, the author prefers the use of either the bovie, scalpel, or rongeur. Dead muscle is quickly debrided with prejudice and sharply with scissors or scalpel or with bovie electrocautery. The muscle of questionable viability is debrided with rongeur, as the consistency and tenacity of healthy muscle will resist the rongeur, whereas necrotic muscle quickly leaves the patient. For the bone, the author prefers the use of a 4 mm high-speed burr, and the "paprika" sign of punctate bleeding from the bone guides the depth of resection. In the author's experience, the bone end associated with open fracture and extruded through skin is *not* viable beyond a cm or so from that stripped of periosteum. Although difficult for the bone surgeon to acquiesce to the debridement of substantial quantities of bone, particularly of the bone surrounding or supporting a joint, there is no excuse for abscess secondary to residual dead—(non-bleeding)—tissue.

For those massive open fractures which require radical resection, the dissection is begun deliberately through normal tissue planes. Those injuries which result in the loss of an entire compartment require a debridement in which the surgeon and patient must anticipate loss of a degree of function in order to an attempt to preserve their limb (and possibly life). All non-critical structures are removed through a normal plane. This includes the skin, muscle, bone, artery, and vein if necessary. These tissues are deemed to be non-critical. There are reliable methods for reconstruction. These efforts, although challenging and protracted, are either doubled or rendered impossible if infection ensues. Nerve is generally the only structure not sharply debrided. Critical nerves are isolated both proximal and distal to the zone of injury and carefully dissected from the proposed resection. Nerve may remain viable and functional for 15–20 to cm or more, even if devoid of surrounding soft tissue. Reversed vein grafts for arterial reconstruction of 20 cm or more are readily employed for a period of 24–48 hours, provided that a soft tissue envelope can be restored, as discussed in subsequent chapters. In every case where infection ensues, the surgeon must assume responsibility and admit that an inadequate debridement was completed. In some instances, the only adequate debridement is that of amputation.

The author would suggest that the surgeons' favorite "anti-biotic" should be stainless steel (or other means of accomplishing effective debridement), as no bacteria has yet found to be resistant. Further, no antibiotic is found capable of compensating for an inadequate debridement. Finally, in accomplishing debridement, provided adequate hemostasis, the surgeons' instruments do not impart toxicity to the patient, nor is there any known allergy.

Skeletal Fixation (Foundation)

Initiating reconstruction of the traumatized and mangled limb requires a foundation, first and foremost. Regardless of injury mechanism, stability must be achieved in order to achieve any further reconstructive efforts [21]. The injured skeleton, lacking normal alignment and rigidity, will not facilitate or promote subsequent efforts, particularly those involving revascularization (plumbing). Skeletal stability can be achieved through a variety of methods, which in turn will be discussed specific to the upper and lower extremity, in later chapters. Whichever method is chosen, it should provide the necessary framework for subsequent surgical effort, align the skeleton in as close to a physiologic normalcy as possible, and preserve the required vascularity for bone and soft tissue healing. Any experienced home-builder or engineer recognizes that only a "true," plumb, and level foundation will permit aesthetic and functional quality without unnecessary revisions and delays.

Subsequent chapters will elucidate the choices of temporizing vs definitive fixation strategies and the differences between upper and lower extremity salvage.

Arterial Injury (Plumbing)

Ensuring arterial inflow is critical. This assessment will have been initiated prior to the operating room [11], and in many cases, abnormalities such as "kinked" vessels secondary to skeletal malalignment can be corrected with simple reduction maneuvers and skeletal stabilization. In cases in which the arterial inflow of a limb remains questionable, immediate exploration, repair, and/or grafting is indicated. The timing of these interventions may vary from patient to patient. However, in every case, a fractured skeleton must in some way be addressed to prevent the disruption of the rela-

tively fragile vascular reconstruction. In certain cases, arterial inflow may be established as the first surgical maneuver (e.g., shunt) [22]. For the critically or "absolutely" ischemic limb, tissue necrosis is ongoing and time dependent, affecting those tissues most dependent on oxidative metabolism. Thus, shunting may be employed as soon as the two ends of a critical vessel are visualized, prior to any significant debridement or skeletal stabilization.

Nerve Injury (Electrical)

The mangled limb's innervation will often be the primary determinant of overall outcome. Confirming integrity of the injured limb's nerve supply is often complicated by the fact that the severely traumatized patient cannot give an adequate, voluntary exam. These patients are often obtunded, sedated, or intubated by the time an extremity surgeon arrives at bedside. Although infrequently definitively addressed during the index operation, taking inventory of the critical nerves of the upper and lower extremity is mandatory. There is often no better time in making an assessment as to what residual function/dysfunction might ensue than during the initial inspection of the injured limb under tourniquet control to assess nerves that may have been lacerated, avulsed, or crushed. This assessment should proceed carefully when debriding non-viable muscle within the zone of injury, to demonstrate that the nerve remains viable. Frequently, skeletal stabilization maneuvers will interfere with further and repeat assessment of these nerves, and as noted above, clinical examination by the expert consultant may or may not occur in the poly-traumatized patient until after the patient is anesthetized and, in some case, until other life-saving and limb-stabilizing maneuvers. In regard to the severed nerve, it is worth mentioning that nerve reconstruction can be greatly facilitated by maintaining a relative anatomic location of the nerve and

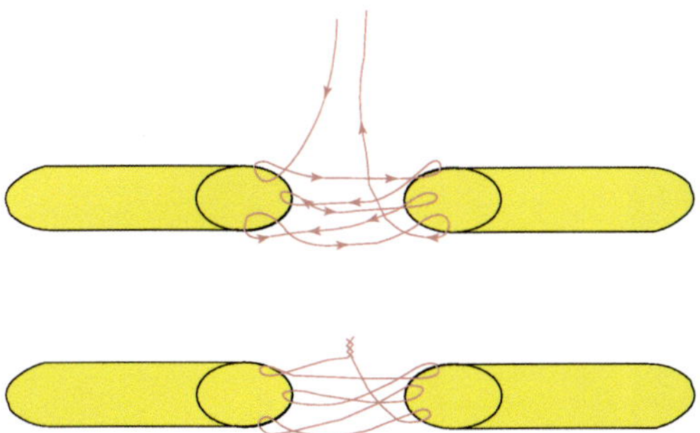 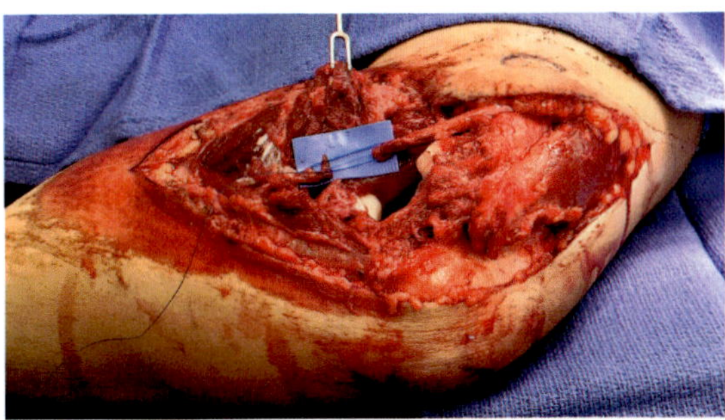

Fig. 1.5 Diagramattic and clinical representation of provisional spanning neurorrhaphy

appropriate tension [23]. "Physiologic tensioning" of the nerve can be achieved by the non-micro surgeon using 6-0 mono-filament poly-propylene suture. In this manner, the surgeon simply "bridges" the ends of a severed nerve with multiple passes of an epineural suture, bringing the nerve ends into relative and reasonable proximity, such that the nerve lays within a single dissection plane. The tension imparted should be "physiologic." This is completed by approximating transected nerves without gap in cases of sharp transection and to a gap distance equal to that of the debridement or that distance expected from the avulsion or loss of tissue. In this way, the nerve ends do not retract unnecessarily, incurring significantly more graft or precluding primary repair until such time that definitive coverage can be achieved and formal nerve repair or reconstruction completed (Fig. 1.5a, b).

Wound Coverage (Fascia/Roof)

Obtaining an appropriate "roof" or coverage for the limb is vital, and a number of soft tissue coverage options will be elucidated in later chapters.

It is worth mentioning, however, that the longevity of any skeletal, nerve, tendon, or vascular reconstruction will only be as successful as the durable barrier to the external environment that prevents desiccation and infection. For this reason, substantial thought and planning must be given to how to achieve skin closure and coverage, preferably with healthy and viable skin or muscle which will also allow permit subsequent planned (or unplanned!) secondary interventions. Temporizing wound coverage methods, such as antibiotic impregnated cement beads contained within an impermeable dressing, a.k.a. "bead-pouch," and vacuum-assisted closure devices, each have their role as temporizing methods [24, 25]. As these are non-physiologic and non-living, they cannot obviously provide durable coverage, immune system constituents, the delivery of peripherally administered antibiotics, or, for that matter, the multitude of other critical cytokines and factors required for successful healing. These methods should be looked upon as only temporary, until such time more advanced and definitive reconstructive options are appropriate.

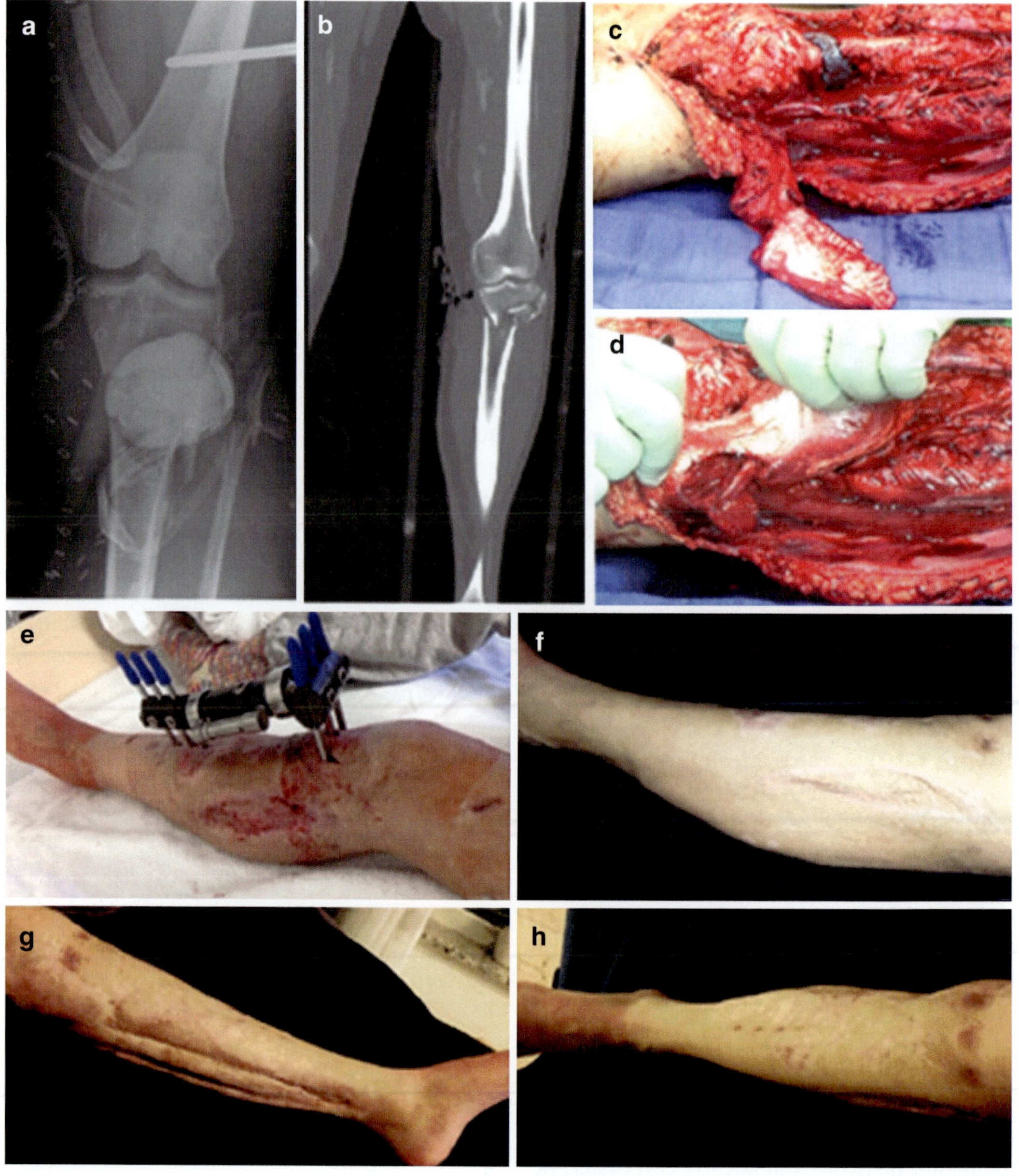

Case 1.1

An 18-year-old female student was struck by a car, sustaining a mangling left leg injury. The thigh and foot appear otherwise intact, with a zone of injury limited to the knee region.

(**a**) Radiographs reveal proximal tibia and fibula fractures, with dislocation of the proximal tibiofibular articulation. (**b**) Coronal cut of the left lower extremity CT scan showing the proximal tibia fracture. CTA confirms disruption of the popliteal artery.

Immediate knee spanning external fixation is completed, and reconstruction of the popliteal artery is completed with reversed ipsilateral saphenous vein graft.

Skeletal and soft tissue debridement results in a large popliteal defect with exposed antibiotic spacer and vein graft.

(**c**, **d**) Careful surgical dissection and appropriate debridement preserved the medial sural artery and the bulk of the medial gastrocnemius, permitting a local rotational medical gastrocnemius flap to provide adequate soft tissue coverage.

Temporizing allograft skin is applied to the open areas, which is then removed at 7 days postoperatively after the vascular reconstruction has matured and swelling partially resolved and replaced with autograft skin. (**e**) Her frame is converted to a non-knee spanning external fixation and bone grafting completed 3 months later, (**f–h**) resulting in a healed tibia and permitting full weight bearing, permitting this young woman to return to dental school

References

1. Salminger S, Sturma A, Roche AD, et al. Functional and psychosocial outcomes of hand transplantation compared with prosthetic fitting in below-elbow amputees: a multicenter cohort study. PLoS One. 2016;11(9):e0162507.
2. Ostlie K, Franklin RJ, Skjeldal OH, et al. Assessing physical function in adult acquired major upper-limb amputees by combining the Disabilities of the Arm, Shoulder and Hand (DASH) outcome questionnaire and clinical examination. Arch Phys Med Rehabil. 2011;92(10):1636–45.
3. Galanakos SP, Bot AG, Zoubos AB, et al. Psychological and social consequences after reconstruction of upper extremity trauma: methods of detection and management. J Reconstr Microsurg. 2014;30(3):193–206.
4. Tennent DJ, Wenke JC, Rivera JC, et al. Characterisation and outcomes of upper extremity amputations. Injury. 2014;45(6):965–9.
5. Chen MW, Narayan D. Economics of upper extremity replantation: national and local trends. Plast Reconstr Surg. 2009;124(6):2003–11.
6. Bosse MJ, MacKenzie EJ, Kellam JF, et al. An analysis of outcomes of reconstruction or amputation after leg-threatening injuries. N Engl J Med. 2002;347(24):1924–31.
7. Pet MA, Morrison SD, Mack JS, et al. Comparison of patient-reported outcomes after traumatic upper extremity amputation: replantation versus prosthetic rehabilitation. Injury. 2016;47(12):2783–8.
8. Doukas WC, Hayda RA, Frisch HM, et al. The Military Extremity Trauma Amputation/Limb Salvage (METALS) study: outcomes of amputation versus limb salvage following major lower-extremity trauma. J Bone Joint Surg Am. 2013;95(2):138–45.
9. Prasarn ML, Helfet DL, Kloen P. Management of the mangled extremity. Strategies Trauma Limb Reconstr. 2012;7(2):57–66.
10. Godina M. Early microsurgical reconstruction of complex trauma of the extremities. Plast Reconstr Surg. 1986;78(3):285–92.
11. Peng PD, Spain DA, Tataria M, et al. CT angiography effectively evaluates extremity vascular trauma. Am Surg. 2008;74(2):103–7.
12. Applebaum R, Yellin AE, Weaver FA, et al. Role of routine arteriography in blunt lower-extremity trauma. Am J Surg. 1990;160(2):221–4.
13. Bernstein ML, Chung KC. Early management of the mangled upper extremity. Injury. 2007;38(Suppl 5):S3–7.
14. Howe HR Jr, Poole GV Jr, Hansen KJ, et al. Salvage of lower extremities following combined orthopedic and vascular trauma. A predictive salvage index. Am Surg. 1987;53(4):205–8.
15. Johansen K, Daines M, Howey T, et al. Objective criteria accurately predict amputation following lower extremity trauma. J Trauma. 1990;30(5):568–72; discussion 572–3.
16. Russell WL, Sailors DM, Whittle TB, et al. Limb salvage versus traumatic amputation. A decision based on a seven-part predictive index. Ann Surg. 1991;213(5):473–80; discussion 480–1.
17. McNamara MG, Heckman JD, Corley FG. Severe open fractures of the lower extremity: a retrospective evaluation of the Mangled Extremity Severity Score (MESS). J Orthop Trauma. 1994;8(2):81–7.
18. Dirschl DR, Dahners LE. The mangled extremity: when should it be amputated? J Am Acad Orthop Surg. 1996;4(4):182–90.
19. Crowley DJ, Kanakaris NK, Giannoudis PV. Irrigation of the wounds in open fractures. J Bone Joint Surg Br. 2007;89(5):580–5.
20. Byrd HS, Spicer TE, Cierney G 3rd. Management of open tibial fractures. Plast Reconstr Surg. 1985;76(5):719–30.
21. Miranda M. Skeletal stabilization in the severely injured limb: fixation techniques compatible with soft tissue trauma. Tech Orthop. 2014;29(4):186–9.
22. Gifford SM, Aidinian G, Clouse WD, et al. Effect of temporary shunting on extremity vascular injury: an outcome analysis from the Global War on Terror vascular injury initiative. J Vasc Surg. 2009;50(3):549–55.
23. Millesi H. Peripheral nerve injuries. Nerve sutures and nerve grafting. Scand J Plast Reconstr Surg Suppl. 1982;19:25–37.
24. Dedmond BT, Kortesis B, Punger K, et al. The use of negative-pressure wound therapy (NPWT) in the temporary treatment of soft-tissue injuries associated with high-energy open tibial shaft fractures. J Orthop Trauma. 2007;21(1):11–7.
25. Bhattacharyya T, Mehta P, Smith M, et al. Routine use of wound vacuum-assisted closure does not allow coverage delay for open tibia fractures. Plast Reconstr Surg. 2008;121(4):1263–6.

The Triage of the Patient with the Mangled Extremity

Anna Romagnoli, Joseph Dubose, and Thomas Scalea

Introduction

A mangled extremity can be classified as any extremity sustaining sufficiently severe injury to a combination of at least three out of four systems of vascular, bony, soft tissue, and/or nerve. From a field triage point of view, patient's exhibiting this injury pattern should be sent to an appropriate facility and evaluated appropriately to optimize the potential for functional outcome. The overarching principle that needs to be followed is always "life over limb." Prompt extraction of the patient and initial stabilization are paramount for the patient's survival. From arrival to the initial hospital, decisions can be made regarding best practices.

Variability in decision-making will be based on local resources and expert consensus opinion. Multiple factors weigh into these decisions. The initial treatment algorithm and accompanying text are designed to address mangled extremities seen in the civilian setting beginning in the emergency department. Many of the same principles apply to battlefield medicine; however wartime nuances are beyond the scope of this chapter.

Field Triage

According to the CDC 2011 field triage guidelines, patients are triaged to trauma centers based according to general physiologic conditions, anatomic conditions, mechanism of injury, as well as certain patient characteristics. Physiologically, the panel recommended transport to a trauma center if any of the following are identified Glasgow Coma Scale (GCS) ≤ 13, or SBP of <90 mmHg, or respiratory rate of <10 or >29 breaths per minute or need for ventilatory support [1].

The panel recognized that even with normal physiologic guidelines, patients with certain anatomical trauma should be triaged to a trauma center if the meet any of the following: all penetrating injuries to head, neck, torso, and extremities proximal to elbow or knee; chest wall instability or deformity (e.g., flail chest); two or more proximal long bone fractures; crushed, degloved, mangled, or pulseless extremity; amputation proximal to wrist or ankle; pelvic fractures; open or depressed skull fractures; or paralysis [1]. In regard to a mangled extremity, this may be in isolation, or part of a polytrauma patient, necessitating multiple specialists at a qualified center. Certain risk factors are associated with the need

A. Romagnoli · T. Scalea
R Adams Cowley Shock Trauma Center, University of Maryland Medical System, Baltimore, MD, USA
e-mail: tscalea@umm.edu

J. Dubose (✉)
Department of Surgery, Uniformed Services University of the Health Sciences,
Baltimore, MD, USA
e-mail: joseph.dubose@umm.edu

© Springer Nature Switzerland AG 2021
R. A. Pensy, J. V. Ingari (eds.), *The Mangled Extremity*, https://doi.org/10.1007/978-3-319-56648-1_2

Table 2.1 Risk factors associated with the need for amputation of a mangled extremity

Risk factors for need for amputation of mangled extremities
Global
Age over 50
High-energy mechanism of injury
Persistent hypotension (<90 mm Hg)
Bony
Gustilo type IIIA tibial fracture with significant tissue loss, nerve injury, accompanying fibular fracture, displacement >50%, comminuted segmental fracture, or high probability of bone graft requirement
Gustilo type III B, III C tibial fractures
Type III open fractures of pilon
Type III B open fractures of ankle
Severe open injury of mid or hindfoot
Vascular
Prolonged warm ischemia time (>6h h)
High degree of vascular segment loss
More proximal the injury
Non-viable distal anastomotic site
Neurologic
Confirmed nerve disruption, particularly high risk is tibial nerve
Soft tissue
Large, circumferential tissue loss
Significant closed soft tissue loss/necrosis
Compartment syndrome with myonecrosis

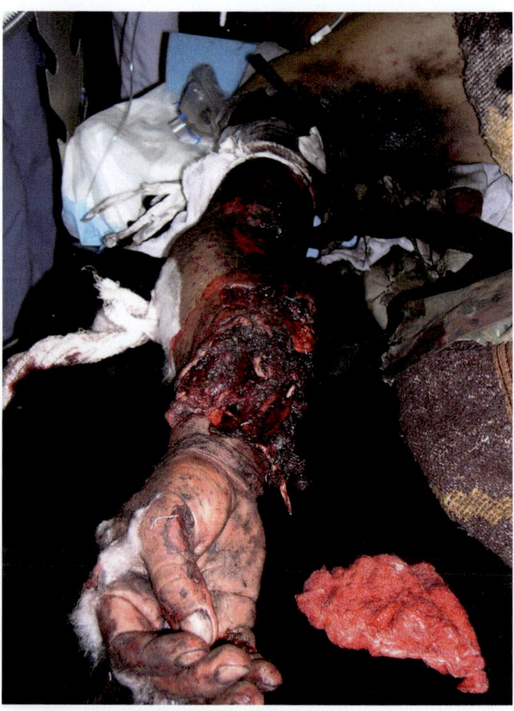

Fig. 2.1 Mangled upper extremity with tourniquet in place. (Courtesy of Dr. Joseph Dubose)

for amputation of a mangled extremity (Table 2.1). Prehospital providers should be familiar with these and attempt to take patients with these characteristics to higher level centers.

Ideally a patient with a mangled extremity will be taken to the nearest appropriate center; however, within the limits of the system, sometimes this does not always happen. In such cases, initial stabilization must be undertaken at the receiving facility. Once stable, the patient can be transferred to a higher level of care.

Initial Field Care

A rapid primary assessment is required by the first responders to identify significant life-threatening injuries. Prehospital Trauma Life Support (PHTLS)/Tactical Combat Casualty Care (TCCC) protocols will aid the responder in rapid examination and intervention. Exsanguinating hemorrhage should be addressed with direct pressure, packing, or a tourniquet (Figs. 2.1 and 2.2). From there, airway, breathing, and circulation can be addressed, and appropriate prehospital interventions can be performed as necessary.

Vascular access is important. It is recommended that this be performed into an uninjured extremity. Intravenous line placement is ideal; however, if there is significant vascular collapse due to shock, intraosseous access may be necessary for initial access. In the absence of head injury, permissive hypotension should be maintained to limit blood loss. En route to the medical facility, the extremity should be monitored as bleeding may resume depending on the patient's hemodynamic status.

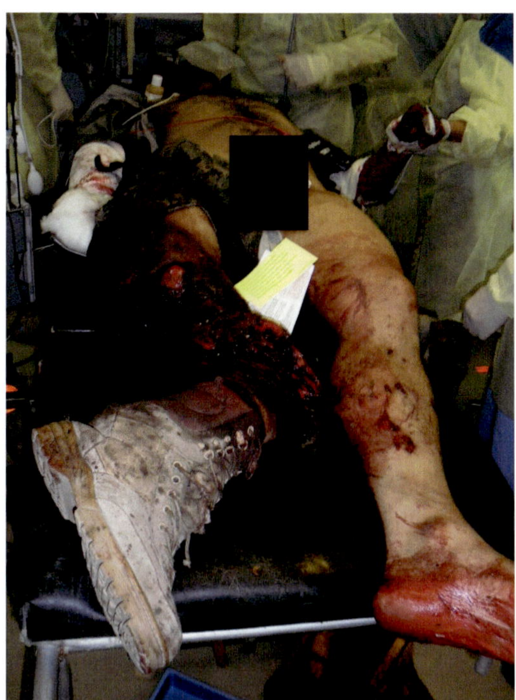

Fig. 2.2 Mangled lower extremity with tourniquet in place. (Courtesy of Dr. Joseph Dubose)

Initial Assessment

Control Active Hemorrhage

It is important to stress that the initial evaluation of a patient with a mangled extremity does not differ from that of any other patients with multiple injuries, with the exception of controlling exsanguination on arrival. In the cases of polytrauma, the adage of "life over limb" holds true. The primary survey and the initial ABC's of standard evaluation take precedence. Providers must resist the temptation to become diverted by the graphic appearance of the extremity and maintain a systematic approach that focuses on the detection and effective treatment of more serious issues. Resuscitation and management of all life-threatening injuries take priority over any extremity problem.

After initial life-threatening injuries have been assessed and addressed or ruled out, attention can be turned to the injured extremity (Table 2.2). A hemorrhage control device, preferably tourniquet (pneumatic or mechanical), can be prepositioned proximal to the injured extremity, if possible, to ensure timely deployment in case of severe hemorrhage when the field dressing is removed. Once in place, the dressing can be removed, and the team member can assess for injury/confirm the mangled extremity. At this point, ongoing extremity hemorrhage may be managed by direct manual pressure, wound packing, pressure dressings, or a tourniquet [2, 3]. If seen, a visible vessel can be controlled with direct clamping and ligature. Blind clamping is not recommended, as this can be potentially harmful. If severe bleeding is noted, the tourniquet can be inflated or tightened or a pressure dressing applied. Further wound exploration in the emergency room is not recommended, as this can precipitate further bleeding and lead to further wound contamination. Tourniquets should be placed as distally possible and be kept to the shortest duration possible to minimize the possibility of worsening ischemia. Operative pneumatic tourniquet systems are preferable to field tourniquets whenever available. It is advisable to provide appropriate inflation of these pneumatic devices for successful arterial occlusion. Pressures below systolic may substantially increase venous pressure (creating a "venous tourniquet"), worsening venous bleeding, worsen subsequent extremity swelling, and potentially increase pressure within the muscular compartments of the extremity.

The only immediately life-threatening aspect of the mangled extremity is external blood loss. An ischemic limb, while an urgent matter, does not represent an immediate threat to life.

It is a common pitfall, among inexperienced providers, to reach for the Doppler probe in an effort to assess distal perfusion as a component of the primary survey. This practice further draws the provider away from the overall care of the patient, focusing only on the extremity. This distraction may result in the delayed diagnosis of truncal hemorrhage, brain injury, or other immediately life-threatening conditions.

Table 2.2 Mangled extremity triage algorithm

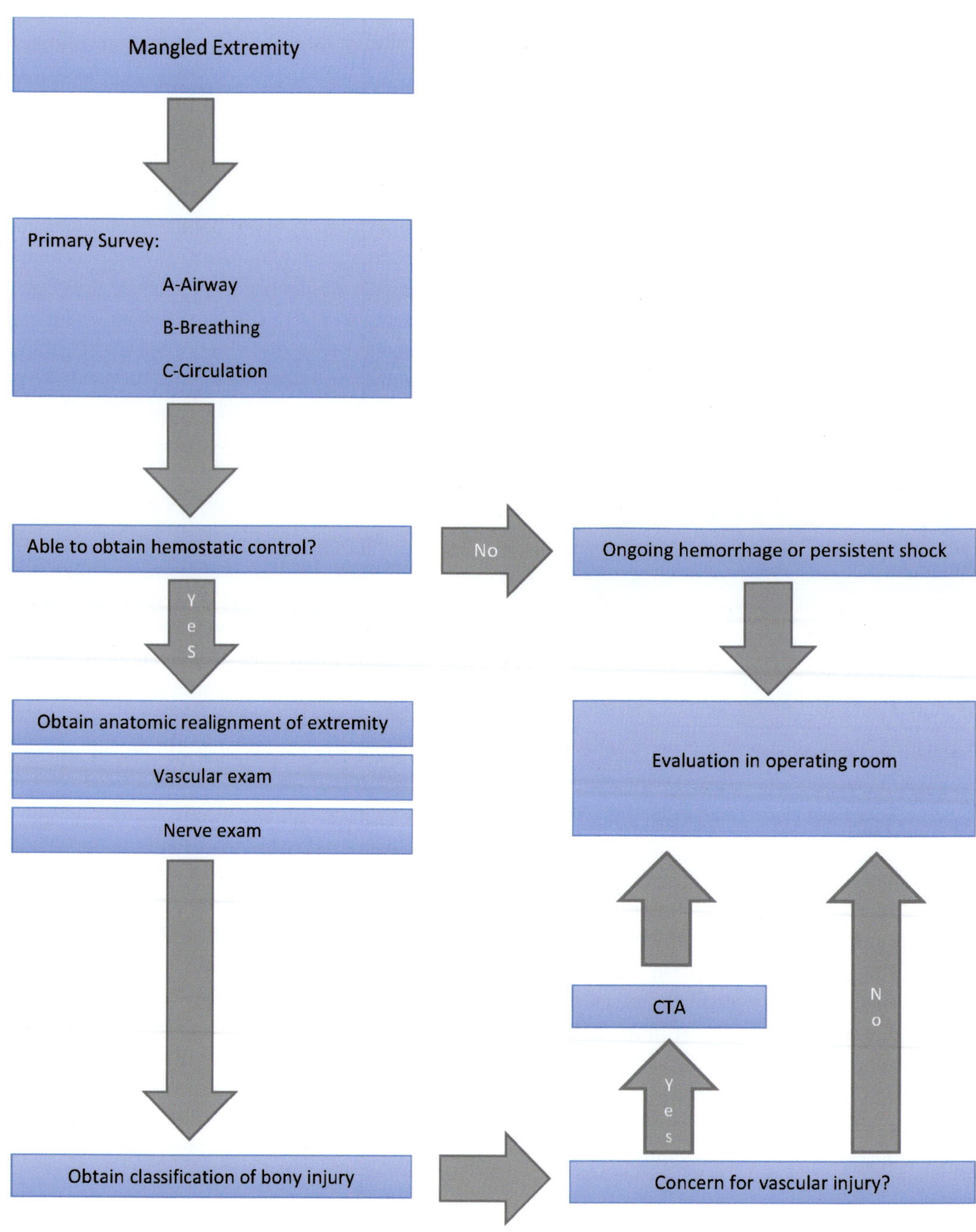

Persistent Hemorrhage or Refractory Hemodynamic Instability

If external bleeding cannot be controlled or the patient remains hemodynamically unstable without other sources despite efforts in the emergency department, the patient should be taken expeditiously to the operating room for surgical control of bleeding. If isolated to a proximal extremity or junctional wound, not amenable to a tourniquet, operative proximal control may need to be obtained.

In the hemodynamically unstable patient, other sources of ongoing blood loss should be entertained. Further imaging with x-ray or ultrasound can help diagnose concurrent chest, abdominal, or pelvic bleeding. If the patient has concomitant intracavitary hemorrhage, it may be advantageous to use two operative teams. If only one team is available, extremity bleeding can be controlled with a tourniquet until cavitary sources of ongoing blood loss are managed. Damage control techniques to intracavitary hemorrhage can allow the extremity to be addressed as early as possible.

Restore Appropriate Alignment of the Extremity

In the patient who remains hemodynamically stable, the most important initial step is to realign the fractured bones with either splinting or traction to alleviate any possible kinking of the vasculature. After reduction, perfusion and further assessment of the bony and soft tissue abnormalities can be performed. Analgesia and sedation are critical to perform good bony alignment. Conscious sedation or endotracheal intubation may be required.

Vascular Evaluation

Blunt vascular extremity injuries may be associated with the need for amputation in as much as 20% of patients [3]. These extremity injuries have an association with multiple additional injuries due to the blunt mechanisms, and competing priorities of initial treatment may delay diagnosis of extremity vascular injury. In addition, pulse examination alterations are common sequelae of displaced fractures in these patients. An early vascular assessment will permit for the rapid identification of these injuries and minimize subsequent ischemic time.

Initial decisions regarding vascular status can be determined by looking for hard signs of vascular injury. These include active hemorrhage; large, expanding, or pulsatile hematoma; bruit or thrill; absent palpable pulses distally; and distal ischemic manifestations (pain, pallor, paralysis, paresthesias, poikilothermia, coolness). All of these require immediate operative intervention.

Soft signs of vascular injury that may be present in a mangled extremity would include history of active bleeding at the scene, proximity of penetrating wound or blunt trauma to major artery, diminished unilateral pulse, small non-pulsatile hematomas, or neurological deficit which are all indications for further evaluation.

After restoration of anatomic alignment and adequate resuscitation, this examination should begin with an attempt to palpate the pulse. If the pulse is not palpable, or weaker than anticipated, then an attempt at bedside Doppler assessment should be undertaken. If a Doppler assessment reveals a signal and tissue loss does not preclude measurement, an Injured Extremity Index can be used to guide the need for additional vascular imaging [4–6]. Doppler indices less than 0.9 or absent/ diminished pulse in the affected extremity indicate the need for additional radiographic characterization, via CT angiography or direct angiography, in appropriately stable patients [6]. Injured Extremity Index can be altered by a number of factors not directly related to vascular injury, including obesity, diabetes, hypotension, and peripheral vascular construction because of hypothermia or hemorrhage. It is imperative to use appropriately sized blood pressure cuffs for this purpose to patient body habitus. Efforts should also be taken to adequately resuscitate and warm the patient to optimize the reliability of Doppler Indices.

Neurologic Evaluation

An adequate neurologic examination of the extremity to assess peripheral nerve function should be conducted. Nerve deficits, particularly

Table 2.3 Peripheral nerve injury findings

Physical exam findings of peripheral nerve injuries	
Upper extremity	
Median nerve	
M: Weak/absent flexion of thumb to index finger	S: Diminished/absent sensation to palmar aspect of thumb, index finger, middle finger
Radial nerve	
M: Weak/absent dorsiflexion of wrist/thumb	S: Diminished/absent sensation dorsal web space of thumb and index finger
Ulnar nerve	
M: Weak/absent abduction and adduction of fingers	S: Diminished/absent sensation to little finger and ulnar aspect of ring finger
Lower extremity	
Femoral nerve	
M: Inability to extend knee	S: Diminished/absent sensation over distal 1/3 of anteromedial thigh
Common peroneal nerve	
M: Weak/absent dorsiflexion of foot/toes, inability to evert foot	
Deep peroneal nerve	
M: Weak/absent dorsiflexion of foot and toes	S: Diminished/absent sensation of dorsal web space between 1st and 2nd toes
Superficial peroneal nerve	
M: Inability to evert foot	S: Diminished/absent sensation of dorsal foot (other than deep peroneal distribution)
Tibial nerve	
M: Weak/absent plantar flexion or foot inversion	S: Diminished/absent sensation of plantar aspect of foot

M motor, *S* sensory

of the tibial nerve, are thought to portend a dire functional outcome. Signs of specific nerve injuries are listed in Table 2.3. A prospective study [7], however, has demonstrated that peripheral nerve deficits are not sensitive predictors for failure of functional limb salvage. This finding may be reflective of the unpredictable natural course of many of these injuries. Differentiating neuropraxia, or temporary deficits, from permanent nerve injury in the acute phases after injury may prove difficult. It is important to document these findings, however, and factor their presence into the decision-making process. Ideally, both detailed sensory and motor function of nerves should be assessed before intubation for a preoperative functional assessment.

Classify Bony/Soft Tissue Injury

Muscular, bony, and soft tissue injury can be assessed by physical exam and imaging. This can be performed initially in the resuscitation area, but more detailed examination should be performed in the operating room. Key elements include evaluation of wound size, contamination of the wound, fracture pattern, soft tissue loss, and association of major arterial injury. The Gustilo Open Fracture Classification System (Table 2.4) takes all of these measures into account for standard wound classification.

As an objective measure, a Mangled Extremity Severity Score (MESS) should be calculated for each patient at the onset of treatment. Consideration of photography to document the severity of the injury should be made for the medical record, to note the initial wounds as well as to document both progress and decline.

Broad-spectrum antibiotics and tetanus should be given to patients with mangled extremities. Balanced resuscitation based on standard trauma algorithms should commence.

Table 2.4 Gustilo open fracture classification system

Gustilo type I
Wound <1 cm with minimal soft tissue injury
Clean wound bed
Fracture is transverse or short oblique fracture with minimal comminution
Gustilo type II
Wound is 1–10 cm with moderate soft tissue injury
Fracture is transverse or short oblique fracture with minimal comminution
Gustilo type IIIA
Wound is >10 cm with extensive soft tissue injury
Soft tissue coverage facilitated by primary suture closure despite soft tissue laceration, flaps, or high-energy trauma, irrespective of wound size
Includes segmental fractures or severely comminuted fractures
Gustilo type IIIB
Extensive soft tissue loss with periosteal stripping and bony exposure, most commonly requiring local or free flap coverage
Usually associated with massive contamination
Gustilo type IIIC
Extensive fracture associated with major arterial injury requiring repair, irrespective of degree of soft tissue injury

Without an algorithmic approach to the mangled extremity, errors in management may occur. Typical errors that might occur include failure to accomplish timely reperfusion of ischemic tissue, delays associated with ineffective communication between surgeons from the necessary specialties, unnecessary delays because of inappropriate vascular imaging requests, inadequate debridement and fracture stabilization, and delays in soft tissue coverage attempts.

Differences arise between the mangled upper and mangled lower extremity, which must be carefully considered. Permissive reperfusion time is longer in the upper (8–10 h) versus the lower extremity (6 h) [8]. Prolonged ischemia time is considered because a transtibial lower extremity amputation carries a much better functional prognosis than a transradial upper extremity amputation, due to the fact that upper extremity prostheses do not function as well as lower extremity prostheses. Proximal shortening of the humerus in the upper extremity to reduce soft tissue defects is tolerated well up to 5 cm, in contrast to the femur in the lower extremity that does not tolerate shortening of more than 2 cm. Upper extremity nerve reconstruction has some reasonable success, whereas in the lower extremity, many consider major nerve injury an indication for primary amputation. The rehabilitation process is also more imperative when the upper extremity is involved [9].

In the absence of an adequate scoring system, the management of the patient with a mangled extremity requires a multidisciplinary approach and careful consideration of complex systemic and limb-related factors. Optimal outcome requires the trauma provider to evaluate these factors systematically to determine the appropriate choice between limb salvage procedures and amputation.

Summary

Patients with mangled extremities remain a significant management challenge in the prehospital environment, initial triage, and ongoing care.

In a polytrauma patient with other priorities, life before limb must always guide the provider. Hemorrhage control in the resuscitation area is of utmost importance with either direct pressure, packing, tourniquet, or direct ligation. From here, additional examination and studies can be undertaken to decide the best course of treatment for the patient. A thoughtful approach to the initial management has the potential to optimize patient outcome after these severe life-altering injuries.

References

1. Sasser S, Hunt R, Faul M, Sugerman D, Pearson W, Dulski T, et al. Guidelines for field triage of injured patients: recommendations of the national expert panel on field triage, 2011. MMWR Recomm Rep. 2012;61(RR01):1–20.
2. Beekley AC, Sebesta JA, Blackbourne LH, 31st Combat Support Hospital Research Group, et al. Prehospital tourniquet use in operation Iraqi freedom: effect on hemorrhage control and outcomes. J Trauma. 2008;64(2 suppl):S28–37; discussion S37.
3. Rozycki GS, Tremblay LN, Feliciano DV, McClelland WB. Blunt vascular trauma in the extremity: diagnosis, management, and outcome. J Trauma. 2003;55:814–24.
4. Mills WJ, Barei DP, McNair P. The value of the ankle-brachial index for diagnosing arterial injury after knee dislocation: a prospective study. J Trauma. 2004;56:1261–5.
5. Nassoura ZE, Ivatury RR, Simon RJ, Jabbour N, Vinzons A, Stahl W. A reassessment of Doppler pressure indices in the detection of arterial lesions in proximity penetrating injuries of extremities: a prospective study. Am J Emerg Med. 1996;14:151–6.
6. Feliciano DV. Management of peripheral arterial injury. Curr Opin Crit Care. 2010;16(6):602–8.
7. Ly TV, Travison TG, Castillo RC, Bosse MJ, MacKenzie EJ, LEAP Study Group. Ability of lower-extremity injury severity scores to predict functional outcome after limb salvage. J Bone Joint Surg Am. 2008;90:1738–43.
8. Togawa S, Yamami N, Nakayama H, Mano Y, Ikegami K, Ozeki S. The validity of the mangled extremity severity score in the assessment of upper limb injuries. J Bone Joint Surg Br. 2005;87:1516–9. https://doi.org/10.1302/0301-620X.87B11.16512. [PubMed] [Cross Ref].
9. Gupta A, Wolff TW. Management of the mangled hand and forearm. J Am Acad Orthop Surg. 1995;3:226–36. [PubMed].

removal of protruding osseous fragments, antiseptic wound dressings, stable reduction, and diligent wound management were core tenants of open fracture management applied by Hippocratic physicians.

Early management of open fractures included the use of a red-hot iron and boiling oil of elder for wound sterilization [10]. Despite these practices, the morbidity and mortality of open fractures remained high, and the practice of amputation became more common in the nineteenth century [10]. Lister's discovery of antisepsis and several more recent discoveries including improved anesthesia, aseptic techniques, advances in prehospital care, and improvements in critical care has advanced the management of open fractures and mangled extremities significantly [10, 11]. A revolution in wound care management and soft tissue transfer has added to the success of treating these injuries.

Timing All open fractures are considered contaminated and at increased risk for infection-related complications. Open fractures cultured in the emergency department are positive 60–70% of the time, highlighting the importance of a thorough and timely debridement [12, 13]. This is of particular concern in the lower extremity, as infection rates related to open fractures of the lower extremity have been demonstrated to be higher than that of their counterparts in the upper extremity [4].

The recommended timing to surgical debridement of complex open fractures has evolved in recent times. While it is largely accepted that an overly prolonged interval between injury and debridement may increase infection rates, the threshold time point at which the risk substantially increases remains a topic of debate [13–16]. While open fractures associated with a mangled extremity are no longer considered an "emergency" unless they are associated with a dysvascular limb, accepted practice is to manage these injuries in an "urgent" fashion when the patient is resuscitated and stable for surgery and a complete complement of surgical support staff is available.

In Practice Initial debridement of the mangled extremity oftentimes begins in the field or emergency department as gross contamination is removed and an initial sterile dressing is applied. More formal surgical debridement typically occurs in the acute or subacute phase of care after initial resuscitation and stabilization have occurred. Prompt assessment and management of life-threatening injuries should be addressed, and appropriate antibiotic therapy with tetanus administration should not be delayed [13, 16–19].

All splints and bandages should be removed from the affected extremity to allow for a complete evaluation of the soft tissue and osseous injury. At the time of initial assessment, the extent of the zone of injury may not be fully appreciated. Surgical exploration is necessary for adequate appreciation of the extent of injury and debridement of damaged and contaminated tissues. Serial debridements may also be indicated to assure that all nonviable tissue is removed. The injured limb is prepped and draped in a standard sterile fashion. A tourniquet should be applied, but we would recommend the judicious use of this device in an effort to avoid further ischemic damage to the limb. Additionally, assessment of tissue viability may be more easily accomplished if perfusion is maintained during debridement by leaving the tourniquet uninflated. The tourniquet may be reserved for those instances where severe and/or uncontrollable hemorrhage is encountered.

Assessment of the wound begins with information provided by medical providers at the scene of the accident and upon arrival in the emergency department. Mechanism of injury, vascular and neurologic status of the limb; size, location, and contamination of wounds; laboratory findings; plain film radiographs; and associated injuries all provide useful information regarding the injury and the patient to which it is attached. Plain film radiographs and computed tomography elucidate the extent of bony injury but also provide useful information regarding the severity of the soft tissue injury. In the awake patient, obtaining and documenting an accurate neurovascular examination should be prioritized as associated injuries to these structures will likely have significant consequence for reconstruction.

Debridement refers to the meticulous resection of devitalized tissue and removal of any foreign material from a wound [9]. The goal of surgical debridement is to minimize the number of remaining bacteria in a viable wound and additionally establish a healthy wound margin and base [10]. This is an absolutely necessary step when managing any open fracture or mangled extremity in an effort to minimize infection and increase potential for bone healing [20–23]. By removing foreign material and dead tissue, the opportunity of any remaining bacteria to proliferate and cause a clinically meaningful infection is minimized. Inadequate debridement will leave behind a large bioburden of bacteria in a wound environment amenable to further proliferation and hence the importance of this process. If a frank infection results, the consequence can be catastrophic as additional soft tissue insult will follow resulting in further tissue necrosis, loss of function, and potential amputation.

The first steps in any surgical debridement should include a methodical evaluation of the injury and vigilant planning with consideration to both the surgical debridement and future procedure to be performed. External wounds which are present in the setting of a mangled extremity often underrepresent the extent or zone of the injury which is present. This is particularly true in proximal extremity segments or areas where there is a larger soft tissue envelope (i.e., the thigh or arm). In these areas the wounds may be small, but the degree of underlying muscle disruption, severity of periosteal stripping, and degree of contamination at the fracture site may be significant [10]. This information is typically evident once the margins of the wound(s) have been extended for complete injury assessment.

While extending the wound is a vital component of debridement, it should be done in a very precise fashion with the goal of defining and exposing the full extent of the closed as well as open elements of the soft tissue injury. This frequently results in an extensile approach to the injured extremity, and care must be taken to avoid creating nonviable tissue flaps or dissecting through tissue planes which create a large dead space. Maintenance of neural and vascular structures should be emphasized. It is important to consider the placement of definitive implants, the need for transfer of local or distant soft tissue, and wound closure options. Balancing these principles with adequate debridement can be one of the most challenging elements of managing the mangled extremity.

The most effective means for completing a debridement utilizes a systematic approach which may vary per physician preference. Some providers utilize a method by which each tissue group (skin, subcutaneous dermis/fat, fascia, muscle/tendon, neurovascular structures, and bone) undergoes sequential debridement in a consistent order. Alternatively working from the peripheral and superficial edge of the wound and progressing in a circular fashion, sequentially moving toward the more central and deep portion of the wound assures that each layer and element of the wound is adequately debrided before moving on to the next. Either method may be successful so long as the surgeon is diligent in their exploration and thorough in their debridement, leaving behind a sterile, viable wound bed (Fig. 3.1). If serial debridements are planned, questionable tissue can be left behind and removed as the injury evolves and various tissues declare their viability. For grossly contaminated wounds, which are frequently associated with the mangled extremity, we advocate the use of antibiotic-impregnated methyl methacrylate bead pouches applied to the wound bed between debridements (Fig. 3.2). These provide for extremely high local concentrations of antibiotics without systemic toxicity, maintain a moist environment surrounding the bony injury which limits desiccation of the periosteum, and generate antibiotic-rich "bead broth" which bathes the entire wound and fracture site. Additionally, the bead pouch is applied in the sterile operating room environment after surgical debridement and

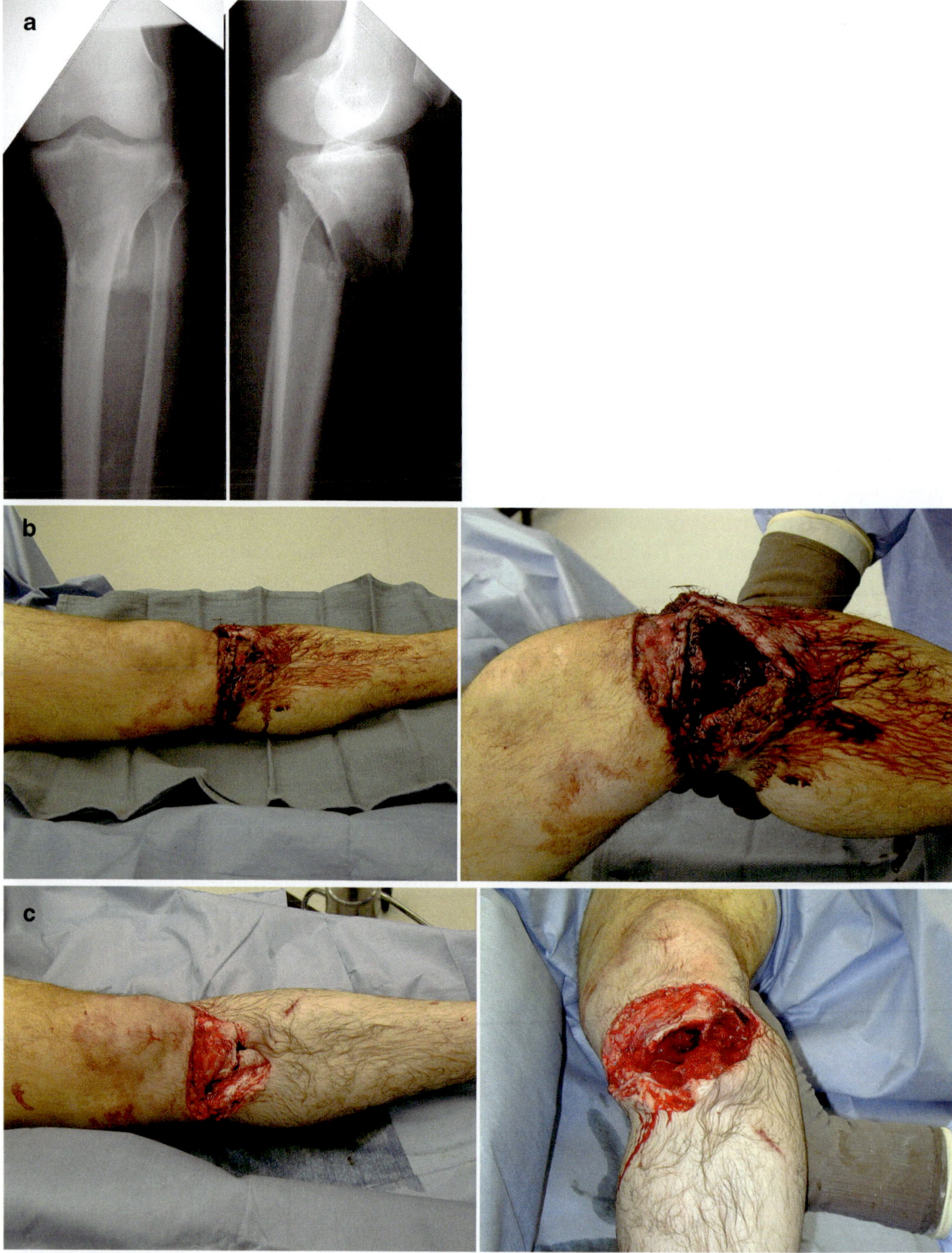

Fig. 3.1 30-year-old male involved in motor vehicle crash, sustained open left proximal tibia fracture. (**a**) AP and lateral injury radiographs of left tibia. (**b**) Predebridement clinical photos of traumatic wound showing gross contamination of soft tissues and fracture site. (**c**) Post-debridement clinical photos depicting conversion to sterile wound bed with healthy, viable tissue remaining. (**d**) Postoperative AP and lateral radiographs after initial debridement, temporizing knee-spanning external fixation, and antibiotic bead insertion. (**e**) Final clinical photos after definitive ORIF and rotational flap coverage demonstrating well-healed soft tissue and return of functional range of motion

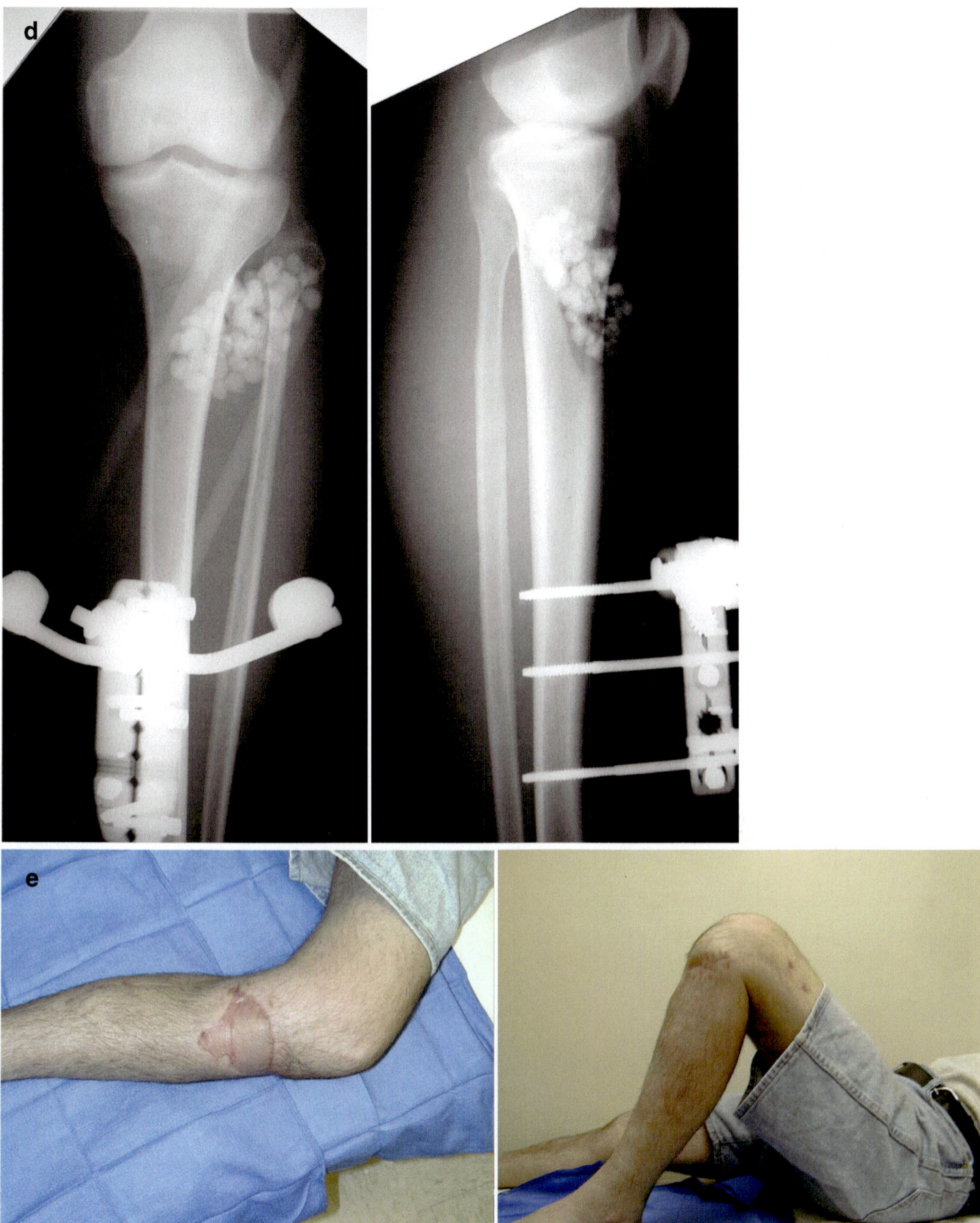

Fig. 3.1 (continued)

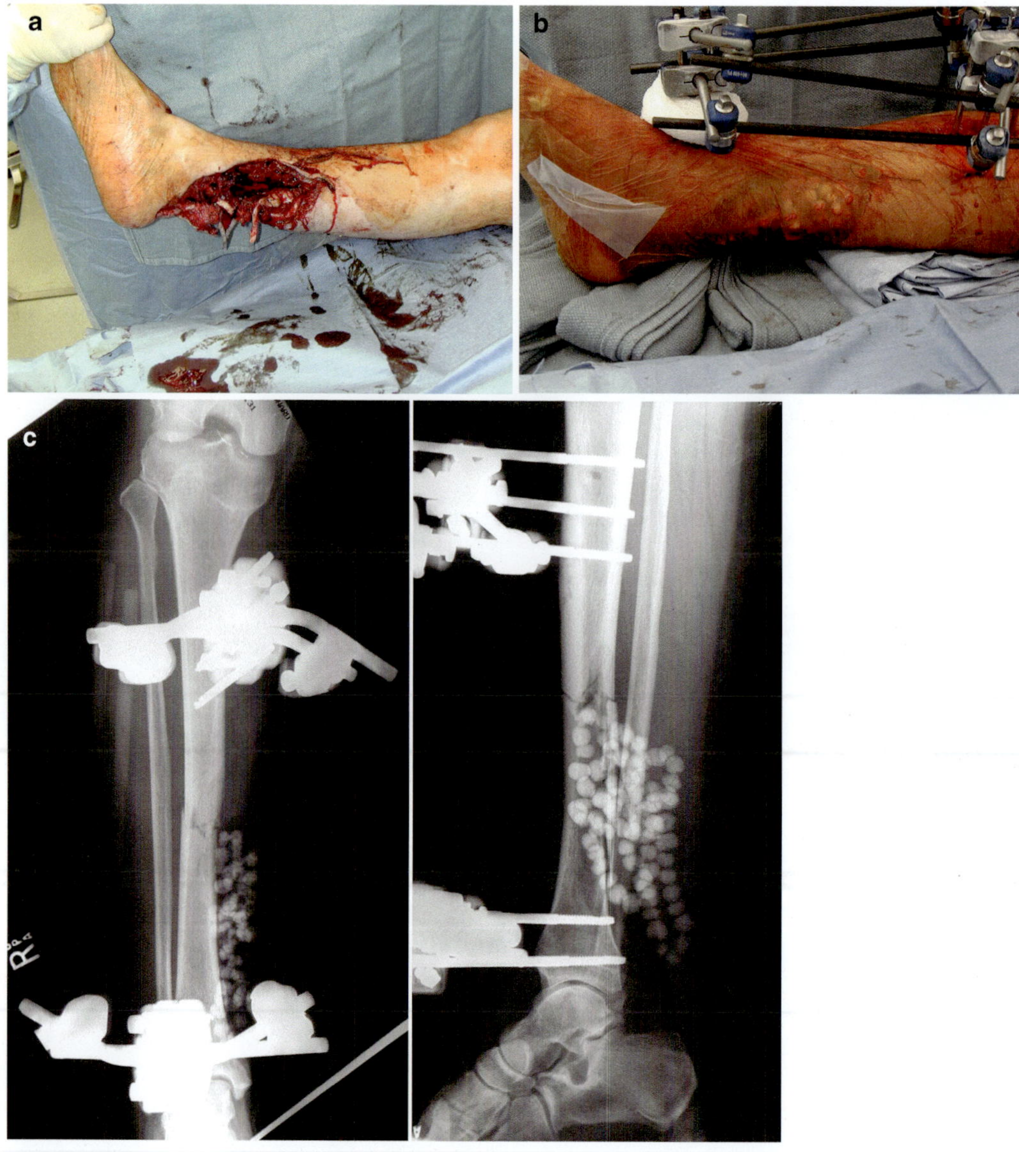

Fig. 3.2 42-year-old male s/p lawn mower injury to right lower extremity. (**a**) Clinical photo demonstrating significant soft tissue injury with multiple tendon lacerations and muscle loss. (**b**) Clinical photo after initial debridement demonstrating temporizing external fixation and antibiotic bead pouch in place. (**c**) AP and lateral radiographs demonstrating provisional reduction and external fixation and antibiotic bead pouch

irrigation and is then sealed in airtight fashion with an adhesive, bio-occlusive dressing, thereby limiting the risk of wound contamination with hospital-acquired pathogens between debridements and allowing longer periods of time between serial debridements. The type and amount of antibiotic agent mixed into the cement vary among surgeons, but our preference is to add 4 grams of vancomycin and 2.4 grams of tobramycin per pack of cement.

The skin should be preserved when able, as this tissue is typically quick to declare and can be removed with future debridements. The skin that is obviously devitalized, macerated, or grossly contaminated should be sharply trimmed. Likewise, subcutaneous tissues and fat should be debrided when necrotic or contaminated. The fascia should be treated in a similar manner. If concern for compartment syndrome is present, the fascia may be released in addition to any debridement to allow for further tissue swelling without risk of impending necrosis.

Muscle should be cleared in a more liberal manner, as nonviable muscle may serve as a fertile culture medium for bacteria [10]. The entire extent of each muscle belly extending through a wound should be evaluated and debrided as needed. Contaminated tendons should be cleared of debris and maintained if possible. The free ends of major bone segments should be delivered into the zone of injury and debrided. Free and devitalized bone pieces are typically removed from the fracture site. Avascular large bone fragments in the lower extremity are generally removed; articular fragments which are essential for limb salvage and reconstruction should be thoroughly cleaned and retained.

Major arteries and nerves are preserved and, if injured, should be repaired as outlined in the chapters pertaining to revascularization and nerve reconstruction. When these structures present themselves within the zone of injury, they are typically identified throughout the length of the wound and protected such that an adequate debridement may ensue. Careful identification and mobilization are necessary to identify surrounding nonviable tissue and wound contamination.

Irrigation

Irrigation with liberal amounts of isotonic fluids will aid in the cleansing of the mangled extremity [20, 23]. While this step is not an acceptable alternative to debridement, it serves to further enhance the process of establishing a satisfactory wound bed. Chronologically irrigation typically follows debridement but can be used as an adjunct at any time point. Fluid irrigation facilitates the removal blood (both fresh and coagulated), foreign contamination, necrotic tissue, and bacteria.

The types of irrigation solution and pressure at which it should be most appropriately applied to the wound have long been sources of controversy [24–32]. Some evidence suggests that high-pressure irrigation may be more effective than low pressure in removing particulate matter and bacteria but at the expense of increased bone and soft tissue damage [27, 29–31]. Basic science studies have suggested that high-pressure irrigation may damage the fractured bone, propagate bacteria into soft tissues and the intramedullary canal, promote stem cell differentiation from bone-forming cells toward the adipocyte cell lineage, and impair in vivo fracture healing [30, 31, 33–35]. Concern about the potential effect this may have on bone healing encouraged further work in this area. Rationale for a low-pressure irrigating fluid is predicated upon the notion that it may avoid bone-healing complications, but at the possible expense of less effective removal of wound contamination and bacteria [23].

The addition of surfactants such as castile soap to irrigation fluid has also been advocated [20, 23, 32, 36–40]. The biologic rationale for using surfactants is based upon the nonpolar and polar molecules of these solutions which act as an emulsifier. Additionally, soap is inexpensive, does not confer any risk of antibiotic resistance, and was thought to be associated with minimal tissue toxicity [36, 39, 41, 42].

In a randomized study of 2551 patients, the FLOW Investigators helped clarify many of the controversies regarding wound irrigation in open fractures [23]. Rates of reoperation were similar between groups of patients treated with high and low pressure, suggesting that physician preference may be used in this regard. However, reoperation rates were higher in the soap group as compared to the plain saline group. Contrary to the results from previous smaller studies, the FLOW trial does not support the use of soap in irrigation fluid.

External Fixation

External fixators have been used to treat fractures for over a century; however, their application has evolved significantly in the past several decades [43–47]. As the techniques and implants used for internal fixation have advanced, the role of external fixation in both the temporary and definitive stages of treatment has changed. This is particularly true when considering the use of external fixators for the management of the mangled extremity. In the setting of severe musculoskeletal trauma, an external fixator is often required for temporary stabilization, soft tissue rest, and particularly in the setting of serial debridements to allow for limb stability (Figs. 3.1 and 3.2). This strategy keeps deep hardware out of the wound during initial management, and if needed, the frame can be easily disassembled and reassembled. This facilitates a thorough inspection and debridement of the fracture site and soft tissues in these complex injuries. Definitive fracture care with an external fixator is also more common for the mangled extremity, where soft tissue compromise and the need for tissue transfer for coverage may make internal fixation less appealing.

External fixators offer many benefits for both the temporary and definitive fixation of fractures with significant soft tissue injury [43–47]. These devices provide osseous stability without additional soft tissue dissection. When applied properly, the half-pins and/or wires are inserted at a distance from the injury site without placing hardware directly in the zone of injury. In the case of periarticular fractures, temporizing external fixation may also be applied in a knee- or ankle-spanning construct to allow pin placement well away from the zone of injury (Fig. 3.3). The ability to appropriately apply and utilize these devices is a requisite skill for management of the mangled extremity.

External fixation is a dynamic tool which can be adjusted to fit a variety of clinical situations and assembled to accommodate a multitude of conditions. The versatility in the configuration of these constructs is a result of their simple application, easy removal/replacement, and ability to combine seamlessly with other fixation constructs. Furthermore, straightforward modifications in frame design and application allow the stability of individual constructs to be easily modified.

Form and Function External fixators, as the name implies, provide osseous stability through the use of threaded or smooth wires that traverse the bone and are joined by clamps, rods, and/or rings which are external to the body. A variety of fixator designs allow application for a diverse range of injuries.

There are three primary types of external fixators: (1) unilateral/monolateral uniplanar, (2) bilateral uniplanar, and (3) multiplanar. Unilateral constructs are positioned on one side of the limb and provide maximal stability in a single plane. Bilateral fixators do the same but with components on either side of the limb and in parallel. Multiplanar fixators have components oriented in multiple planes resulting in increased multiplanar control and stability. External frames may be simple or modular in configuration. Large bone segments may be controlled through large threaded pins, while smaller fragments can be captured with the use of thin wires. Dynamization or compression can be achieved if needed, adding to the utility of these devices. Furthermore, the amount of stability provided by the frame can be adjusted by a variety of factors.

The primary component of an external fixator is the pin. The pin connects the external components of the fixator to the bone. Pins may be terminally threaded, centrally threaded, or smooth and range in size from 2.0 mm to 6.0 mm in diameter. Pins may be coated in an effort to improve bone integration and/or decrease the rate of infection. The most commonly applied coating is hydroxyapatite; however, the benefit of this coating is not clear [48–53]. Pins are then connected to external rods or rings through the use of simple or multiplanar clamps. Alternatively, tensioned wires may be used to connect the bone to external rings. These wires range from 1.5 to 2.0 mm in diameter and are smooth. Tensioning the wires adds rigidity to the construct and prevents pin migration. Finally, rods are used to connect and unitize the external fixator. Rods attached to the pins or rings through the use of clamps can be stainless steel, aluminum alloy, or carbon fiber.

Basic Application The final frame construct may be simple or complex in nature depending on the number of bone fragments and overall complexity of injury (Table 3.1). When managing mangled extremities, the provider must balance the need for bony stability with the potential impact on the soft tissues, ultimate reconstructive plan, and construct cost. Given the complex nature of these injuries, modular frames are often needed to provide multiplanar stability and allow for flexibility of frame application. Modular frames allow for pins and wires to be applied prior to reduction and rod attachment. This affords ease of application. Our preference is to

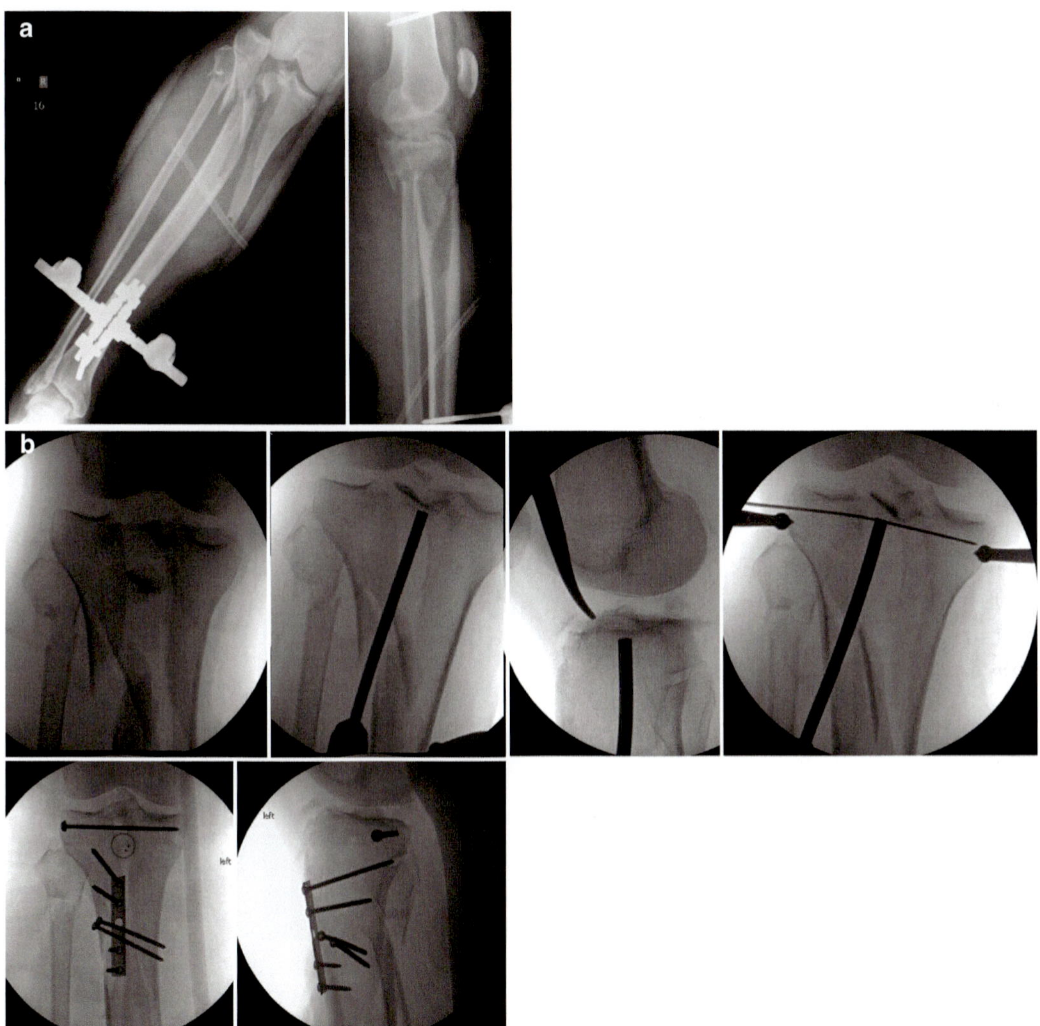

Fig. 3.3 45-year-old male s/p motorcycle crash who sustained complex bicondylar tibial plateau fracture with compartment syndrome. Transferred from outside facility after undergoing 4-compartment fasciotomy and application of temporizing knee-spanning external fixator. (**a**) AP and lateral radiographs demonstrating complex tibial plateau, poor provisional reduction. (**b**) Intraoperative fluoroscopic images at time of external fixator revision and limited ORIF. (**c**) Clinical photo of right lower extremity immediately prior to definitive ORIF and manipulation of knee under anesthesia at 2 months post-injury and AP and lateral radiographs of right tibia demonstrating healed fracture 2 months after definitive surgery. (**d**) Clinical photos of right lower extremity 2 months s/p definitive ORIF demonstrating healed soft tissue envelope and return of functional knee ROM

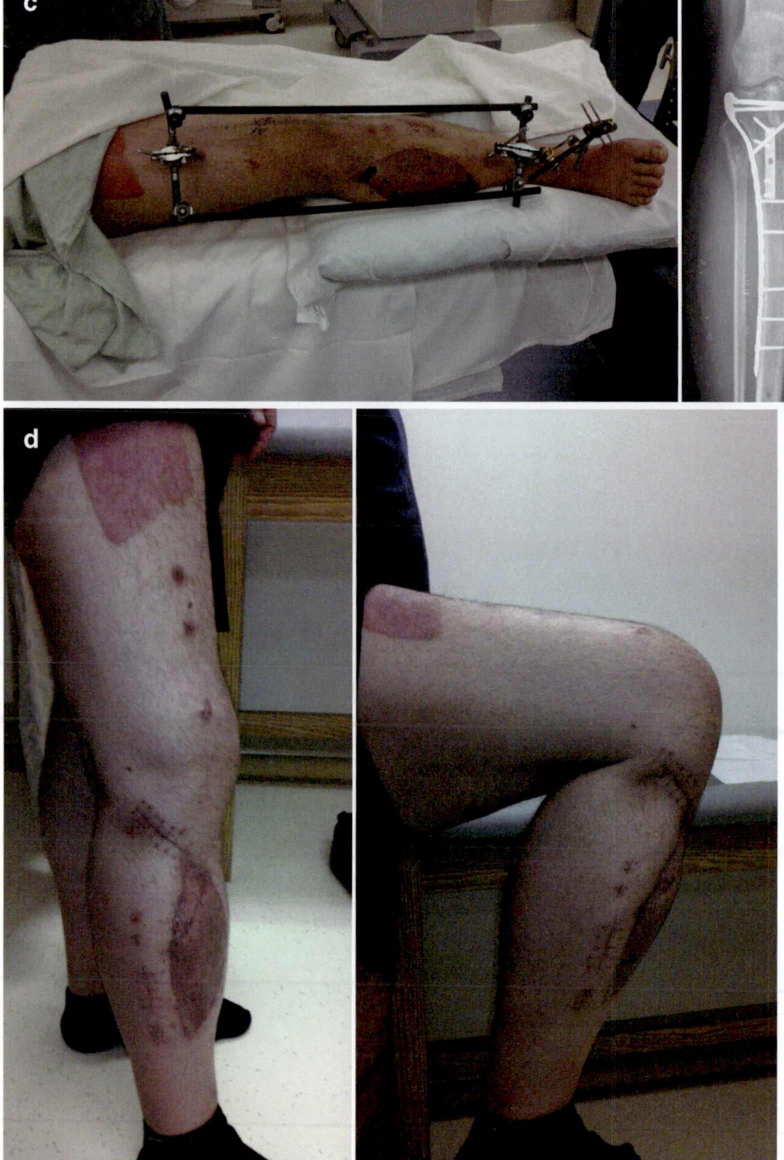

Fig. 3.3 (continued)

provide stability to the extremity but minimize fixation in temporizing circumstances when the frame is not being used for definitive care. In this setting we prefer the use of pins as compared to wires, as threaded pins can achieve bicortical purchase without passing completely through the lower extremity. Furthermore, pins do not necessitate the use of a tensioning device.

When the external fixator is applied as a temporizing device, several basic principles should be followed. The fractures, and therefore limb, should be held in as near anatomic alignment as possible. This provides the benefit of reestablishing normal anatomy, providing appropriate tissue tension to ease in definitive fixation at a later date, and stabilizes the soft tissue envelope. The

Table 3.1 Standard temporizing external fixators

Application	Pin size	Pin number	Pin location

Femur	5.0 mm	Proximal fragment: 2 or 3 Distal fragment: 2 or 3	Anterior
			  Pro: Ease of placement
			  Con: Through the quadriceps muscle/tendon, may prohibit hip flexion, risk to neurovascular structures with proximal placement
			Anterolateral
			  Pro: Muscle/tendon sparring
			  Con: Technical placement
			Lateral
			  Pro: Ease of placement
			  Con: Through the vastus lateralis, prohibits decubitus patient positioning

Knee spanning	Femur: 5.0 mm Tibia: 5.0 mm	Femur: 2 or 3 Tibia: 2 or 3	Femur
			  Anterior or anterolateral (see above)
			Tibia
			  Anteromedial

Tibia	5.0 mm	Proximal fragment: 2 or 3 Distal fragment: 2 or 3	Anteromedial
			  Pro: Ease of placement, muscle/tendon sparring
			  Con: Subcutaneous nature of tibia at this level risks osteomyelitis with pin tract infection

Ankle spanning	Tibia: 5.0 mm Calcaneus: 5.0 mm Midfoot/ forefoot: 4.0 mm or 3.0 mm	Tibia: 2 or 3 Calcaneus: 1 or 2 Midfoot/ forefoot: 1 or 2	Tibia
			  Anteromedial (see above)
			Calcaneus
			  Medial to lateral centrally threaded transfixion pin (protect neurovascular structures)
			Midfoot (optional, 1 pin, transcuneiform)
			  Dorsal-medial (muscle/tendon sparring)
			Forefoot (optional, 2 pins, first metatarsal)
			  Dorsal-medial (muscle/tendon sparring)

burden of hardware applied to the limb should be minimized but balanced appropriately by providing enough stability to the limb that the reduction can be maintained. As previously mentioned, a primary benefit of external fixation is minimal soft tissue insult for the placement of pins and wires in bone segments; however, soft tissue management, fixator care, and radiographic imaging become more challenging as additional fixation is added to each construct.

Ring Fixator Ring fixators are a type of modular, multiplanar fixators that are most frequently used along the definitive treatment pathway. These fixators use external rings or semicircles which are attached to the bone by tensioned wires or half pins. The rings are then joined to one another by stainless steel rods or telescoping struts. These fixators are more onerous to apply and are significantly more expensive but do offer great versatility. These multiplanar fixators can be used to make gradually correct angular malalignment, rotational deformity, or length disparity. They offer excellent mechanical stability and can effectively capture and stabilize small fragments.

Our preference has been to avoid the application of ring fixators in the acute setting, given the complexity of application and the significant limit they place on soft tissue access. However, these constructs are frequently used for the definitive treatment of the mangled extremity, especially once the soft tissues have been adequately addressed. Some modern modular external fixation systems afford the opportunity to convert a provisional or temporizing external fixator into a hybrid construct. This is a desirable treatment strategy for injuries which may require several soft tissue procedures or debridements in the

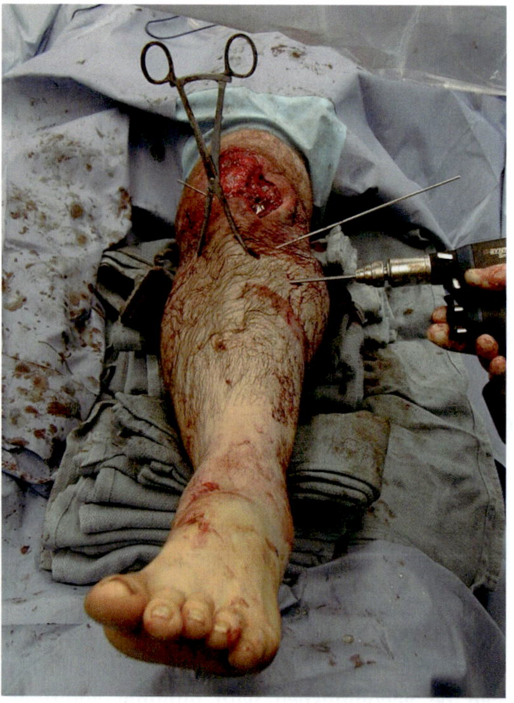

Fig. 3.4 Intraoperative clinical photo demonstrating minimally invasive plate osteosynthesis technique with percutaneous clamp placement and submuscular plating of tibial plateau fracture

etal stability. Advances in plate technology, including the evolution of locked plating, have improved the capacity to use plates in many challenging settings [80–82]. Locking plates are of particular value in the setting of complex periarticular injuries with metaphyseal comminution. The benefit of locked plating when caring for these injuries is the creation of a fixed-angle, toggle-free device. Furthermore, these plates may be applied using minimally invasive techniques (Fig. 3.4) with potentially improved bone healing and lower incidence of wound complications. While immediate plate fixation of the tibia in association with open wounds has been associated with relatively high infection rates, a "fix and flap" approach can be successfully employed in certain clinical scenarios. Our preference is to use this strategy, when appropriate, only after serial debridements with provisional external fixation and immediately preceding flap coverage although some authors have reported success with doing this in the acute setting [99].

Plates used to bridge areas of comminution, whether traditional or locked, are often bulky. This should be a consideration prior to placement as soft tissue coverage of these devices can be challenging. It is our preference to minimize the profile and overall hardware load of deep implants when managing skeletal injuries in conjunction with severe soft tissue injury. The use of small or mini-fragment plating systems to aid in the reduction and stabilization of key fracture fragments or intraarticular injuries can be useful in achieving this goal (Figs. 3.5 and 3.6). These systems offer a variety of plate options and even the ability for locked fixation when necessary. The stability of the construct can be increased with the adjunctive application of an external fixator or intramedullary nail. These devices may be used to span areas of bone loss or large, segmental regions of comminution which would otherwise require the application of a larger plate.

Plate Failure Another matter of importance when considering plate application for the mangled extremity is longevity of the implants. Internal fixation may be viewed as a race between biology and mechanics, in other words, a race between fracture healing and implant failure. Plates applied to inherently unstable fracture patterns, such as those fractures with segmental comminution, bone loss, or cortical gap opposite the plate, are at particular risk. In these instances, the plate is exposed to repeated cyclical loading by physiologic muscle forces and/or weight bearing. Typically the bone and implant share this load, but in unstable fracture patterns, the implant may be subject to a majority of the stress. As cyclical bending stresses continue, the risk of plate failure increases. If the area of comminution or fracture gap is able to heal with callus, the plate may maintain its integrity. But if this process is delayed secondary to the amount of bone loss or degree of soft tissue compromise limiting healing capacity, the plate will reach its fatigue limit and fail. This concept highlights the importance of recognizing the degree of soft tissue injury and making surgical plans for skeletal stabilization accordingly. Bone fragments that are devascularized by the injury or surgical stripping have impaired healing capacity, therefore changing the timeline for the race between healing and implant failure.

Intramedullary Nail Fixation

Some of the skeletal injuries associated with mangled extremities will not be amenable to intramedullary nail fixation. Fracture patterns which are primarily intraarticular in nature or involve compromised soft tissue around the nail entry site are not ideal for intramedullary treatment. Intramedullary nails function as internal fixation devices to bridge long bone injuries. These devices allow for fracture micromotion and healing through callus. However, for comminuted diaphyseal fractures, the intramedullary nail remains an attractive treatment option as they can oftentimes be placed through an incision remote from any soft tissue injury, require very little soft tissue dissection/stripping, and involve minimal extramedullary hardware burden.

Nail Considerations In routine application, the nail is placed across a fracture using closed manipulation and reduction techniques. In the mangled extremity, however, reduction may often be facilitated through the open soft tissue injury. Bumps, fluoroscopy, traction, percutaneous clamps, Schanz screws, Steinmann pins, and blocking screws are all reduction tools and

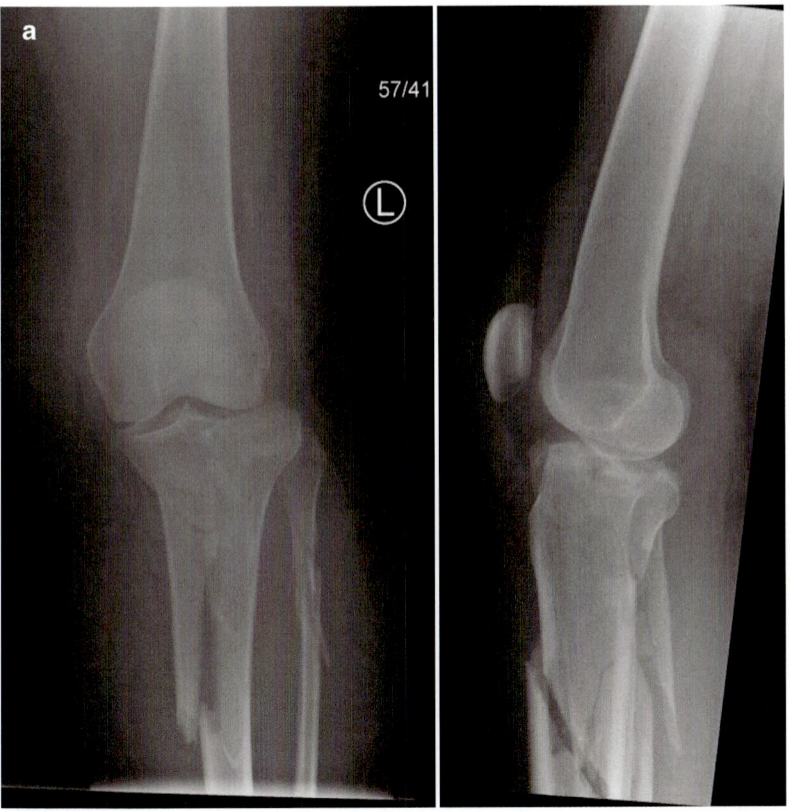

Fig. 3.5 63-year-old female s/p fall from counter with complex left bicondylar tibial plateau fracture. (**a**) AP and lateral injury radiographs demonstrating complex left bicondylar tibial plateau fracture with segmental meta-diaphyseal comminution. (**b**) Intraoperative fluoroscopic images demonstrating provisional mini-fragment fixation of the medial column and articular injury at the time of temporizing knee-spanning external fixation. Use of mini-fragment fixation affords early articular reduction and augments ability of spanning external fixator to maintain length with minimal hardware load in acute phase of soft tissue injury. (**c**) Final AP and lateral radiographs 7 months post-injury demonstrating healed fracture in near-anatomic alignment

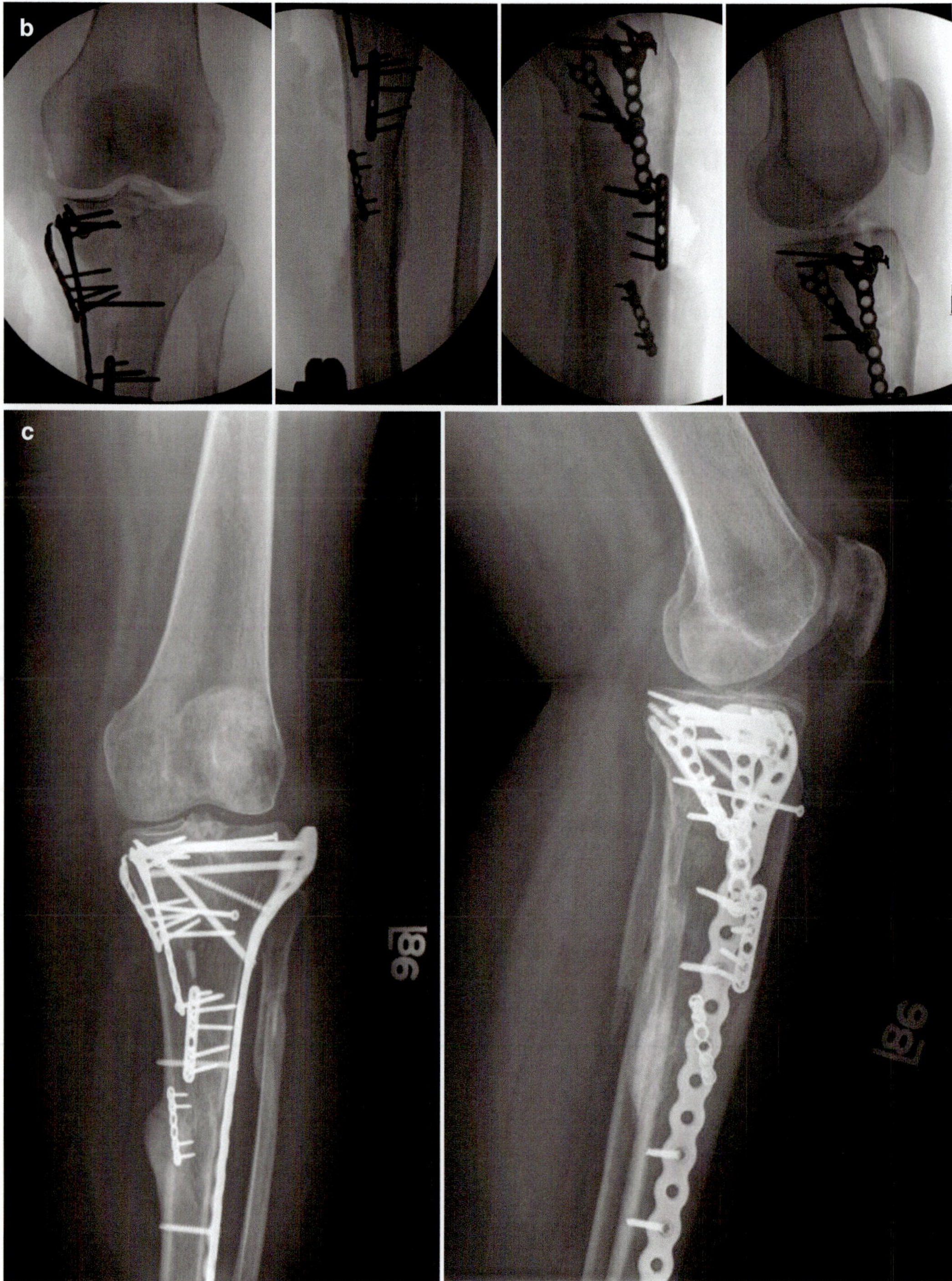

Fig. 3.5 (continued)

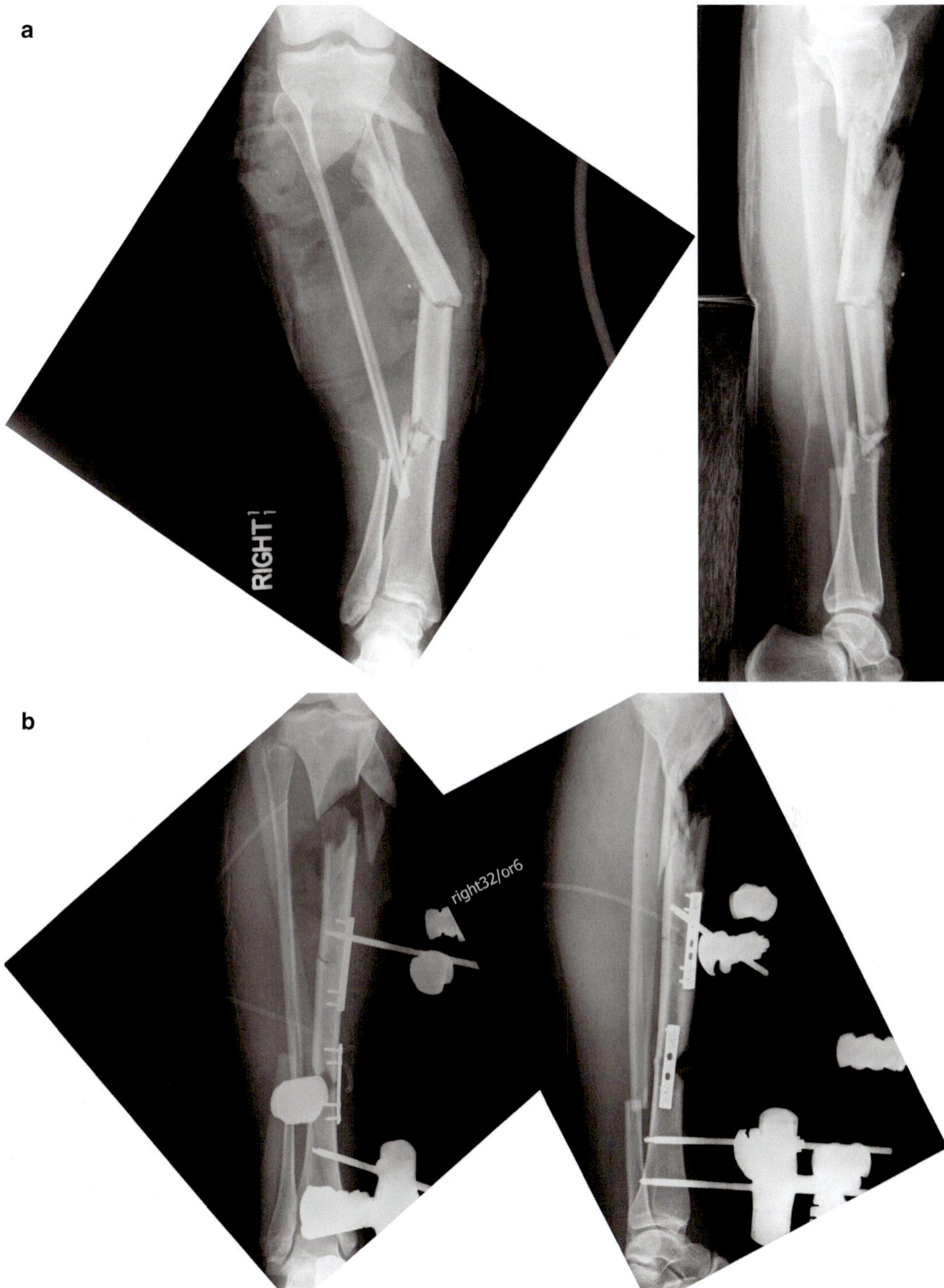

Fig. 3.6 47-year-old female s/p motorcycle crash with open segment right tibia shaft fracture. (**a**) AP and lateral injury radiographs demonstrating complex, multi-segmental tibial shaft fracture. (**b**) AP and lateral postoperative radiographs after initial debridement, provisional mini-fragment fixation, and external fixation. (**c**) Clinical photos demonstrating complex soft tissue injury and restoration of overall alignment following initial debridement and mini-fragment internal fixation prior to external fixator application. (**d**) Final construct after staged definitive ORIF. (**e**) Clinical photos demonstrating final outcome with bony and soft tissue healing and restoration of functional range of motion

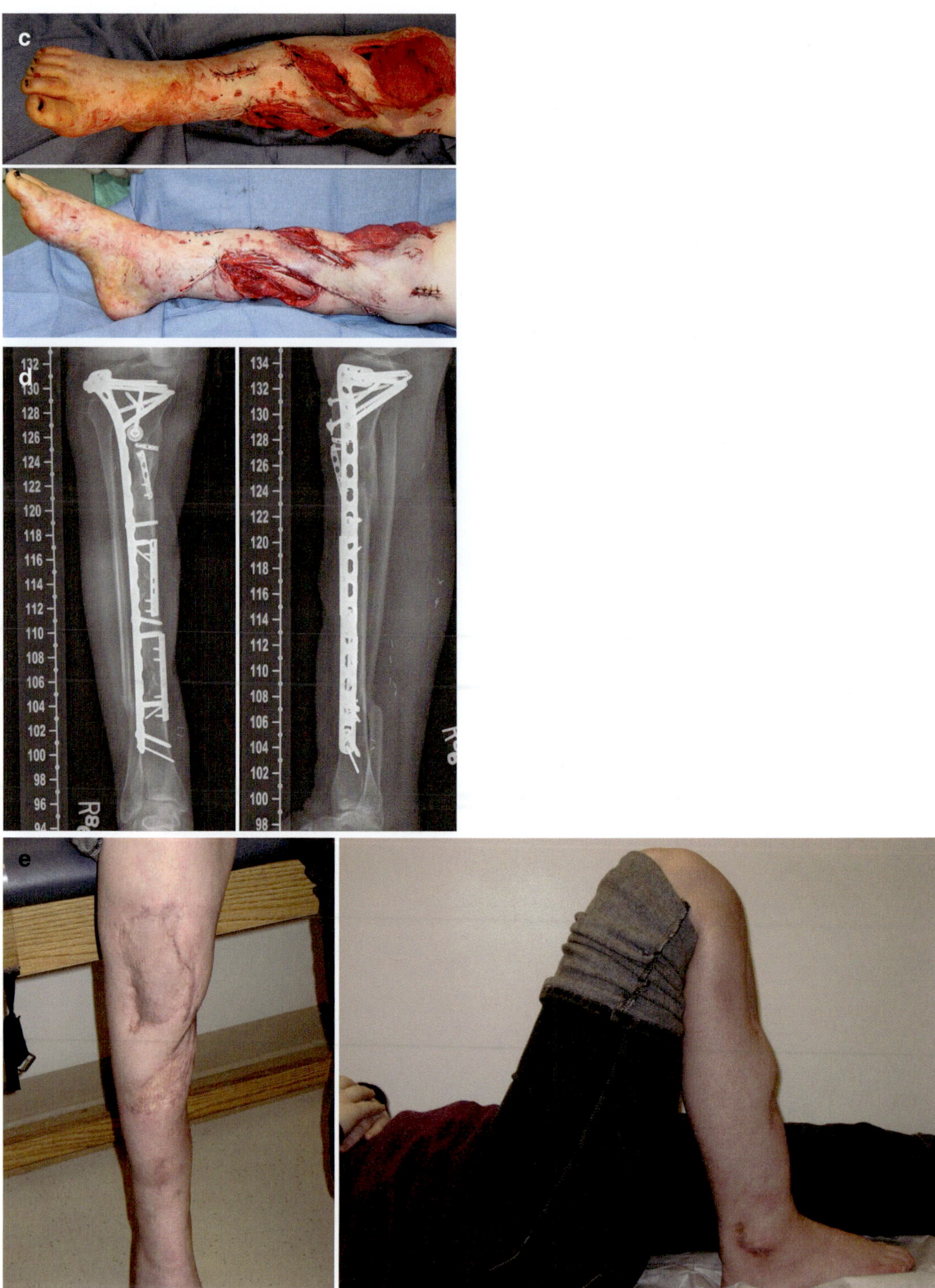

Fig. 3.6 (continued)

adjunctive techniques at the surgeon's disposal to facilitate reduction in intramedullary nailing procedures, either open or closed. These techniques can serve to minimize the need for direct surgical exposure of the fracture site. As a result, the overlying soft tissue envelope is left intact, and the periosteal vascular supply of the bone may be preserved. This is of particular advantage when managing the mangled extremity.

Intramedullary implants also provide another "layer" of protection against infection. Because of their position within the medullary canal, these implants are typically further from any associated soft tissue injury. This is a significant benefit of these devices as they may be less likely to be affected by a superficial soft tissue infection. Additionally, it has been our experience that implant infections involving intramedullary nails are more easily managed than those associated with plate/screw constructs.

Achieving reduction with an intramedullary implant requires the provider to remain aware of fracture alignment in the coronal, sagittal, and axial (rotational) planes. For simple fractures at the diaphysis of the long bone, the implant will aid in the reduction by achieving intramedullary "fit" proximal and distal to the fracture site. In this case, achieving a functional reduction prior to reaming and implant placement is less important. However, during nailing of more distal or proximal patterns, a keen understanding of anatomy and alignment is needed to avoid common pitfalls.

Reaming The use of reaming to enlarge the intramedullary canal was developed by Kuntscher in an effort to produce a space of more uniform canal diameter and increased contact between the endosteum and implant [10, 83, 84]. The enlargement of the intramedullary canal also offered the ability to insert a larger diameter nail with greater fatigue strength. While the process of reaming is relatively straightforward, it causes an increase in the medullary pressure and an elevation in cortical temperature [85–87]. Additional concern that reaming destroys medullary contents, including the endovascular blood supply, and may there-fore decrease healing capacity was also present for many years [88–94]. However, the only prospective multicenter trial to evaluate the effect of reaming on open and closed tibia fractures found no difference in the need for bone grafting, implant exchange, or dynamization in reamed and unreamed nails [95] (Table 3.3).

Osseous Union

Open fractures and mangled extremities have been reported to have non-union rates up to 60% [96, 97]. Injury factors such as the amount of fracture displacement, degree of comminution, severity of soft tissue insult, amount of bone loss, and presence of infection all influence the rate of union in these injuries (Table 3.4). Injury management strategies including appropriate antibiotic therapy, thorough surgical debridement, and temporizing/definitive skeletal fixation likely also contribute to the ultimate healing of these injuries. The ability to achieve osseous union is critical for restoration of limb function [61, 98]. Furthermore, a stable union can allow patients to begin rehabilitation sooner and likely increase their ability to return to gainful employment. When a stable union is not achieved, several interventions may be used to increase the likelihood of healing. These include the use of dynamization, bone grafting, distraction osteogenesis, and vascularized bone grafting. Discussion of each of these techniques is beyond the scope of this chapter, but they may be considered as soon as the soft tissue permits.

Conclusion

Fractures with significant soft tissue injury represent some of the most challenging injuries to treat. Coordination of care with other teams is often necessary to manage associated injuries in these patients and also plan for appropriate soft tissue reconstruction. The extremity surgeon's responsibility is to organize care for the local injury and understand how it is best managed in the setting of the patient's overall condition and

Table 3.3 Comparison of definitive treatment strategies for the MANGLED EXTREMITY

Technique	Pros	Cons	Commentary
External fixator	Low burden of hardware Minimal required soft tissue dissection/stripping Application for periarticular injuries Versatility of application Ability to make gradual correction to angular malalignment, rotational deformity, length disparity	Complexity of application Unfamiliarity of use (for many surgeons) Pin site infections Pin loosening Patient dissatisfaction	External fixators are used in both the temporizing and definitive treatment of mangled extremities. Additionally, they can be applied as an adjunct to other forms of skeletal fixation (intramedullary nail, plate and screw fixation)
Plate	Application for periarticular injuries Use in short segment bone fragments Maintenance of anatomic reduction	Hardware burden Soft tissue dissection/stripping Plate failure	The advances in plate technology have furthered their application in treating the mangled extremity. Particularly, small and mini-fragment-type locking plates which can be applied to periarticular injuries or essential fracture fragments with lower hardware burden and surgical dissection
Intramedullary nail	Remote entry site Minimal required soft tissue dissection/stripping Hardware is protected by the bone	Difficulty of placement for proximal or distal fractures Inability to address periarticular fractures	Intramedullary nails may be preferred for treatment of some mangled extremities as they offer some of the benefits of external fixators (minimal soft tissue stripping) but are typically easier to apply and better tolerated by patients

Table 3.4 Factors contributing to skeletal union in mangled extremities

Injury factors	Management factors
Initial displacement	Antibiotic therapy
Degree of comminution	Thorough debridement and irrigation
Severity of soft tissue injury	Fixation strategy
Amount of bone loss	
Presence of infection	

associated injuries. In general, wound debridement and temporizing stabilization of the fracture are the first stages of treatment. This may require multiple debridements and management with antibiotic bead pouches or negative pressure wound dressings. Subsequent to this, secondary wound closure or treatment with local or free tissue transfer typically occurs. The decision to proceed with definitive skeletal stabilization typically occurs immediately preceding or just after the soft tissues have been closed or covered definitively.

It is important to think of treatment of the soft tissues and bone as mutually beneficial. Temporizing stability of the bone preserves length and decreases the mechanical stress transmitted to tenuous soft tissues by ongoing motion and instability. Appropriate care of the soft tissue provides an environment conducive to bony union. The proper timing and overlap of interventions are of essential importance in the reconstructive phase of care. Definitive treatment with external fixation, plates and screws, or an intramedullary implant is dependent upon a multitude of factors. Each construct, when applied appropriately, can be used successfully and provide patients with suitable stability to allow for soft tissue healing, bony union, and functional recovery.

Clinical Pearls
- Treatment of the soft tissue and bone injuries of mangled extremities is interdependent and reciprocally beneficial.
- External fixation is the foundation of temporizing skeletal stability as it allows for access to soft tissues, and these constructs can be easily adjusted, assembled, and disassembled as needed.
- External fixation, plate fixation, or intramedullary nailing can be used for definitive skeletal treatment of the mangled extremity.

Clinical Pitfalls
- Incomplete debridement and/or the lack of serial soft tissue evaluation can increase risk of infection and catastrophic complication.
- Moving toward definitive skeletal fixation with internal devices prior to complete debridement and soft tissue assessment.
- Management planning based upon the skeletal injury in isolation, without consideration of the associated soft tissue injury, will result is suboptimal outcomes.

References

1. Stranix JT, Lee Z-H, Jacoby A, et al. Not all Gustilo type IIIB fractures are created equal: arterial injury impacts limb salvage outcomes. Plast Reconstr Surg. 2017;140(5):1033–41. https://doi.org/10.1097/PRS.0000000000003766.
2. Redett RJ, Robertson BC, Chang B, Girotto J, Vaughan T. Limb salvage of lower-extremity wounds using free gracilis muscle reconstruction. Plast Reconstr Surg. 2000;106(7):1507–13.
3. Katzman SS, Dickson K. Determining the prognosis for limb salvage in major vascular injuries with associated open tibial fractures. Orthop Rev. 1992;21(2):195–9.
4. Dellinger EP, Miller SD, Wertz MJ, Grypma M, Droppert B, Anderson PA. Risk of infection after open fracture of the arm or leg. Arch Surg. 1988;123(11):1320–7.
5. Hansen ST. The type-IIIC tibial fracture. Salvage or amputation. JBJS. 1987;69(6):799–800.
6. Caudle RJ, Stern PJ. Severe open fractures of the tibia. JBJS. 1987;69(6):801–7.
7. Keeley SB, Snyder WH, Weigelt JA. Arterial injuries below the knee: fifty-one patients with 82 injuries. J Trauma Injury Infect Crit Care. 1983;23(4):285–92.
8. O'Donnell TF, Brewster DC, Darling RC, Veen H, Waltman AA. Arterial injuries associated with fractures and/or dislocations of the knee. J Trauma Injury Infect Crit Care. 1977;17(10):775–84.
9. Mukherjee GD. The rise of surgery: from empiric craft to scientific discipline. Plast Reconstr Surg. 1980;65(4):531.
10. Browner BD. Skeletal trauma. Gulf Professional Publishing; Houston, TX 2003.
11. Müller ME, Allgöwer M, Willenegger H. Manual of internal fixation. Berlin, Heidelberg: Springer Science & Business Media; 2012. https://doi.org/10.1007/978-3-642-96065-9.
12. Patzakis MJ. Management of open fractures and complications. Instr Course Lect. 1982;31:62–4.
13. Patzakis MJ, Wilkins J. Factors influencing infection rate in open fracture wounds. Clin Orthop Relat Res. 1989;243:36–40.
14. Skaggs DL, Kautz SM, Kay RM, Tolo VT. Effect of delay of surgical treatment on rate of infection in open fractures in children. J Pediatr Orthop. 2000;20(1):19–22.
15. Skaggs DL, Friend L, Alman B, et al. The effect of surgical delay on acute infection following 554 open fractures in children. JBJS. 2005;87(1):8–12. https://doi.org/10.2106/JBJS.C.01561.
16. Bednar DA, Parikh J. Effect of time delay from injury to primary management on the incidence of deep infection after open fractures of the lower extremities caused by blunt trauma in adults. J Orthop Trauma. 1993;7(6):532–5.
17. Patzakis MJ, Wilkins J, Moore TM. Considerations in reducing the infection rate in open tibial fractures. Clin Orthop Relat Res. 1983;178:36–41.
18. GUSTILO RB, Anderson JT. JSBS classics. Prevention of infection in the treatment of one thousand and twenty-five open fractures of long bones. Retrospective and prospective analyses. J Bone Joint Surg. 2002;84-A:682.
19. Schurman DJ, Hirshman HP, Burton DS. Cephalothin and cefamandole penetration into bone, synovial fluid, and wound drainage fluid. JBJS. 1980;62(6):981–5.
20. Anglen JO. Wound irrigation in musculoskeletal injury. J Am Acad Orthop Surg. 2001;9(4):219–26.

21. Gustilo RB, Anderson JT. Prevention of infection in the treatment of one thousand and twenty-five open fractures of long bones: retrospective and prospective analyses. JBJS. 1976;58(4):453–8.

22. Foote CJ, Guyatt GH, Vignesh KN, et al. Which surgical treatment for open tibial shaft fractures results in the fewest reoperations? A network meta-analysis. Clin Orthop Relat Res. 2015;473(7):2179–92. https://doi.org/10.1007/s11999-015-4224-y.

23. Flow Investigators, Bhandari M, Jeray KJ, et al. A trial of wound irrigation in the initial management of open fracture wounds. N Engl J Med. 2015;373(27):2629–41. https://doi.org/10.1056/NEJMoa1508502.

24. Petrisor B, Jeray K, Schemitsch E, et al. Fluid lavage in patients with open fracture wounds (FLOW): an international survey of 984 surgeons. BMC Musculoskelet Disord. 2008;9(1):7. https://doi.org/10.1186/1471-2474-9-7.

25. Crowley DJ, Kanakaris NK, Giannoudis PV. Irrigation of the wounds in open fractures. J Bone Joint Surg Br. 2007;89(5):580–5. https://doi.org/10.1302/0301-620X.89B5.19286.

26. Bhandari M, Thompson K, Adili A, Shaughnessy SG. High and low pressure irrigation in contaminated wounds with exposed bone. Int J Surg Investig. 2000;2(3):179–82.

27. Bhandari M, Schemitsch EH, Adili A, Lachowski RJ, Shaughnessy SG. High and low pressure pulsatile lavage of contaminated tibial fractures: an in vitro study of bacterial adherence and bone damage. J Orthop Trauma. 1999;13(8):526–33.

28. Gross A, Cutright DE, Bhaskar SN. Effectiveness of pulsating water jet lavage in treatment of contaminated crushed wounds. Am J Surg. 1972;124(3):373–7.

29. Bhhaskar SN, Cutright DE, Runsuck EE, Gross A. Pulsating water jet devices in debridement of combat wounds. Mil Med. 1971;136(3):264–6.

30. Hassinger SM, Harding G, Wongworawat MD. High-pressure pulsatile lavage propagates bacteria into soft tissue. Clin Orthop Relat Res. 2005;439:27–31.

31. Polzin B, Ellis T, Dirschl DR. Effects of varying pulsatile lavage pressure on cancellous bone structure and fracture healing. J Orthop Trauma. 2006;20(4):261–6.

32. Anglen JO, Apostoles S, Christensen G, Gainor B. The efficacy of various irrigation solutions in removing slime-producing Staphylococcus. J Orthop Trauma. 1994;8(5):390–6.

33. Bhandari M, Schemitsch EH. High-pressure irrigation increases adipocyte-like cells at the expense of osteoblasts in vitro. J Bone Joint Surg Br. 2002;84(7):1054–61.

34. Bhandari M, Adili A, Lachowski RJ. High pressure pulsatile lavage of contaminated human tibiae: an in vitro study. J Orthop Trauma. 1998;12(7):479–84.

35. Adili A, Bhandari M, Schemitsch EH. The biomechanical effect of high-pressure irrigation on diaphyseal fracture healing in vivo. J Orthop Trauma. 2002;16(6):413–7.

36. Tarbox BB, Conroy BP, Malicky ES, et al. Benzalkonium chloride. A potential disinfecting irrigation solution for orthopaedic wounds. Clin Orthop Relat Res. 1998;346:255–61.

37. Conroy BP, Anglen JO, Simpson WA, et al. Comparison of castile soap, benzalkonium chloride, and bacitracin as irrigation solutions for complex contaminated orthopaedic wounds. J Orthop Trauma. 1999;13(5):332–7.

38. Burd T, Christensen GD, Anglen JO, Gainor BJ, Conroy BP, Simpson WA. Sequential irrigation with common detergents: a promising new method for decontaminating orthopedic wounds. Am J Orthop. 1999;28(3):156–60.

39. Gainor BJ, Hockman DE, Anglen JO, Christensen G, Simpson WA. Benzalkonium chloride: a potential disinfecting irrigation solution. J Orthop Trauma. 1997;11(2):121–5.

40. Huyette DR, Simpson WA, Walsh R, et al. Eradication by surfactant irrigation of Staphylococcus aureus from infected complex wounds. Clin Orthop Relat Res. 2004;427:28–36.

41. Kaysinger KK, Nicholson NC, Ramp WK, Kellam JF. Toxic effects of wound irrigation solutions on cultured tibiae and osteoblasts. J Orthop Trauma. 1995;9(4):303–11.

42. Sprung J, Schedewie HK, Kampine JP. Intraoperative anaphylactic shock after bacitracin irrigation. Anesth Analg. 1990;71(4):430–3.

43. Behrens F. General theory and principles of external fixation. Clin Orthop Relat Res. 1989;241:15–23.

44. Behrens F, Johnson W. Unilateral external fixation. Methods to increase and reduce frame stiffness. Clin Orthop Relat Res. 1989;241:48–56.

45. Chapman MW, Madison M. Operative orthopaedics. Philadelphia: Lippincott Williams & Wilkins; 1993.

46. Dabezies EJ, D'Ambrosia R, Shoji H, Norris R, Murphy G. Fractures of the femoral shaft treated by external fixation with the Wagner device. JBJS. 1984;66(3):360–4.

47. Velazco A, Fleming LL. Open fractures of the tibia treated by the Hoffmann external fixator. Clin Orthop Relat Res. 1983;180:125–32.

48. Moroni A, Pegreffi F, Cadossi M, Hoang-Kim A, Lio V, Giannini S. Hydroxyapatite-coated external fixation pins. Expert Rev Med Devices. 2005;2(4):465–71. https://doi.org/10.1586/17434440.2.4.465.

49. Moroni A, Toksvig-Larsen S, Maltarello MC, Orienti L, Stea S, Giannini S. A comparison of hydroxyapatite-coated, titanium-coated, and uncoated tapered external-fixation pins. An in vivo study in sheep. JBJS. 1998;80(4):547–54.

50. Pizà G, Caja VL, González-Viejo MA, Navarro A. Hydroxyapatite-coated external-fixation pins. The effect on pin loosening and pin-track infection in leg lengthening for short stature. J Bone Joint Surg Br. 2004;86(6):892–7.

51. Caja VL, Pizǎ G, Navarro A. Hydroxyapatite coating of external fixation pins to decrease axial deformity during tibial lengthening for short stature. JBJS. 2003;85-A(8):1527–31.
52. Akilapa O, Gaffey A. Hydroxyapatite pins for external fixation: is there sufficient evidence to prove that coated pins are less likely to be replaced prematurely? Acta Orthop Traumatol Turc. 2015;49(4):410–5. https://doi.org/10.3944/AOTT.2015.14.0206.
53. Saithna A. The influence of hydroxyapatite coating of external fixator pins on pin loosening and pin track infection: a systematic review. Injury. 2010;41(2):128–32. https://doi.org/10.1016/j.injury.2009.01.001.
54. Halsey D, Fleming B, Pope MH, Krag M, Kristiansen T. External fixator pin design. Clin Orthop Relat Res. 1992;278:305–12.
55. Kasman RA, Chao EY. Fatigue performance of external fixator pins. J Orthop Res. 1984;2(4):377–84. https://doi.org/10.1002/jor.1100020410.
56. Johnson KD, Tencer AF. Biomechanics in orthopaedic trauma. Taylor & Francis; Philadelphia, PA 1994.
57. Lavini FM, Brivio LR, Leso P. Biomechanical factors in designing screws for the Orthofix system. Clin Orthop Relat Res. 1994;308:63–7.
58. Kowalski M, Schemitsch EH, Harrington RM, Chapman JR, Swiontkowski MF. Comparative biomechanical evaluation of different external fixation sidebars: stainless-steel tubes versus carbon fiber rods. J Orthop Trauma. 1996;10(7):470–5.
59. Behrens F. A primer of fixator devices and configurations. Clin Orthop Relat Res. 1989;241:5–14.
60. Behrens F, Johnson WD, Koch TW, Kovacevic N. Bending stiffness of unilateral and bilateral fixator frames. Clin Orthop Relat Res. 1983;178:103–10.
61. Behrens F, Searls K. External fixation of the tibia. Basic concepts and prospective evaluation. J Bone Joint Surg Br. 1986;68(2):246–54.
62. Egan JM, Shearer JR. Behavior of an external fixation frame incorporating an angular separation of the fixator pins. A finite element approach. Clin Orthop Relat Res. 1987;223:265–74.
63. Huiskes R, Chao EY. Guidelines for external fixation frame rigidity and stresses. J Orthop Res. 1986;4(1):68–75. https://doi.org/10.1002/jor.1100040108.
64. Thordarson DB, Markolf KL, Cracchiolo A. External fixation in arthrodesis of the ankle. A biomechanical study comparing a unilateral frame with a modified transfixion frame. JBJS. 1994;76(10):1541–4.
65. Aro HT, Chao EY. Biomechanics and biology of fracture repair under external fixation. Hand Clin. 1993;9(4):531–42.
66. Briggs BT, Chao EY. The mechanical performance of the standard Hoffmann-Vidal external fixation apparatus. JBJS. 1982;64(4):566–73.
67. Pettine KA, Chao EY, Kelly PJ. Analysis of the external fixator pin-bone interface. Clin Orthop Relat Res. 1993;293:18–27.
68. Byrd HS, Cierny G, Tebbetts JB. The management of open tibial fractures with associated soft-tissue loss: external pin fixation with early flap coverage. Plast Reconstr Surg. 1981;68(1):73–82.
69. Green SA. Complications of external skeletal fixation. Clin Orthop Relat Res. 1983;180:109–16.
70. Wade PA, Campbell RD. Open versus closed methods in treating fractures of the leg. Am J Surg. 1958;95(4):599–616.
71. Nowotarski P, Brumback RJ. Immediate interlocking nailing of fractures of the femur caused by low- to mid-velocity gunshots. J Orthop Trauma. 1994;8(2):134–41.
72. Chapman MW, Mahoney M. The role of early internal fixation in the management of open fractures. Clin Orthop Relat Res. 1979;138:120–31.
73. Chapman MW. The role of intramedullary fixation in open fractures. Clin Orthop Relat Res. 1986;212:26–34.
74. Chapman MW. The use of immediate internal fixation in open fractures. Ortho Clin North Am. 1980;11(3):579–91.
75. Holbrook JL, Swiontkowski MF, Sanders R. Treatment of open fractures of the tibial shaft: ender nailing versus external fixation. A randomized, prospective comparison. JBJS. 1989;71(8):1231–8.
76. Brumback RJ, Ellison PS, Poka A, Lakatos R, Bathon GH, Burgess AR. Intramedullary nailing of open fractures of the femoral shaft. JBJS. 1989;71(9):1324–31.
77. Biliouris TL, Schneider E, Rahn BA, Gasser B, Perren SM. The effect of radial preload on the implant-bone interface: a cadaveric study. J Orthop Trauma. 1989;3(4):323–32.
78. Clancey GJ, Hansen ST. Open fractures of the tibia: a review of one hundred and two cases. JBJS. 1978;60(1):118–22.
79. Olerud S, Karlström G. Tibial fractures treated by AO compression osteosynthesis. Experiences from a five year material. Acta Orthop Scand Suppl. 1972;140:1–104.
80. Augat P, Rüden v C. Evolution of fracture treatment with bone plates. Injury. 2018;49(Suppl 1):S2–7. https://doi.org/10.1016/S0020-1383(18)30294-8.
81. MacLeod AR, Pankaj P. Pre-operative planning for fracture fixation using locking plates: device configuration and other considerations. Injury. 2018;49(Suppl 1):S12–8. https://doi.org/10.1016/S0020-1383(18)30296-1.
82. Haidukewych GJ, Ricci W. Locked plating in orthopaedic trauma: a clinical update. J Am Acad Orthop Surg. 2008;16(6):347–55.
83. Küntscher G. Intramedullary nailing of pseudarthrosis. Zentralbl Chir. 1973;98(29):1041–7.
84. Lentz W. The history of intramedullary nailing. A brief look backwards. Der Chirurg; Zeitschrift fur alle Gebiete der operativen Medizen. 1990;61:474–80.

85. Green J. History and development of suction-irrigation-reaming. Injury. 2011;41:S24–31. https://doi.org/10.1097/BOT.0b013e318238b22b.

86. Robert Y Wang 1, Ru Li, Rad Zdero, David Bell, Michael Blankstein, Emil H Schemitsch. The physiologic and pathologic effects of the reamer irrigator aspirator on fat embolism outcome: an animal study. J Orthop Trauma. 2012 Sep;26(9):e132–7. https://doi.org/10.1097/BOT.0b013e318238b22b.

87. Thomas F Higgins 1, Virginia Casey, Kent Bachus. Cortical heat generation using an irrigating/aspirating single-pass reaming vs conventional stepwise reaming. J Orthop Trauma. 2007 Mar;21(3):192–7. https://doi.org/10.1097/BOT.0b013e318038d952.

88. Olerud S, Strömberg L. Intramedullary reaming and nailing: its early effects on cortical bone vascularization. Orthopedics. 1986;9(9):1204–8.

89. Hupel TM, Aksenov SA, Schemitsch EH. Cortical bone blood flow in loose and tight fitting locked unreamed intramedullary nailing: a canine segmental tibia fracture model. J Orthop Trauma. 1998;12(2):127–35.

90. Schemitsch EH, Turchin DC, Kowalski MJ, Swiontkowski MF. Quantitative assessment of bone injury and repair after reamed and unreamed locked intramedullary nailing. J Trauma Injury Infect Crit Care. 1998;45(2):250–5.

91. Schemitsch EH, Kowalski MJ, Swiontkowski MF. Soft-tissue blood flow following reamed versus unreamed locked intramedullary nailing: a fractured sheep tibia model. Ann Plast Surg. 1996;36(1):70–5.

92. Grundnes O, Utvåg SE, Reikerås O. Restoration of bone flow following fracture and reaming in rat femora. Acta Orthop Scand. 1994;65(2):185–90.

93. Rhinelander FW. Tibial blood supply in relation to fracture healing. Clin Orthop Relat Res. 1974;105:34–81.

94. Forster MC, Bruce ASW, Aster AS. Should the tibia be reamed when nailing? Injury. 2005;36(3):439–44. https://doi.org/10.1016/j.injury.2004.09.030.

95. Study to Prospectively Evaluate Reamed Intramedullary Nails in Patients with Tibial Fractures Investigators, Bhandari M, Guyatt G, et al. Randomized trial of reamed and unreamed intramedullary nailing of tibial shaft fractures. J Bone Joint Surg Am. 2008;90(12):2567–78. https://doi.org/10.2106/JBJS.G.01694.

96. Rosenthal RE, MacPhail JA, Oritz JE. Non-union in open tibial fractures. JBJS. 1977;59(2):244–8.

97. O'Halloran K, Coale M, Costales T, et al. Will my tibial fracture heal? Predicting nonunion at the time of definitive fixation based on commonly available variables. Clin Orthop Relat Res. 2016;474(6):1385–95. https://doi.org/10.1007/s11999-016-4821-4.

98. Prasarn ML, Helfet DL, Kloen P. Management of the mangled extremity. Strategies Trauma Limb Reconstr. 2012;7(2):57–66. https://doi.org/10.1007/s11751-012-0137 4.

99. Gopal S, Majumde S, Bathcelor AG, De Boer O, Smith RM. Fix and flap: the radial orthopaedic and plastic treatment of severe open fractures of the tibia. J Bone Joint Surg Br. 2000;82(7):959–66.

Temporizing and Definitive Skeletal Fixation for the Mangled Upper Extremity

Steven A. Horton and W. Andrew Eglseder

On initial assessment, the decision to amputate is made clear in cases where the limb is connected only by subcutaneous tissue with severe destruction of the distal part. More commonly, it is a multifactorial assessment. Surveying the limb for associated soft tissue damage is performed first with a focus on neurovascular injury. If the indication for limb salvage is obvious or there is no definitive decision for amputation, the dysvascular limb is treated initially with vascular repair and subsequently reassessed for ongoing tissue viability versus evolving necrosis [1]. Often, the mangled upper extremity will have significant soft tissue degloving and vascular injury that may not be immediately apparent, thus requiring temporizing methods of fixation which are soft tissue "friendly." A thorough assessment of skin color, turgor, and extent of degloving is made during the index procedure and along with thorough exploration of the wound bed and an active inventory of critical structures, specifically the involved vascular and neurologic structures.

If performing a vascular repair, skeletal fixation is often coordinated simultaneously. The importance of reperfusion via either a shunt or arterial repair is paramount. Reperfusion cannot be performed in a vacuum excluding skeletal stability, which provides not only soft tissue stabilization but protection of the arterial repair. The fixation strategy, whether definitive or temporizing, must involve a careful determination of the length of potential vein graft and/or arterial reconstruction. In these cases, either a single surgeon experienced in both vascular and skeletal surgery will complete these simultaneous efforts, or the individual vascular and orthopedic surgeons will work closely together for the best result. A lack of careful coordination between these surgical teams is a recipe for imminent disaster.

In regard to the timing of the extent of skeletal interventions for a mangled upper extremity, the condition of the patient must be assessed. Age, smoking status, comorbidities, resuscitation status, intraoperative stability, and host of other factors come into play. An 80-year-old 50 pack-year smoker may not tolerate the repeated procedures from a medical perspective, so it is advantageous to obtain definitive fixation in the initial operative encounter. Similarly, the hemodynamically unstable patient, who will benefit from skeletal stability but not the blood loss or time required for extensive fixation efforts, may benefit from an entirely different fixation strategy.

The options for skeletal stabilization include some level of open reduction internal fixation, external fixation, intramedullary fixation, and

S. A. Horton
Department of Orthopaedics, University of Maryland Medical Center, Baltimore, MD, USA

W. A. Eglseder (✉)
Department of Orthopaedics, University of Maryland Medical System, Baltimore, MD, USA
e-mail: aeglseder@umoa.umm.edu

R. A. Pensy, J. V. Ingari (eds.), *The Mangled Extremity*, https://doi.org/10.1007/978-3-319-56648-1_4

splints. Locked, intramedullary fixation is rarely utilized because of the technical nuances of the starting point, imaging, locking, and device considerations. Splinting is also not appealing because this limits access to soft tissue for monitoring as well as not providing adequate bony stabilization.

On first glance, it is frequently touted that the best decision will be to rapidly instrument with external fixation and return when stable. However, the surgeon may choose to quickly employ limited internal fixation, specifically in cases where compartment releases are indicated, as the exposure for the release in the upper extremity is similar to that required for fixation, or in those periarticular injuries where stabilizing and reducing grossly malaligned joint fragments will be important to long term success.

Limited internal fixation of diaphyseal fractures facilitates patient care, as it decreases the need for splinting, and thus allows for venous access and elevation of the injured extremities. Another benefit is to avoid the financial cost and small but potential morbidity of external fixation. No one treatment best serves all patients. Each patient has different injuries, risk factors, and medical comorbidities that will guide treatment and the timing of any treatment.

External fixation has some degree of attractiveness because of the apparent ease and expediency in application. This is not always the case depending on the level of injury particularly to proximal arm injuries. Because of the need for access to the arterial system, brachial, radial, and ulnar arteries, the approach will frequently afford the opportunity to gain skeletal access. Shunting will provide the opportunity for definitive fixation as well as at least limited provisional fixation. Depending on the nature of the arterial injury, sometimes definitive arterial repairs can be performed after open reduction and internal fixation particularly if collateral flow exists and back flow is present.

Scapula and Clavicle

Treatment of scapular fractures varies significantly based on location. The majority of closed fractures of the scapular body have historically been treated non-operatively secondary to their excellent functional recovery and the avoidance of a highly morbid surgical approach. These fractures are missed on initial trauma evaluation and are usually found on chest CT scan as part of the trauma workup. Higher energy trauma and the history of a motorcycle accident or ejected passenger should raise the suspicion for scapular fracture. Fractures involving the glenohumeral joint are more likely to need operative intervention as they are more directly responsible for shoulder motion. Scapulothoracic dissociations can be seen with near amputations of the extremity, and we have seen commonly with vascular and nerve issues (injury/complications, etc.). Open injuries involving the scapular spine, AC joint, or scapula body represent some of the most devastating upper extremity injuries and, in certain cases, are life-threatening. In cases where either skeletal or ligamentous stability is severely compromised, unusual fixation options may be useful to provide adequate stability for patient mobilization, soft tissue repairs, and/or vascular reconstruction, such as the implementation of a AC joint spanning locking plate construct. See Fig. 4.1 for an example of this technique realizing that hardware prominence is sometime unavoidable in the mangled shoulder.

Humerus

Each bone in the upper extremity relies on its osseous and ligamentous support surrounding for stability. The glenohumeral joint benefits from a robust ligamentous and muscular tether to maintain joint reduction. However, the glenohumeral osseous anatomy provides only minimal intrinsic restraint, predisposing the joint to high rates of dislocation compared to those of the lower extremity. Dislocations of the glenohumeral joint are common in high-energy trauma, and reduction is generally uncomplicated. Although rotator cuff tears are common [2], these rarely warrant urgent treatment. In cases where the joint will not reduce, open reduction is required and may be performed concomitantly with proximal humerus fixation. This fixation is preferentially performed

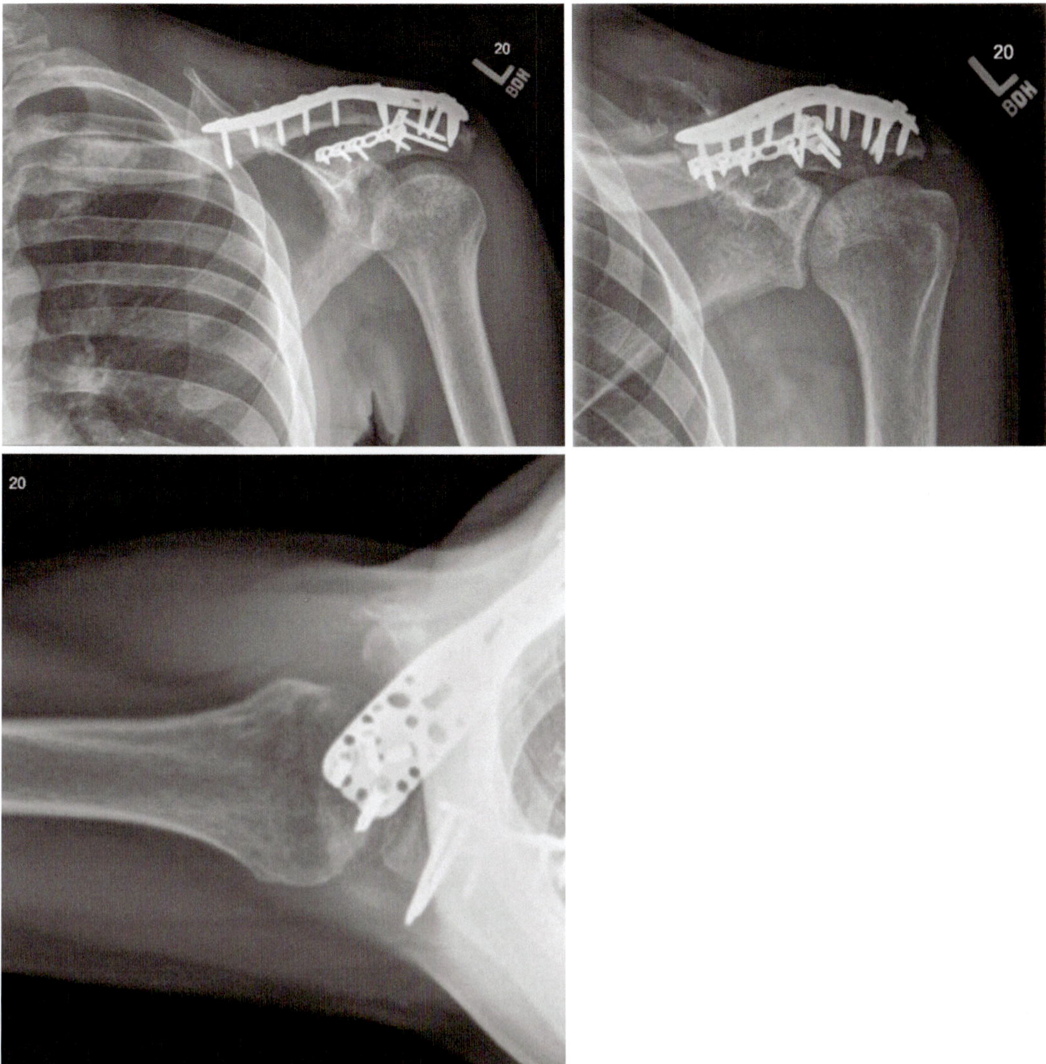

Fig. 4.1 Scapular fixation using a contoured proximal humerus plate applied in reverse fashion to align locking screws over acromion

through the deltopectoral approach, as it can be extended to the anterolateral exposure of the humerus, allowing concomitant brachial artery and other soft tissue reconstructions via large, extensile exposures through releasing the pectoralis major if necessary. In cases involving posterior glenoid fractures, a posterior exposure to the scapula, such as the Judet or modified Judet, can be helpful.

Where the proximal shaft or metaphyseal region is involved and external fixation is indicated, pin placement is performed ~15 cm from the anterolateral edge of the acromion along the anterolateral humerus, as it represents a relative safe zone [3]. This essentially localizes to, or proximal to, the deltoid tubercle and proximal to the course of the radial nerve. The authors prefer the use of a 5 mm half-pins that are placed with predrilling the holes and pins which are inserted by hand, allowing for more manual control and less likelihood of iatrogenic neurologic or vascular injury. The authors also prefer a four-pin clamp, with the first and last pin slots used. We recommend predrilling with a soft tissue protector and then inserting blunt tipped pins for maximum control.

For fractures of the shaft, several factors about the mangled extremity and the patient must be considered. In a closed wound where damage control orthopedics is the goal, the purpose of an intervention is to support patient resuscitation. Displaced humeral shaft fractures can be a source of extraluminal blood loss but should not be considered equal to femoral shaft in this regard. Coaptation splints can provide the necessary stability and be used to achieve acceptable reduction. These can be applied quickly in the trauma bay.

Most mangled upper extremities are, however, open by definition. The location of the skin defect and the location of the fracture may lead the surgeon toward a particular approach. If there is concern for radial nerve laceration, then the nerve is commonly visualized posteriorly through a lateral paratricipital approach. If the fracture is amenable to definitive fixation at this time, this approach can give excellent access to both the traversing radial nerve for repair and a mid-shaft humeral shaft fracture. Choices of fixation hinge on the available time and overall plan.

Generally, through open exposure, the surgeons will be able to achieve reduction with traction and manipulation for more simple patterns. For more complex fracture patterns that are unstable or comminuted, the use of mini-fragment plates can maintain the initial, provisional reduction prior to the contouring and application of the more definitive small or large fragment plate fixation. The use of mini-fragment plates may also aid in stability in conjunction with external fixation if the patient is unable to tolerate longer procedures or when reduction can be partially completed and when a need to revisit the wound exists. Mini-fragment uni-cortical screws will provide stout purchase and can be done rapidly to achieve and temporarily hold an anatomic reduction without the delay of measuring and are preferred when placing mini-plates for provisional reduction, as discussed above. The use of four or five-hole mini-plates may be used to better control large, mobile fragments compared with k-wire fixation alone. The authors prefer to place two screws both proximal and distal to the fracture in these temporizing settings for rotational

control as well as fixation strength. These small plates are generally placed orthogonal to the planned larger plate and do not require future removal.

As mentioned above, standard external fixation of humeral shaft injuries with distal metaphyseal and proximal metaphyseal performs well with mid-shaft fractures in the appropriate setting [3]. Figure 4.2 demonstrates the use of this technique for a transverse humeral shaft fracture.

Elbow Joint

Open elbow dislocations, fracture dislocations, and other associated open periarticular distal humerus fractures in the unstable patient with a mangled limb often present a challenge to the surgeon. In the non-acute patient, many treatment options exist for achieving anatomic reduction and stability of the fractured or dislocated, unstable elbow, but these procedures are technically demanding and time-consuming. Floating elbow joints are paired with high-energy trauma, and initial temporizing efforts may be limited by patient factors such as hemodynamic lability, accessibility of large c-arm image intensification, and inability to rapidly employ technically demanding maneuvers. Splinting will not stabilize the joint effectively, and when an arterial injury exists, skeletal fixation is needed to protect the repair and maintain length. In these cases, careful consideration is given to temporizing fixation strategies.

In the emergent situation where a floating elbow or distal humeral fracture exists, a temporary 6.5 mm transfixion screw starting from the proximal ulna proximally into the distal humeral shaft may provide an internal brace, with the small compromise of joint and cartilage injury at the entry point. This method is infrequently used due to its potential morbidity; however, it is a fast and reliable method to have in the surgeons' armamentarium.

The presence of brachial or antebrachial neurovascular injury with concomitant distal humerus fracture is commonly encountered. The approach or approaches chosen are matched to

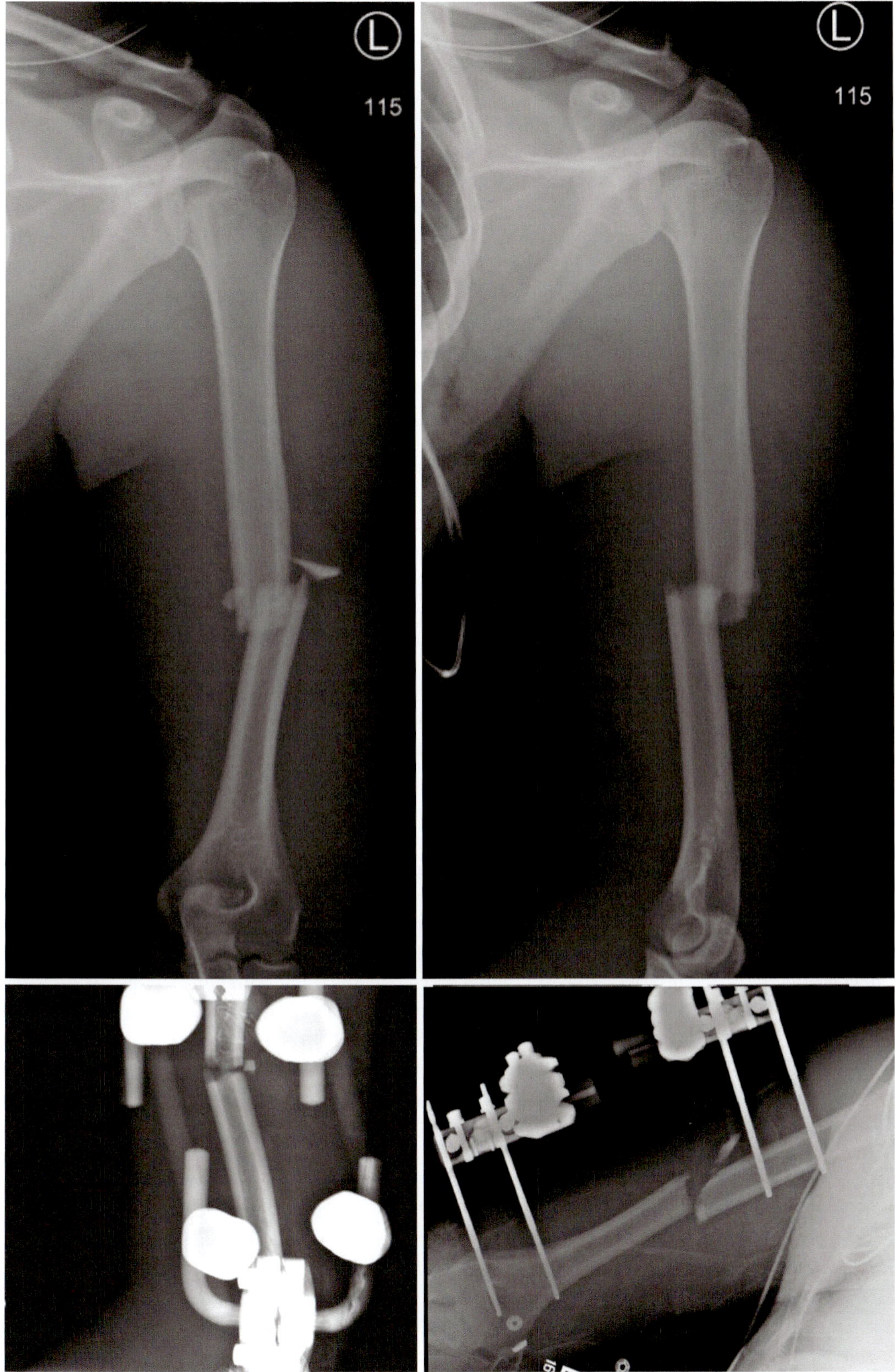

Fig. 4.2 Example of humeral shaft external fixation in a closed fracture in a polytrauma patient

the location and extent of the presenting neurovascular injuries. An anterolateral approach may allow for either a transcondylar external fixation pin for temporizing external fixation or a transcondylar lag screw for suitable nondisplaced articular fracture types. The medial approach to the brachial artery can be used for medial plate fixation in distal humerus fractures. In the setting of complex distal humerus fractures and elbow dislocations and the unstable patient, external fixation is utilized to provide bony stability, soft tissue stability, and length restoration and maintenance for arterial reconstruction. For placement of external fixation pins, an open exposure for pin placement is recommended for the placement of external fixation pins within the supracondylar metaphysis of the distal humerus to avoid injury to the radial nerve. This incision is made inferior to the expected location of the nerve, and careful dissection is used to avoid the radial nerve, remembering that the nerve courses through the lateral intermuscular septum approximately 10 cm above the lateral epicondyle. Having made this incision, two separate, parallel, 5.0 mm halfpins are placed through separate incisions anteriorly, after predrilling with a 4.0 mm drill and utilization of the appropriate soft tissue protecting drill sleeves. These pins are placed in the distal lateral supracondylar ridge, with the distal pin occasionally placed distal to the olecranon fossae to achieve control of a distal fragment.

Anterior approaches to the distal humerus and/or proximal radioulnar joint are helpful in certain definitive fixation techniques involving articular or periarticular injuries. However, in the initial surgical encounter, this approach is not usually chosen until after patient stabilization, as these fixation strategies are also time-consuming and complex. Nonetheless, brachial artery injury at the antecubital fossa level is common in open elbow dislocations and fracture dislocations [4]. If the arterial repair occurs prior to definitive fixation, care must be taken to avoid reinjury of the tenuous vascular repair during subsequent fixation or operative interventions to the extremity.

Fractures about the olecranon are commonly encountered in the mangled extremity and we find that when amenable, an intramedullary, partially threaded cancellous screw serves as an excellent option to stabilize and compress simple olecranon fracture patterns. This fixation method, seen in Fig. 4.3, relies upon endosteal purchase of the outer threads of the intramedullary screw within the diaphyseal ulna; therefore, careful "sounding" of the canal using the appropriately sized tap is critical to choose the appropriate length and diameter screw. We prefer this method over plate fixation as the screw has a low subcutaneous profile and its presence is not commonly a complaint from patients postoperatively. For more comminuted fractures, resisting the pull of the triceps and restoring the articular surface are accomplished using either small plate fixation in combination with either tension banding or, if necessary, bridge plate constructs. Spanning fixation can provide an external support to protect tenuous fixation in more comminuted cases or in those injuries with massive soft tissue defects.

Radius and Ulna

Forearm trauma resulting in segmental fractures or severe comminution presents a creative challenge to the treating surgeon. A combination of internal and external fixation is routinely used on initial presentation. The restoration of length, alignment, and rotation of the fractured radius and ulna deserves specific attention, as most surgeons agree that these parameters are critical to successful outcomes [5]. In the mangled forearm, where both bones are usually fractured (often segmentally), temporizing external fixation has limited ability to approximate the fracture ends anatomically. By its design, spanning external fixation results in segmental fragment instability, and therefore supplementing with plating or intramedullary fixation is common practice. While the employed external fixation may be temporary, the initial plating may be left in situ. The use of mini-fragment system plates is routinely employed temporarily in this role as a stabilizing adjuvant in both radius and ulna shaft injuries. In either the humeral or forearm injury, if there is segmental bone loss, anti-biotic cement spacers placed around intramedullary threaded

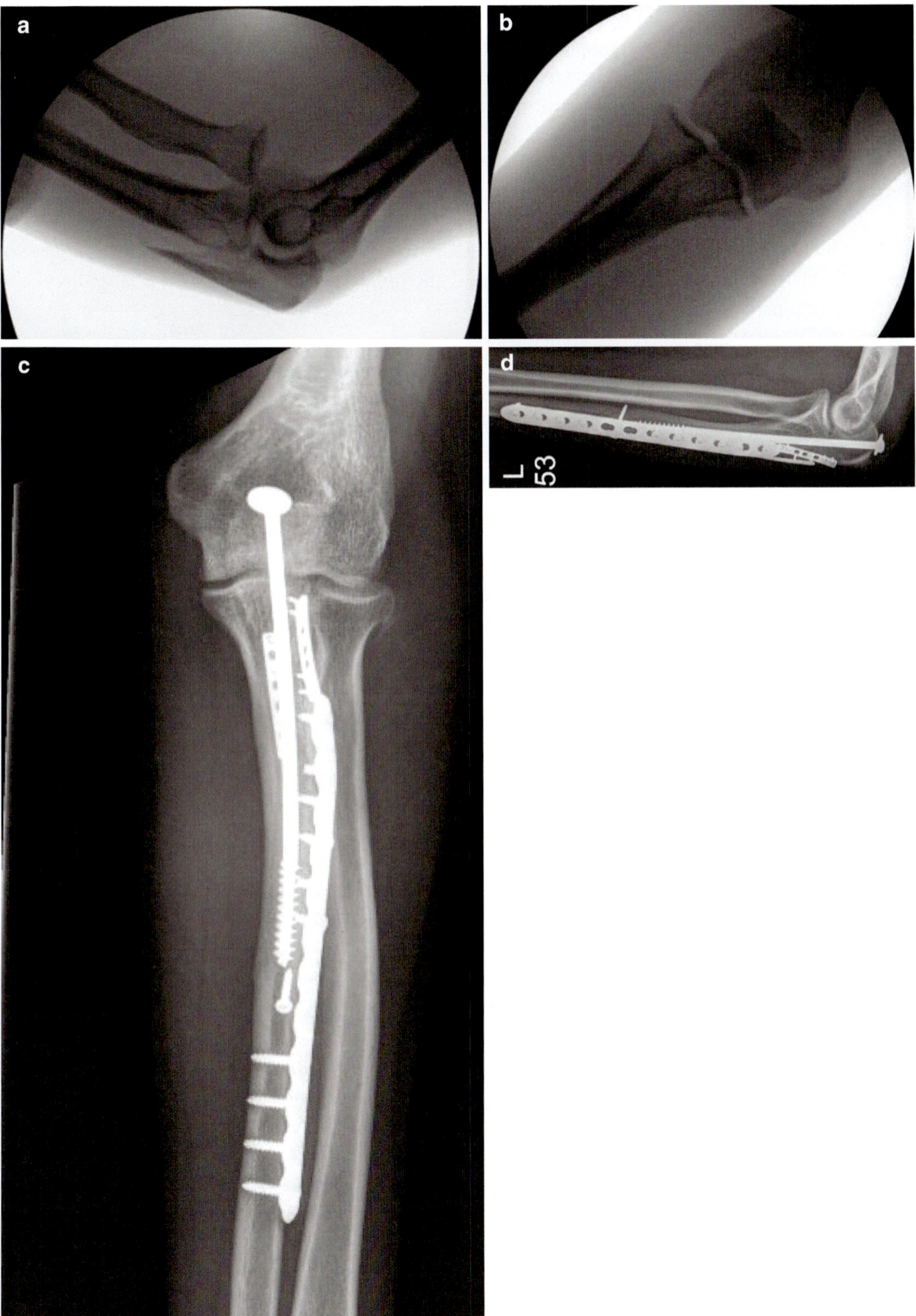

Fig. 4.3 Intraoperative discovery of a Monteggia variant Bado type 1 in an intubated MCC polytrauma patient (**a/b**). Initial fixation was performed rapidly with mini-fragmentary plate/screws and 6.5 mm cancellous screw to restore the joint followed by subsequent shaft fixation with LCP plate (**c/d**)

Steinmann pins can be utilized which affords soft tissue access, length restoration, relative stability, delivery of local anti-biotics, and soft tissue volume maintenance for later bone grafting, as indicated.

In regard to external fixation of the ulna, the proximal ulna is subcutaneous, and external fixation pins are thus placed percutaneously with soft tissue which guides to avoid major neurovascular structures. Distally, access is found through the flexor carpi ulnaris (FCU) and the extensor carpi ulnaris (ECU) interval. Pins are placed in the posteromedial cortex distally with the forearm in supination. For forearm fractures treated with temporizing external fixation, we recommend the use of two 4 mm half-pins in the proximal ulna and distal ulna, with consideration of the final plate construct and its length, so as to avoid blocking final, definitive fixation. Pins placed within the radial shaft must be placed under direct visualization to avoid the superficial cutaneous branch of the radial nerve. We prefer an open technique, through which we identify the interval between the extensor carpi radialis longus and brevis [6], noting that the superficial branch of the radial nerve exits between the brachioradialis and the extensor carpi radialis longus. Proximally, the pins are again inserted under direct visualization through an interval of the mobile wad and the ECU. Insertion of these pins puts the posterior interosseous nerve at significant risk, as they penetrate the supinator muscle. The proximal most pin should be distal to the radial neck to reduce risk of posterior interosseous nerve injury.

Plating these fractures definitively is usually performed with a standard 3.5 mm plate, and the plates may benefit from a small coronal bend for ideal conformity. Bridge plate and locking plate techniques are used in comminuted patterns to overcome significant bone loss, with reference to the contra-lateral, uninjured forearm if available for length assessment. We have also found that in particular situations, the use of intramedullary nail fixation of the ulna may have a role. In cases where there may be missing diaphyseal bone and the soft tissue surrounding the ulna is tenuous, one option can be to place a flexible nail from the olecranon anterograde as performed in pediatrics commonly with the addition of bone or cement spacers to restore a length of shaft. This can be a creative approach to aligning the ulna, maintaining the proximal and distal radioulnar joint congruity, or creating an internal brace for secondary osteosynthesis. Figure 4.4 demonstrates a case utilizing an ulnar nail in a hand replantation after close-range shotgun injury for the forearm.

Hand and Wrist

In the distal upper extremity, fractures and associated soft tissue injuries that involve the distal aspects of either the radius or ulna or extend into the carpal bones and hand structures are usually treated in a delayed fashion. These are usually amenable to splinting in the trauma bay where reasonable alignment can be achieved. Internal and external fixation strategies frequently are employed in cases of the mangled extremity in the interest of monitoring the surrounding soft tissues closely. External fixation principles in this area depend on metacarpal fixation, preferably bicortical fixation of the 2nd or 3rd metacarpals (MC) with 3.0 mm half-pins, while positioning the wrist in slight ulnar deviation and while maintaining neutral wrist flexion. With careful dissection over the 2nd MC, one avoids sensory branches more readily. When placing the index metacarpal half-pins, flexing the index metacarpophalangeal joint to 90 degrees moves the extensor hood distally while translating the relevant extensor tendons ulnarly, giving the surgeon safer access to the bone so as to not ensnare the hood or tendon. Similarly, the pins are inserted 45 degrees in reference to the sagittal plane to avoid the extensor tendons. Initial pins should be placed in the metacarpals, and then attention should be shifted proximally to the distal radius. To improve any remaining articular deformity, Kirschner wire percutaneous fixation can aid in reduction.

Common pitfalls include over-distraction of the radiocarpal joint while applying the external fixator, which has been shown to increase carpal

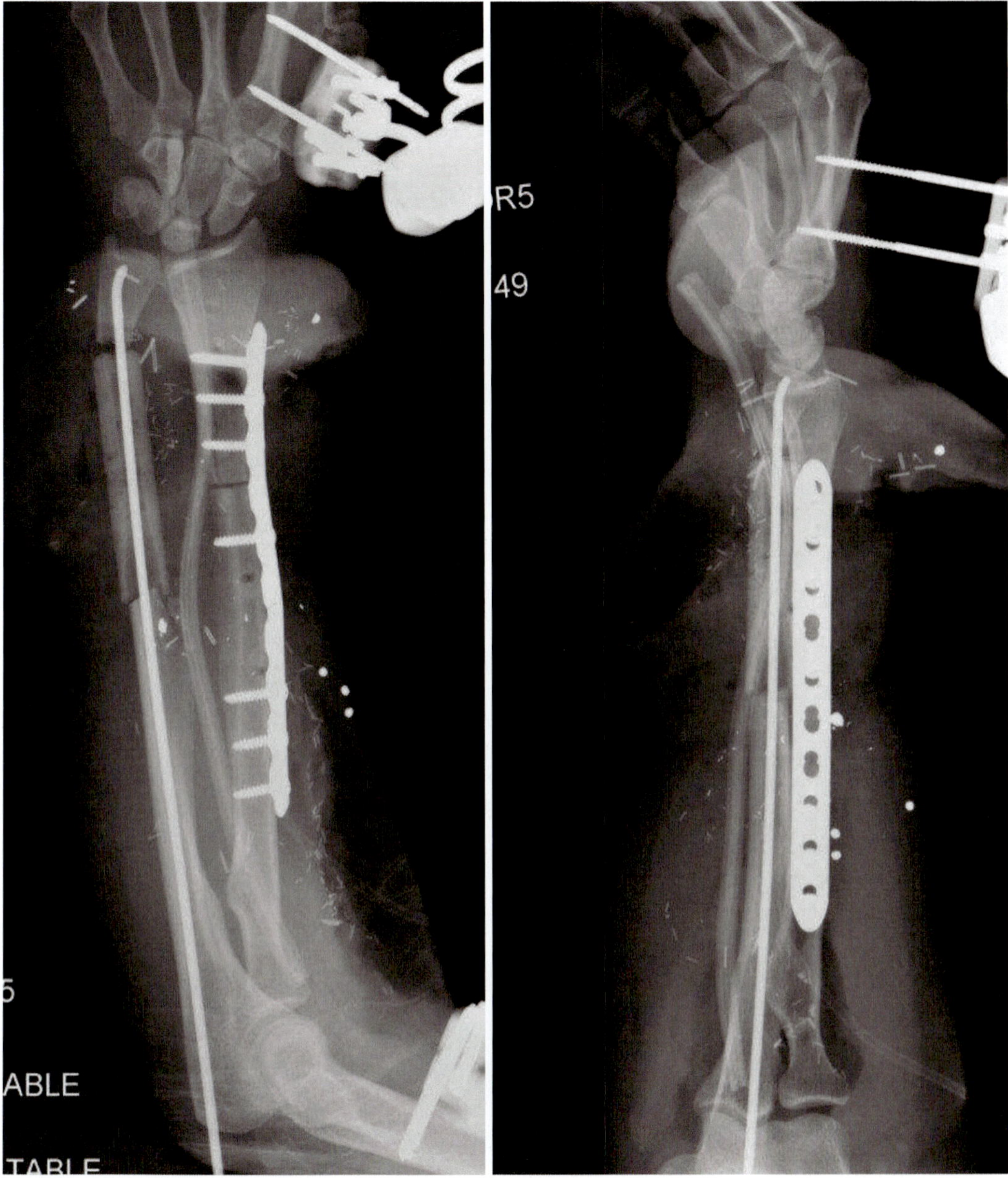

Fig. 4.4 Use of an intramedullary nail for ulnar fixation with a spacer in the distal diaphysis after a shotgun injury amputated the right hand

tunnel pressures [7] and has been associated with increased risk of CRPS [8]. Similarly, flexion and ulnar deviation of the wrist (Cotton-Loder position) to achieve reduction of the distal radius are to be avoided, as wrist flexion similarly induces increased carpal tunnel pressure and increased tension upon the extrinsic extensors, limiting both MPJ and IPJ flexion, resulting in finger stiffness. Spanning plate fixation (dorsal bridge plate) for comminuted intraarticular distal radii or carpal injuries has gained in popularity [9] and is typically left in place for 2–3 months if adequate reduction is achieved. This technique is also helpful in patients with severely osteoporotic bone that cannot maintain reduction with standard palmar plating techniques.

Summary

When choosing the optimal skeletal fixation strategy, remembering that not all options are available or recommended for a given patient may require a unique combination of options to achieve the best possible result. The use of temporizing hardware should be employed readily when applicable, and it can be done safely and quickly. External fixation can be used alone or in combination with these techniques but has its own advantages and limitations. With careful planning, the temporizing and definitive fixation methods should balance the needs of the patient, revascularization requirements, soft tissue, and flap considerations, in line with the anticipated long-term demands of the extremity. This will ensure that the patient will achieve the best outcome possible outcome with maximum functional return.

Case Examples

1. 41M involved in an MVC sustained an open type IIIC proximal humerus fracture. Two field tourniquets were placed in the patient's axilla, and the patient was brought emergently into the OR upon presentation. Severe soft tissue damage was present, and there was a high degree of earthy contamination in the wounds. His brachial artery and basilica vein were found to be avulsed along with his median ulnar and radial nerves. The brachial artery was addressed first using a flexible carotid shunt to restore distal flow, while debridement was carried out. The humerus fracture was an oblique pattern with minimal comminution. When initial debridement of soft tissue and

   osseous structures was completed, compartments were released down to the wrist, and the bone was approximated using an 8-hole 2.0 mm DCP plate on the medial side, followed by a 12-hole proximal humerus locking plate placed through the deltopectoral interval. Nerve repair of the median nerve was performed with the unsalvageable ulnar nerve as autograft and neural tubing. The cephalic vein was found to be intact, and therefore the avulsed basilic vein was used as vein graft for the brachial artery.

   The patient's family was counseled on the likely events to follow which would include two more debridements, an above elbow amputation, and ultimately a revision amputation at the proximal humerus level 14 days post injury.

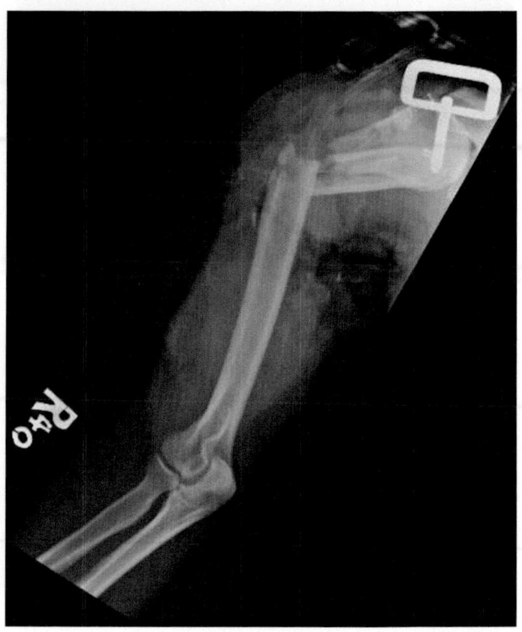

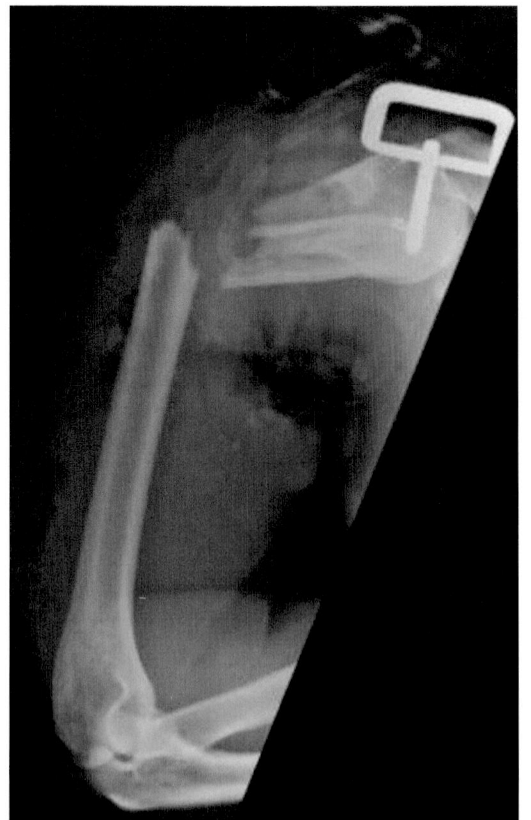
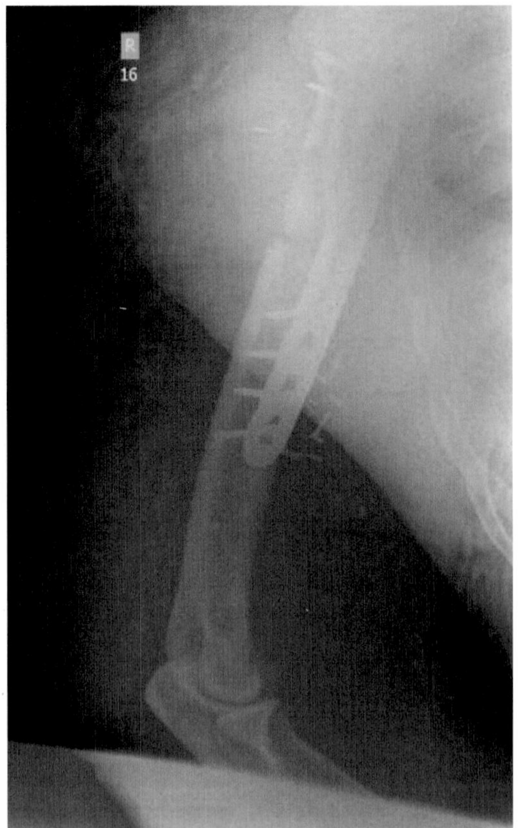
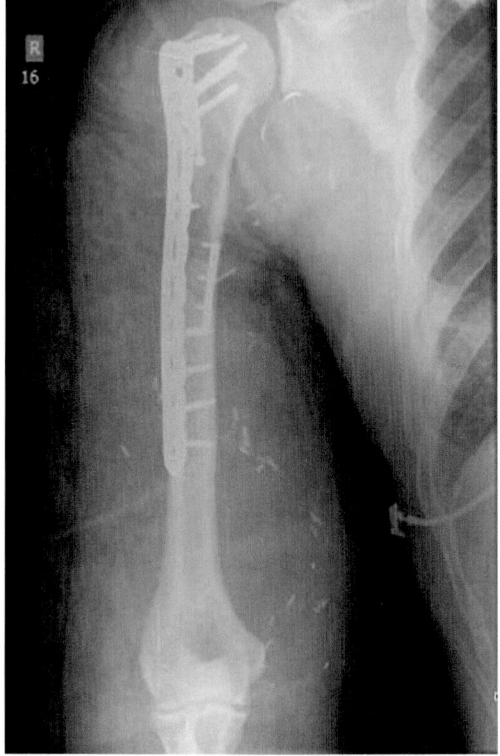

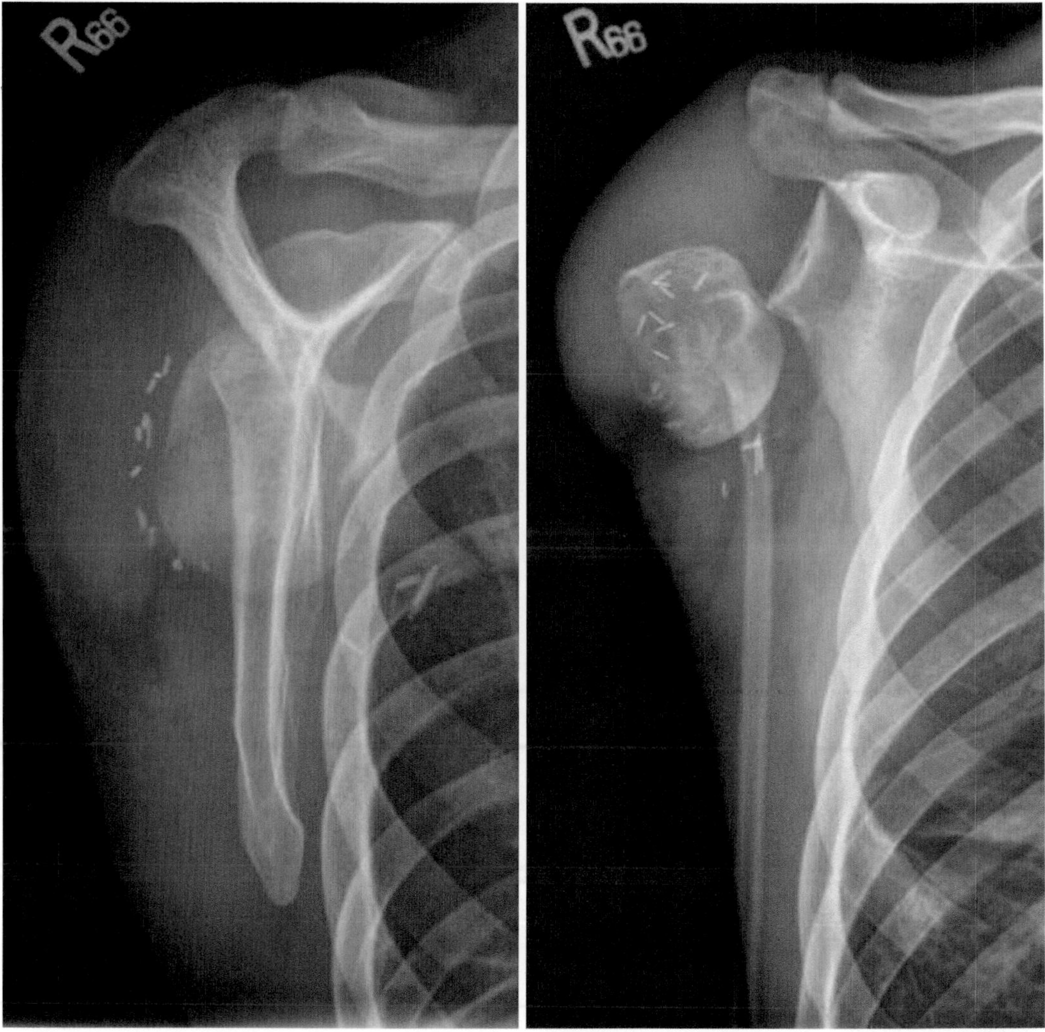

2. 28M trapped underneath industrial washing machine, presented to trauma unit with a cold and pulseless hand. He was noted to have a humeral shaft fracture on presentation and was taken emergently to the OR for exploration and revascularization. The images demonstrate the anterior approach to the humerus to visualize the brachial artery, and it was discovered to be transected at the level of the fracture. It underwent immediate shunting, definitive fixation with a plate and screws, vein grafting, and then nerve repair.

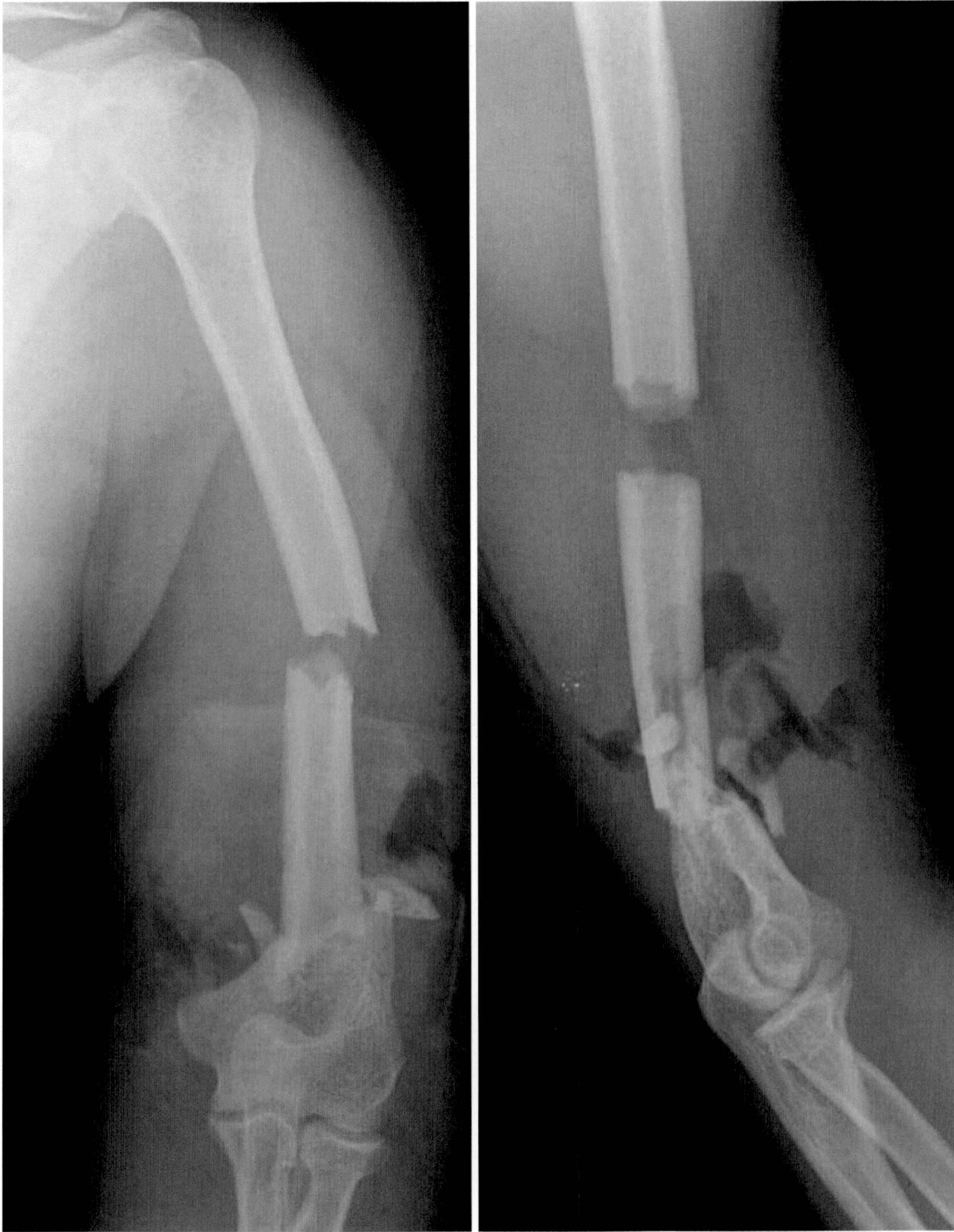

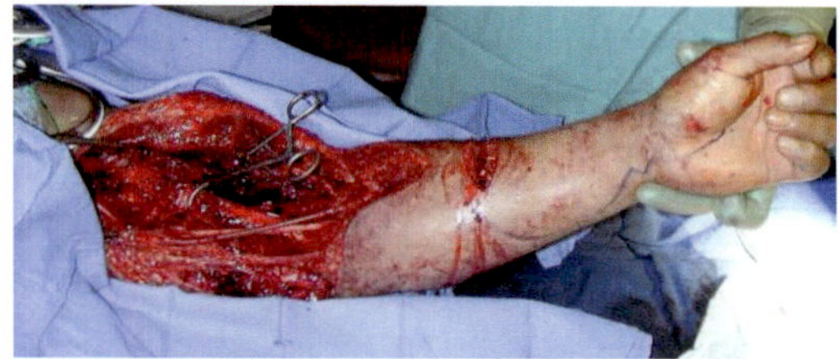
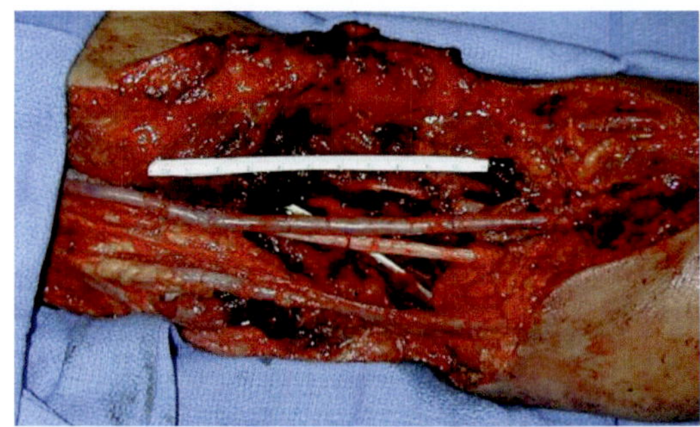
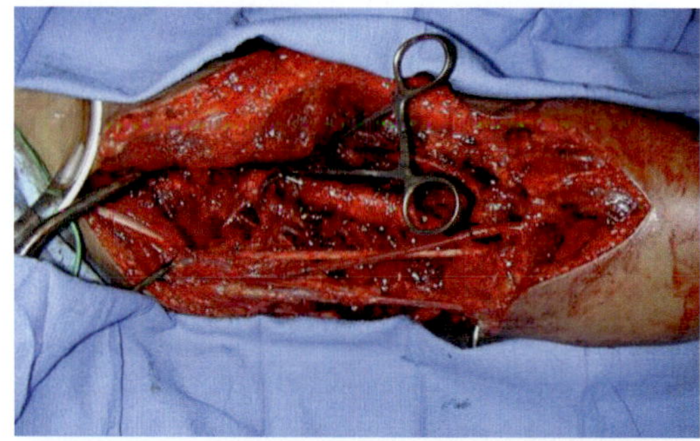
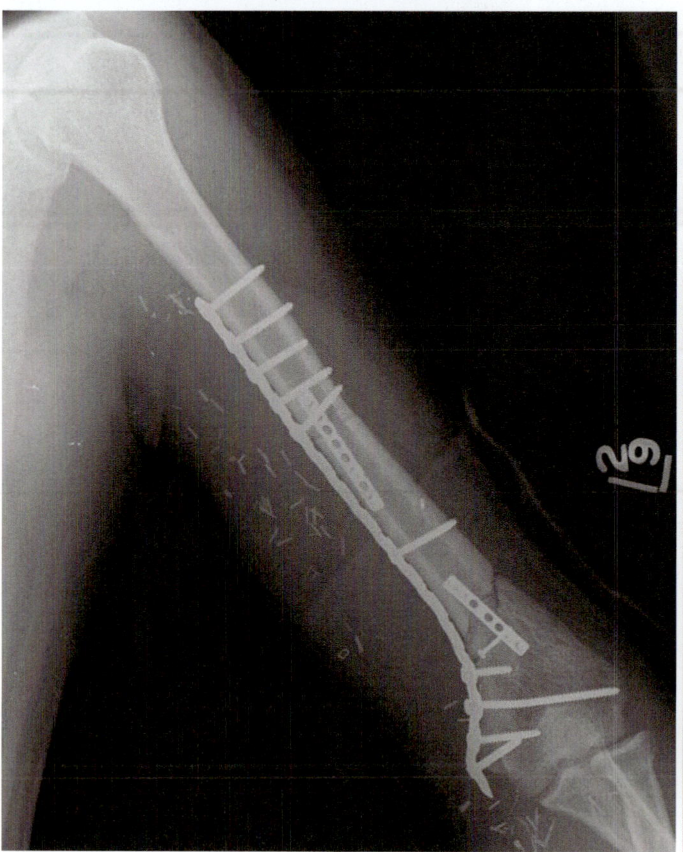
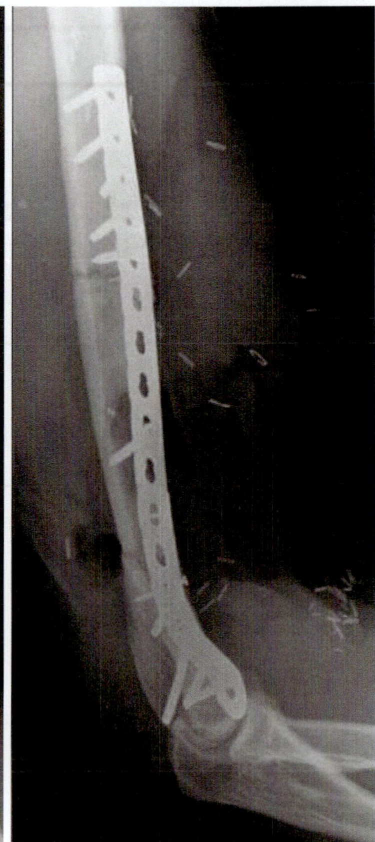

3. 47M involved in MCC sustained an open pelvis fracture, multiple visceral injuries, right thigh and gluteal compartment syndrome, and open left forearm fractures. He had his pelvis stabilized and debrided and was safe for debridement and irrigation of his left arm. The patient had an anterior incision that was extended between the flexor carpi radialis and the brachioradialis where the proximal shaft was visualized under the pronator teres. The flexor pollicis longus and part of the pronator were elevated to visualize distally. The ulnar butterfly fragment was mobilized and secured. The plan was established to debride and provisionally stabilize both bones with subsequent definitive fixation. The radial butterfly fragment was reduced and held with 2.0 mm lag screw. A 12-hole DCP plate was applied radially this with two screws proximally and distally. The ulna was reduced with minifragment plates and lag screws similarly to the radius.

The patient returned 5 days later for revision debridement and definitive fixation. The radial plate was secured with more screws proximally and distally. A 14-hole 3.5 mm plate was selected and placed in a sub-extensor carpi ulnaris fashion. Provisional closure was performed, and the patient underwent skin closure at a later date.

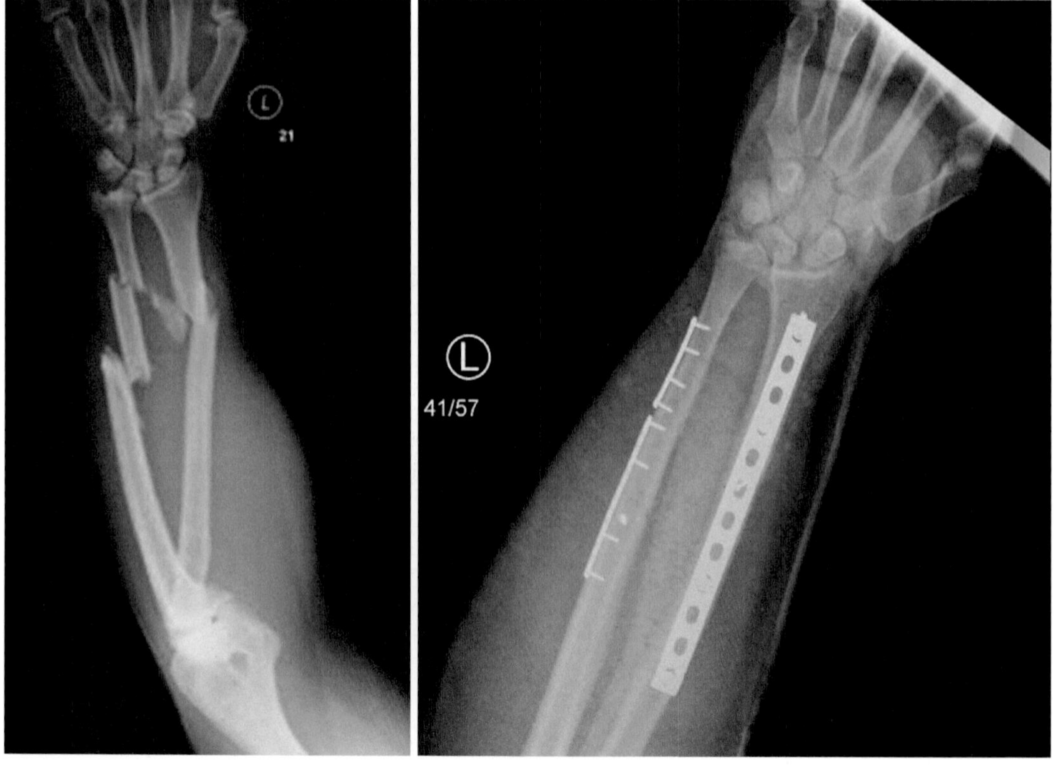

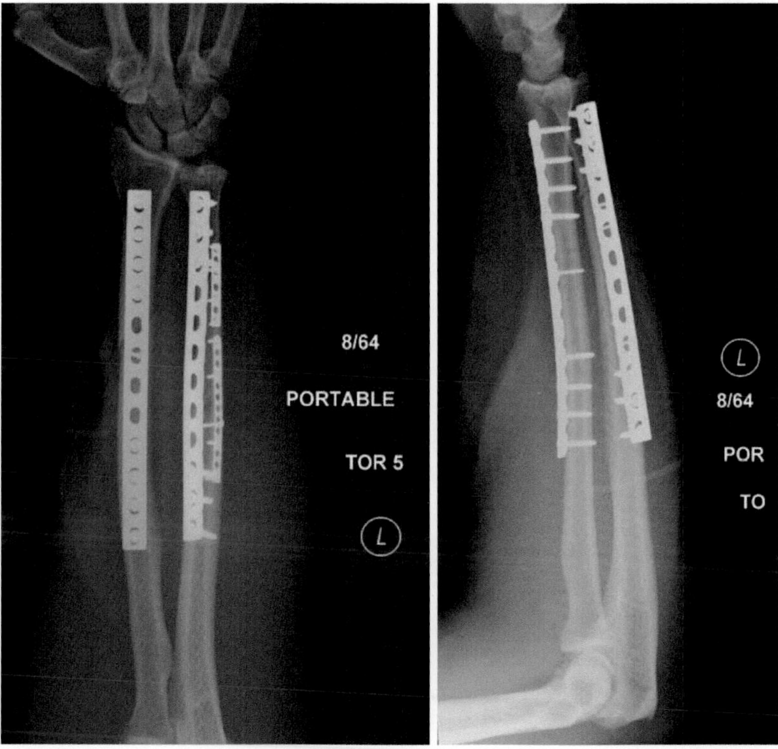

References

1. Scalea TM, DuBose J, Moore EE, West M, Moore FA, McIntyre R, et al. Western Trauma Association critical decisions in trauma: management of the mangled extremity. J Trauma Acute Care Surg. 2012;72(1):86–93.
2. Neviaser TJ, Neviaser RJ, Neviaser JS. Incomplete rotator cuff tears. A technique for diagnosis and treatment. Clin Orthop Relat Res. 1994;306:12–6.
3. Eglseder WA. Atlas of upper extremity trauma: a clinical perspective, vol. 920. Cham: Springer International Publishing; 2018.
4. Ayel JE, Bonnevialle N, Lafosse JM, Pidhorz L, Al Homsy M, Mansat P, et al. Acute elbow dislocation with arterial rupture. Analysis of nine cases. Orthop Traumatol Surg Res. 2009;95(5):343–51.
5. Dumont CE, Thalmann R, Macy JC. The effect of rotational malunion of the radius and the ulna on supination and pronation. J Bone Joint Surg Br. 2002;84(7):1070–4.
6. Eglseder WA, Hay M. Open half-pin insertion for distal radial fractures. Mil Med. 1993;158(11):708–11.
7. Baechler MF, Means KR Jr, Parks BG, Nguyen A, Segalman KA. Carpal canal pressure of the distracted wrist. J Hand Surg Am. 2004;29(5):858–64.
8. Mathews AL, Chung KC. Management of complications of distal radius fractures. Hand Clin. 2015;31(2):205–15.
9. Brogan DM, Richard MJ, Ruch D, Kakar S. Management of severely comminuted distal radius fractures. J Hand Surg Am. 2015;40(9):1905–14.

Revascularization of the Mangled Limb

5

Naji Madi and Ray Pensy

Mangling injuries of the limb are, by virtue of their severity, urgent conditions. However, injury resulting in limb ischemia represents the most time-dependent and reversible condition the extremity surgeon will encounter. Ischemia, defined as a lack of adequate oxygen delivery to the affected tissues, is generally the result of interruption of the arterial tree. For the purposes of this chapter, we will discuss ischemia as the result of extremity trauma, and not the result of the generally insidious condition of peripheral arterial disease.

The importance of ischemic time, as it relates to successful limb salvage, cannot be overstated [1]. For the extremity surgeon, ischemia is the one diagnosis which should prompt the surgical team to move with haste. The treatments aimed at mitigating ischemia should precede any other treatment, other than those that are compromising airway, ventilation, or circulation, as outlined in the first chapter. In many cases, addressing ischemia will occur in conjunction with the appropriate and timely management of these conditions, as severe extremity trauma infrequently occurs in isolation.

In defining ischemia as it relates to trauma, and particularly as it relates to the mangled limb, it is important to categorize tissue perfusion into three general levels: level I, no ischemia or viable; level II, threatened (marginally or immediately) or non-critical (relative) ischemia; and level III, major irreversible or critical ischemia [2]. Clinically, the difference between non-critical and critical ischemia in the acute care setting can be difficult to discern. Accurate distinction of the two, however, has enormous impacts on the overall management and outcome of the patient, as well as the sequence of interventions for any given mangled limb. In order to gain a basic understanding of ischemia, a brief discussion of physiology is warranted.

Physiology

The tissues of the extremities are variably affected by ischemia, with muscle being the most dependent on aerobic metabolism [3]. Other tissues such as the skin and bone can tolerate significant ischemia times. In the presence of arterial occlusion or disruption, characteristic metabolic changes occur within skeletal muscle as the result of anoxia/hypoxia. At the molecular level, decreased adenosine triphosphate synthesis occurs as the result of the inhibition of the oxidative pathway. During the first 3–4 hours of ischemia, adenosine triphosphate (ATP) levels within skeletal muscle are

N. Madi (✉)
Department of Orthopaedic Surgery,
Rutgers University, Newark, NJ, USA
e-mail: nm88@aub.edu.lb

R. Pensy
R Adams Cowley Shock Trauma Center, 22 South Greene St, Baltimore, MD 21201, USA
e-mail: rpensy@som.umaryland.edu

© Springer Nature Switzerland AG 2021
R. A. Pensy, J. V. Ingari (eds.), *The Mangled Extremity*, https://doi.org/10.1007/978-3-319-56648-1_5

maintained through anaerobic activities utilizing glycogen stores and the phosphocreatine pathways [4]. Within approximately 4 hours, these reserves are exhausted, and irreversible muscle death begins to occur and is complete at approximately 6 hours. During muscle ischemia, metabolites of the anaerobic pathway accumulate and are responsible for the creation of free radical and reactive oxygen species that are deleterious to muscle viability and limb function upon reperfusion.

During prolonged ischemia, depletion of ATP results in mitochondrial membrane instability and alterations in the balance of sodium and calcium ions. This imbalance results in enzymatic dysfunction, ending in apoptosis [5]. Upon cell lysis, the products of anaerobic metabolism (lactate), potassium, and the proteins of muscle cell structure (myoglobin) are released into general circulation, which can cause alterations in serum pH, as well as cardiac and renal function [6]. The degree of metabolic and systemic disturbances is proportional to the volume of ischemic muscle and can be life-threatening to the patient after reperfusion. Not surprisingly, the overall health and comorbid status of the patient is correlated with limb survival when treating ischemic disease, in part due to the patient's physiologic capacity to manage the aforementioned perturbations [7].

Large volumes of muscle necrosis can be lethal, secondary to the metabolic disruption noted above. Efforts to mitigate these effects through renal dialysis and continuous veno-venous hemofiltration (CCVH) are employed but represent a reactionary and less effective method of treatment, compared to restoring perfusion in a timely fashion [8].

Assessment

The experienced clinician will use a constellation of physical exam findings to determine the degree of ischemia: palpable or non-palpable (dopplerable) pulses, skin color, turgor, temperature, capillary refill, and active motion of the involved extremity are all important descriptors [9]. These variables supplement the obvious hard signs commonly used to diagnose vascular trauma requiring intervention: pulsatile bleeding, expanding hematoma, bruits, and thrills [10]. "Soft signs," such as

neurologic deficit, or history of moderate hemorrhage, in and of themselves, do not warrant further evaluation or exploration [11].

These physical examination findings, however, must be assessed in the context of the overall condition of the patient [12]. An absent radial pulse and dusky hands or feet are frequent findings in those patients with a systolic pressure below 80 mmHg—or in those patients who are receiving vasopressors. Further, identifying a vascular insult requiring immediate intervention is made much more difficult in the cool or cold patient, who presents in a state of peripheral vasoconstriction. Appropriate warming, through blankets and "bear hugger," occurring immediately after appropriate Advanced Trauma Life Support (ATLS) protocols, is indicated, to ensure that the vascular tree is afforded the opportunity to vasodilate. Appropriate splinting and alignment of the fractured limb will often reduce the degree of arterial vasospasm, and potential kinking, improving the odds of meaningful perfusion. In sum, the diagnosis of traumatic limb ischemia is best made in the normotensive, warm, and properly aligned limb.

Traumatic critical ischemia, defined as an interruption of oxygenation which will result in immediate tissue loss, manifests physical examination hard signs that are often obvious: a pale hand or foot, with no appreciable pulse and no capillary refill. In these cases, immediate treatment is indicated, occurring secondary only to the requirement of life-saving measures. Relative ischemia is much more difficult to discern and is the more common scenario. It is common for a patient with severe extremity trauma to present without palpable pulses and yet maintain some degree of capillary refill.

Quantification of the perfusion deficit in relative ischemia, and thus the elucidation of the immediacy of the injury, is challenging even for the experienced clinician. In the absence of hard signs, ankle-brachial, brachial-brachial, or wrist-brachial indices are employed, as they provide an objective and reliable method of assessing relative perfusion [11]. In patients who are cool, volume depleted, and/or under-resuscitated or have other systemic factors complicating the exam, the contralateral, uninjured limb provides an "internal control." In cases where the arterial pressure index of the limb in question is less than 0.9 of the control, vascular injury is suspected, and further study indicated [13]. A hand-held doppler can be used to evaluate for audible pulses in the extremity as well. Treatable vascular injury resulting in relative ischemia requires triage and prioritization in the overall management of the patient, as discussed in more detail later. This prioritization is dependent on an understanding of the overall picture for the individual patient: the mechanism of injury; the type, quantity, and location of ischemic tissue; the "salvage ability" of the injured extremity; comorbidities; and more critical system involvement.

Anatomy

Relative ischemia can occur in cases of compartment syndrome. Varying degrees of swelling and edema occur within compartments dependent on the mechanism of injury: direct muscle contusion or crush, skeletal injury such as fracture or dislocation that has been reduced, hemorrhage associated with bone, or soft tissue disruption all result in altered compartment pressures [14]. These factors invariably result in wide ranges of increased pressure, typically measured in mmHg, within the described compartments of the upper and lower limb. These changes manifest as paresthesia, painful passive stretch of the affected muscles within the compartment in question, increased tone, loss of motor function, and, less reliably, firmness of the compartments. Therefore, knowledge of the anatomy of the compartments of the forearm and leg is essential (Fig. 5.1).

Maintaining adequate perfusion of the involved tissue and compartment requires an arterial inflow pressure that exceeds that of the impedance (Fig. 5.2). When this does not occur, even in the absence of obvious and named vessel injury, ischemia ensues, resulting in further edema and pressure increase [14]. This relative

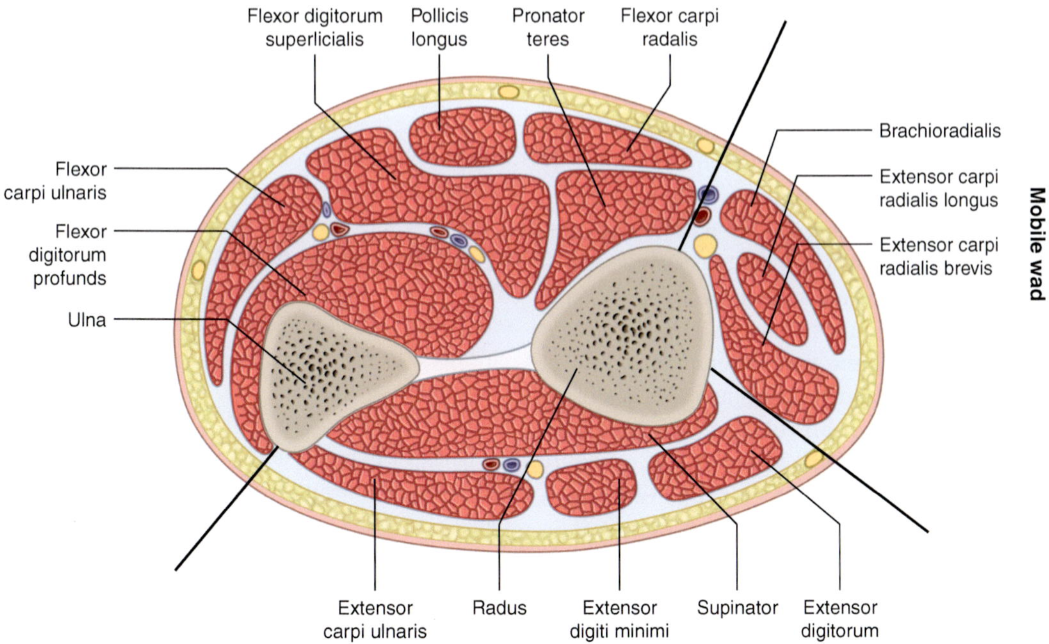

Fig. 5.1 A schematic illustration of the forearm compartments. Three main compartments are differentiated: volar compartment divided into superficial and deep. Dorsal compartment and the mobile wad

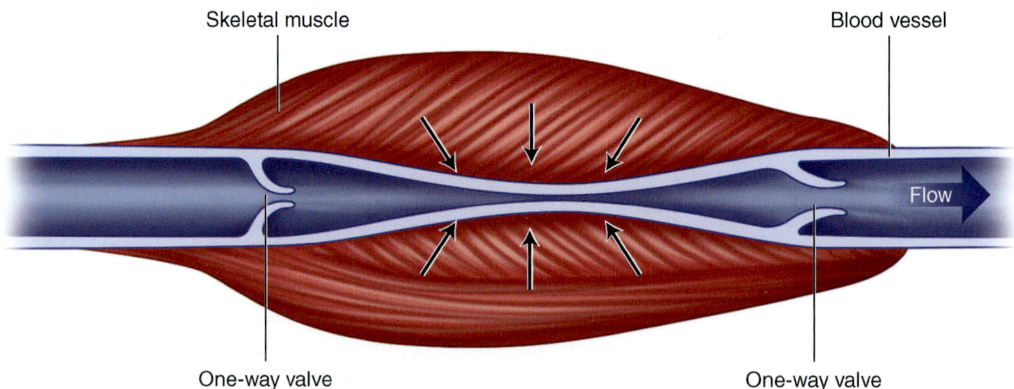

Fig. 5.2 An illustration showing the effect of intra-compartmental pressure on the arterial blood flow. An increase in the compartment pressure will increase the impedance; hence tissue perfusion will be endangered

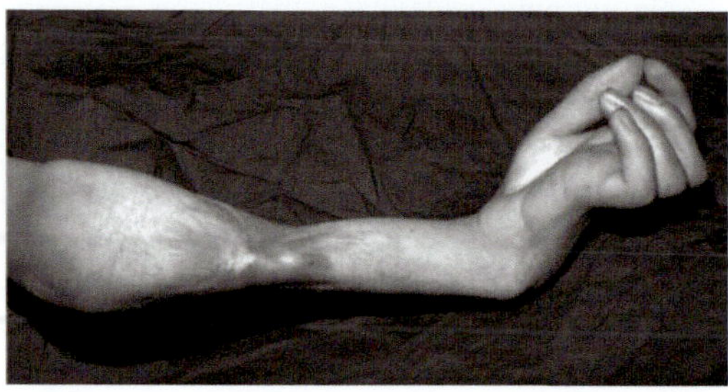

Fig. 5.3 A photograph of a severely contracted forearm in a young patient with chronic compartment syndrome. Volkmann's ischemic contracture. (*From Green's Operative Hand Surgery, 5th Ed.*)

ischemia, left untreated, has the exact same result as that of a muscle rendered absolutely ischemic: paralyzed, then necrotic, then fibrotic, and finally contracted [15] (Fig. 5.3).

It is not uncommon for the muscle compartments of the forearm and leg to undergo significant and frequently complete necrosis. Yet, the skin, bone, and joints remain, as they are far less sensitive to ischemic time. Therefore, the lower limb will often end in amputation, as restoring muscle function is difficult and maintaining an insensate, nonfunctional lower limb is generally less favorable than amputation [16]. Preservation of the upper limb is generally preferred, even in the presence functional muscle loss [17].

The student of anatomy will understand the significant and robust collateral systems of the shoulder girdle, arm, forearm, and hand. Connections between the subclavian artery and the circumflex scapular artery, via the transverse cervical artery, can maintain limb viability (Fig. 5.4) even in cases of complete subclavian artery thrombosis/occlusion. Similarly, perfusion to the upper limb can be maintained in cases of axillary artery injury via the collaterals present between the suprascapular artery and the anterior and posterior circumflex humeral arteries. More obvious is the collateral flow provided via the profunda brachii artery in cases of brachial artery injury via the connections of the anterior and posterior radial collateral arteries to the radial recurrent artery and the connections between the superior and inferior ulna collateral arteries to the ulnar recurrent artery [18] (Fig. 5.5).

The most clinically relevant fact is that the arm enjoys a more robust collateral system at the elbow level than the lower limb at the level of the knee. Whereas the forearm can maintain viability in a large percentage of cases with brachial artery injury at a level distal to the profunda brachii artery via the collaterals mentioned above, an injury to the popliteal artery will result in a nonviable leg in the vast majority of cases (Fig. 5.5).

Thus, in many cases of upper extremity arterial injury, the resulting ischemia is relative, secondary to the relatively robust collateral flow, whereas in the leg, the ischemia is much commonly absolute. This fact is critically important in prioritizing treatment and expediency, particularly in those cases requiring the integration of differing subspecialties such as orthopedics and vascular surgery.

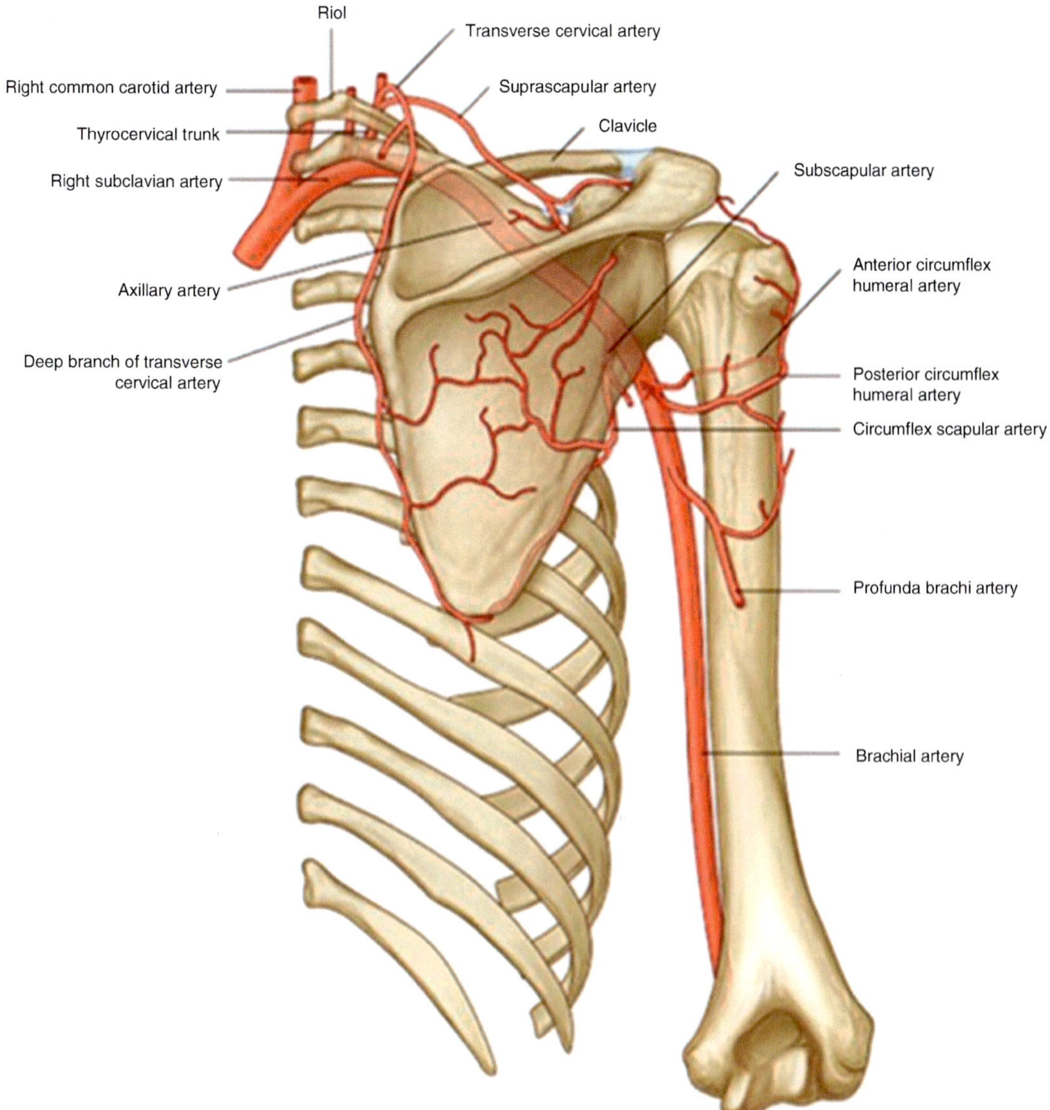

Fig. 5.4 An illustration demonstrating the blood supply of the arm with the rich collateral system. (*From: Gray's anatomy for Students, 2nd Edition. Copyright © 2009 by Churchill Livingstone, an imprint of Elsevier, Inc. All rights reserved*)

Imaging

It is imperative that standard extremity radiographs are obtained in any patient with clinical exam findings consistent with traumatic ischemia. Visualizing and understanding the spatial relationship of displaced normal anatomy can be quickly done with standard, orthogonal radiographs. A prime example of this is the dislocated knee in an obese patient. Although physical examination is often sufficient for the diagnosis of the dislocated knee, the obese patient presents significant challenges to physical examination. A plain radiograph will confirm the displacement (Fig. 5.6). Abundant literature describes the tethered nature of the anterior tibial artery as it passes through the interosseous membrane, frequently resulting in its avulsion and thrombosis of its ori-

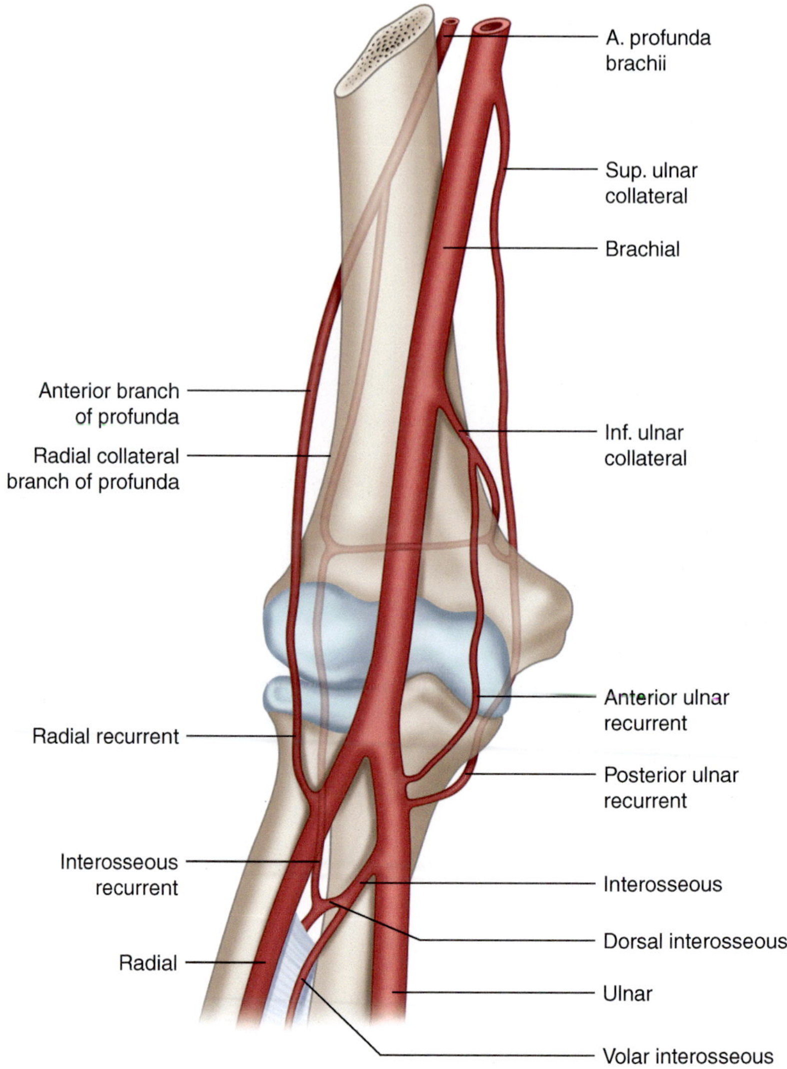

Fig. 5.5 An illustration demonstrating the blood supply of the forearm with the rich collateral system at the elbow

gin and of the associated tibioperoneal trunk, causing critical ischemia of the leg and occasional amputation [19].

Similarly, it is possible for the dislocated elbow or fractured humerus to result in occlusion of the brachial artery. The simple maneuver of reducing and splinting the elbow, or aligning the fractured humerus, may restore normal circulation or, at the very least, provide the opportunity for some degree of collateral flow to return. Simultaneously, it mitigates further muscle injury and edema subsequent to the lack of normal skeletal "foundation." Thus, for an experienced clinician, associating a standard radiograph, which can be communicated by the emergency physician or resident staff via electronic messaging, with the report of a pulseless limb, can yield an enormous amount of information.

A high-velocity weapon can impart an enormous amount of energy and, therefore, disruption to all the affected tissues. In some cases, the amount of soft tissue destruction is obvious by the magnitude of the skin loss and underlying defect. A radiograph showing markedly comminuted fracture of dense, healthy bone reflects quickly the "high-energy" nature of such injury. Unlike the isolated laceration of the brachial artery, with an intact profunda brachii collateral flow, from a stab or even open fracture, the rifle injury seen on radiograph indicates a vast damage reaching the collateral flow.

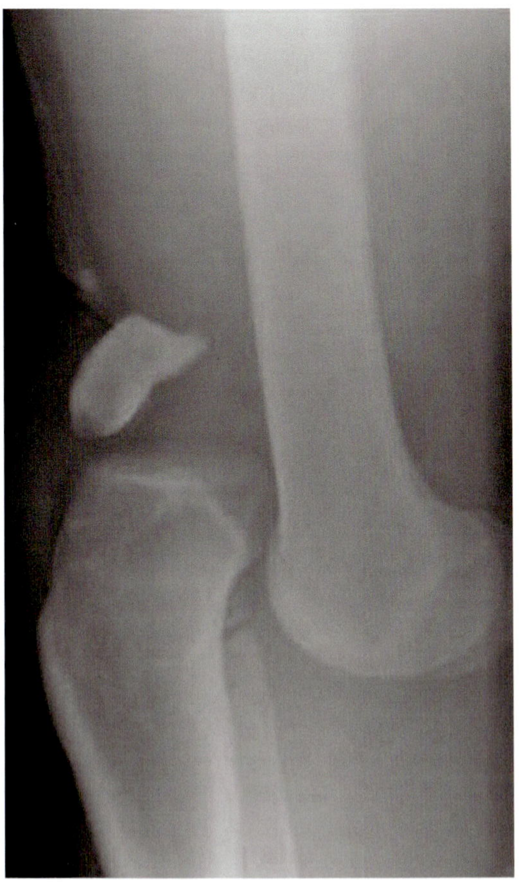

Fig. 5.6 A lateral radiograph of the knee showing an anterior knee dislocation. This is the most common type of knee dislocation and usually causes intimal tear of the popliteal artery

ing angiogram as the modality of choice in discerning abnormalities of the extremity axial vessels, as it can be obtained rapidly in the trauma setting. CTA does not require the advanced technical skills necessary of standard angiography and only requires a peripheral IV, rather than that of direct cannulation of the arterial tree and selective administration of dye. CTA has been found to be as sensitive and specific as standard angiography for injuries to axial vessels, and furthermore, the images can be reformatted to provide sagittal, coronal, and three-dimensional representations of the extremity in question [11].

In certain instances, however, standard angiography is preferred. In the author's experience, detailing the small, distal vessels of the foot and hand are better visualized with standard angiography. Additionally, the presence or absence of atherosclerosis of the vessels can be better assessed with angiography [16].

MRA, when combined with magnetic resonance venography (MRV), permits an even more comprehensive approach for limb salvage, particularly when considering free tissue transfer, but is rarely used in cases of acute vascular trauma secondary to time and logistical requirements [20].

Treatment

The clinician, hopefully armed with a thorough history, examination, and imaging studies, has to make determination as to whether the ischemia is relative or critical, as the treatment options will vary accordingly. Those options are best divided according to the anatomical location into upper extremity and lower extremities [21].

Tourniquet utilization has become increasingly widespread and has resulted in decreased mortality [22]. First responders across the developed world employ tourniquets appropriately for many mangled limbs, whether or not the affected limb is critically ischemic, in order to stem life-threatening loss of blood. However, by definition, a properly applied tourniquet causes critical limb ischemia, with no collateral flow and no oxygenation potential to the affected muscles. In the

In the former, the collateral flow makes the ischemia relative instead of absolute, hence, less risk of significant muscle loss. Whereas in the latter, as the ischemia is critical, the muscle loss is imminent if not ongoing. In many cases, ischemia requiring repair or reconstruction can be determined based on a thorough history and physical examination and plain radiographs, without advanced imaging. In questionable cases, or if the mechanism of injury (e.g., motor vehicle ejection) dictates obtaining advanced imaging, the latter should be finished expeditiously.

A variety of vascular imaging studies are now available: computed tomographic angiography (CTA), standard angiography, and magnetic resonance angiography (MRA). CTA has rapidly gained in popularity over the last decade, replac-

author's opinion, this represents an absolute urgency for limb survival. Upon arriving at the receiving medical center, ATLS protocols are employed. Only after blood pressure, pulse, and resuscitation status of the patient has been determined, with large-bore IV access secured, should the tourniquet be removed. It is imperative to have another tourniquet, immediately available, preferably a pneumatic tourniquet which provides accurate pressure. Following tourniquet removal the clinician must make an immediate assessment of bleeding and restoration of pulses. If bleeding cannot be controlled with a moderate pressure dressing and appropriate splinting, the tourniquet should be reapplied, with a judicious pressure and the time marked. Once again, the limb now becomes critically ischemic, and ongoing muscle injury is definite with increasing likelihood of limb and life loss with each passing hour [23].

In cases where the tourniquet has been applied to the remaining part of a completely amputated limb, the tourniquet should be left in place until such time that replantation or revision amputation is completed. Additionally, in those cases where the traumatized limb is deemed non-salvageable, leaving the tourniquet in place until the patient is in the operating room to complete amputation is recommended.

In many cases, a field tourniquet is applied to a limb that has not sustained a vascular injury resulting in critical ischemia. In these cases, the clinician must carefully consider the risk/benefit of tourniquet removal prior to the operating room. The advantages to tourniquet removal cannot be overlooked: in many well-established trauma centers, the time from presentation to exploration and revascularization is measured in the range of 3–4 hours. Secondary to collateral flow, brachial artery injury distal to the profunda brachii artery results in amputation in the minority (25%) of cases [24]. In cases of brachial artery disruption without significant hemorrhage, muscle viability can be maintained through collateral flow in the absence of tourniquet. In the arm and brachial artery injuries, the mechanism is often predictive of the degree of ischemia. A narrow zone of injury, secondary to a laceration from stab or low-velocity gunshot wound, will often result in preservation of the collateral flow via the radial and ulnar collateral systems (Fig. 5.5). In these cases, although a hard sign of a pulseless wrist will be evident, the hand will maintain capillary refill, and in the non-obtunded patient without any respective neurologic injury, the preservation of muscle perfusion will permit adequate voluntary control. Hence, vascular reconstruction is indicated but may occur in a manner that does not require haste. Reversed interposition vein grafting, often from the same extremity, can be accomplished. Sources for vein can include the basilic, cephalic, or associated venae comitantes, as indicated [25].

Similarly, in the forearm, the injury will often affect either the radial or ulnar artery, permitting sufficient flow to the hand that will not require revascularization. However, in a minority of cases, exposure of the injured arteries is warranted.

In those injuries secondary to crush, shot gun, high-velocity projectile (bullet), or severe open fractures, the zone of injury is large, and the collateral flow is affected. Therefore, the hard signs of absent pulse, along with absent capillary refill, and motor deficit of the hand and forearm will be noted. In these cases, the ischemia can be assumed to be absolute, requiring immediate and emergent revascularization [10]. It depends on the clinical scenario whether to start with the vascular repair or the orthopedic stabilization: fracture stability and comminution and cold ischemia time are the main factors to be considered [26]. An arterial shunt can be used temporarily once the patient is in the operating room. It will perfuse the distal segment while the bony fixation is being performed. Studies did not show an inferiority of these shunts as compared with primary repair [27].

In case of a venous injury, three options are proposed: primary repair, vein graft repair, or vein ligation [16].

Fasciotomy

The fasciotomy rate has been more common in lower extremity arterial trauma as compared to upper extremity. It can be done prior to the vascular repair in questionable limbs to evaluate the muscles viability or post repair either prophylactically or to release a high compartment pressure [28]. In the author's experience, upper limb/forearm fasciotomy should be considered when the following are present: crush injury, high velocity or shot gun ballistic injuries to the arm, lack of back bleeding from the distal brachial artery, evidence of critical forearm muscle ischemia upon release of the lacertus fibrosis (lack of contractility, dusky appearance, non bleeding) and in the awake patient, abscence of voluntary muscle activity in the forearm. Those injuries resulting from stab/sharp penetraring or low energy mechanism about the elbow will frequently NOT require fasciotomy after having carefully assessed and documented the above clinical parameters. For the lower extremity, injury to the superifical femoral artery of popliteal artery should nearly universally be accompanied by urgent prophylactic fasciotomy, as the collateral flow about the knee is far less robust than that of the elbow.

Postoperative Care

The vascular repair postoperatively should be assessed on hourly basis for the first 24 hours. A loss of preexisting peripheral pulse (by hand or Doppler) requires urgent reassessment of the patient condition and a decision of secondary intervention to be made [16]. The rehabilitation postoperatively will depend mostly on the orthopedic injury and fixation. Although in peripheral vascular disease the routine use of anticoagulant postoperatively is widely recommended, in acute upper extremity arterial injury, the literature will support diversified protocols ranging from multiple anticoagulants to none [25].

The following upper extremity cases represent suggested algorithms:

[**Case 2.1**] Upper Extremity Brachial Artery Injury with Associated Humeral Shaft Fracture: **Absolute Ischemia**

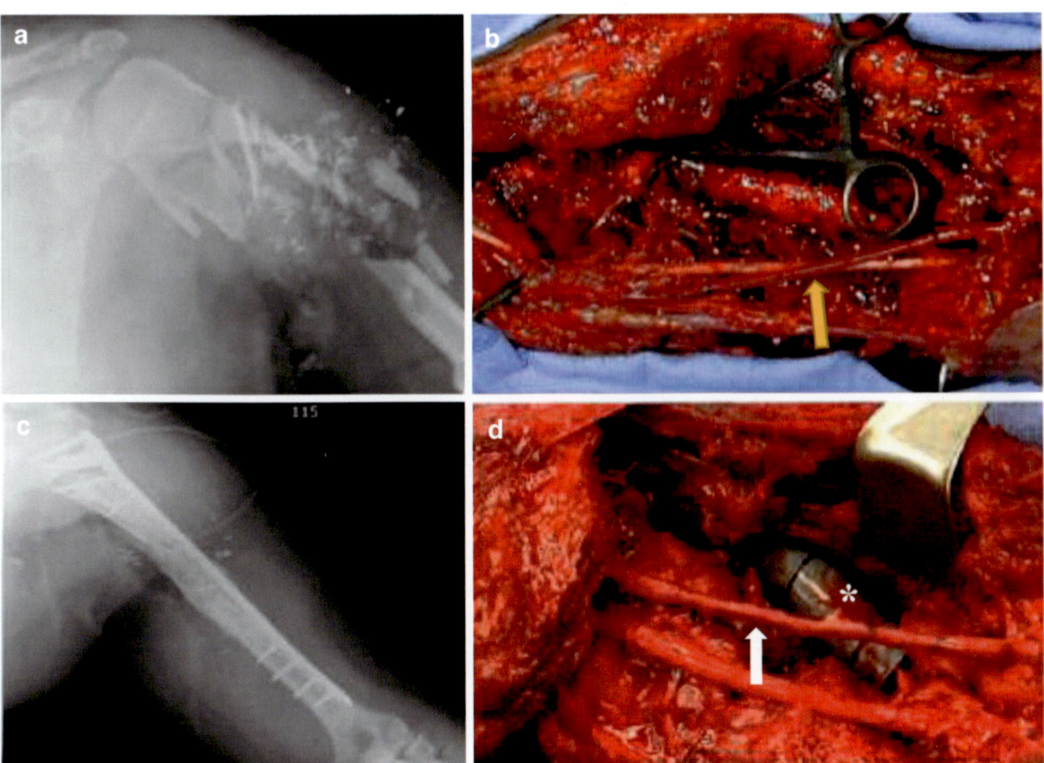

[**Case 2.1**]: A 65-year-old male presents with a high caliber ballistic injury to his left humeral diaphysis. (**a**) Severely comminuted proximal humerus facture. (**b**) Vascular shunt (*yellow arrow*) employed immediately after identification of median nerve and resection of injured arterial segment. (**c, d**) With shunt in place, definitive debridement and plating with antibiotic spacer (*) placed, for future planned bone grafting. (**d**) Interposition vein graft (*white arrow*)

The patient demonstrates a cold, pale, and pulseless hand without capillary refill. The alert and oriented patient opts for attempts at limb salvage. After appropriate airway control and IV access is established, he is taken emergently to the operating room.

Based upon the examination demonstrating a critically ischemic hand, with a time from injury of approximately 3 hours, decision is made to rapidly shunt the brachial artery. A large, anterior deltopectoral exposure is completed, with elevation of the pectoralis muscle from the humerus insertion. Rapid exposure of the distal axillary artery and brachial artery is completed, in conjunction with assessment of the forearm muscles after release of the lacertus fibrosus. No back bleeding is identified in the distal arterial stump, and the forearm muscles are dusky and not contractile. After resecting the brachial artery to healthy levels, a Fogarty thrombectomy catheter is used to dilate and provide thrombec-

tomy to the proximal and distal arteries, and a shunt is placed (Case 2.1 - b), immediately demonstrating improved color to the hand and forearm muscles. Formal forearm fasciotomies are completed.

Extensive debridement of nonviable soft tissue and bone is completed after further identification of the median and ulnar nerves, which are found in continuity. The skin incision is elevated laterally to provide access to an anterolateral plating of the humerus (Case 2.1 - c) and placement of an antibiotic spacer (Case 2.1 - d). The shunt is then replaced with a reversed interposition saphenous vein graft (Case 2.1 - d). His forearm fasciotomies require skin grafting, and he is discharged to home on postoperative day 7 with a palpable radial pulse and a wrist splint for his radial nerve palsy.

[Case 2.2] Upper Extremity Brachial Artery Injury with Associated Humeral Shaft Fracture: **Relative Ischemia**

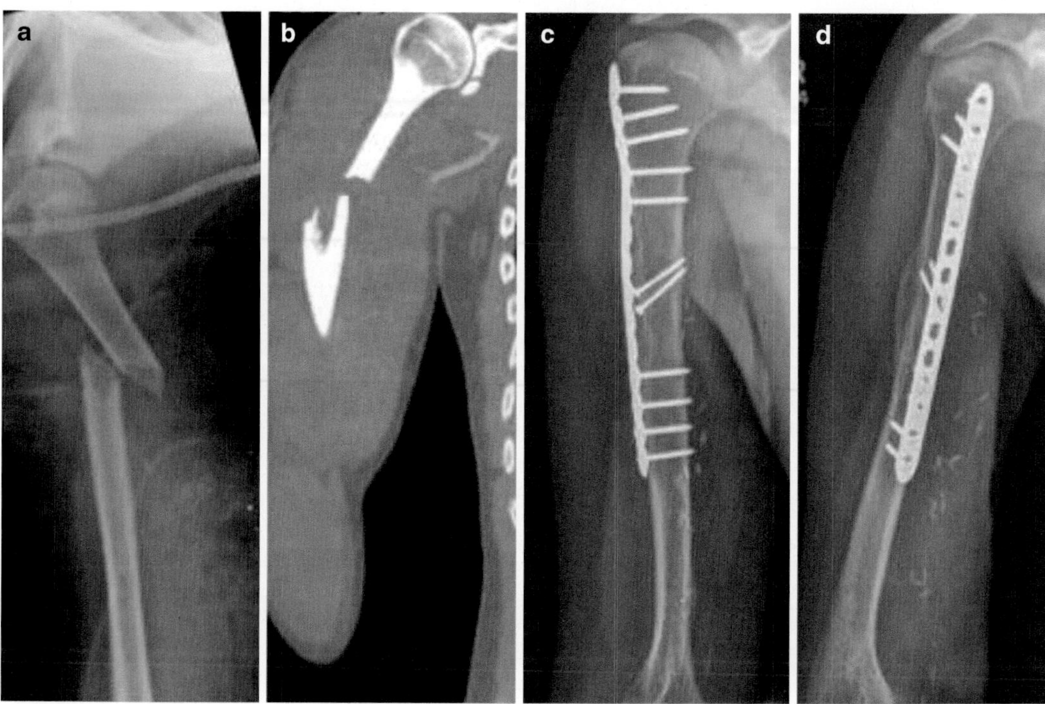

[Case 2.2]: An 18-year-old male sustains (**a**) a right diaphyseal humerus fracture after motor vehicle collision (MVC). (**b**) Coronal reconstruction of a computed tomographic angiogram, showing disruption of the brachial artery. (**c**, **d**) Absolute stability principle applied to achieve definitive fixation of the fracture

The patient presents with a hand that has non-palpable but dopplerable pulses about the wrist. He maintains slow >3 s cap refill and a hand that is cool compared the contra-lateral limb. He maintains weak flexion of the digits and has a large hematoma about the upper right arm. Computed tomographic angiogram reveals disruption of the brachial artery proximally.

The patient undergoes routine workup for a MVC, to include abdominal ultrasound, as well as CT scan of the head, chest, and pelvis, which are normal.

He is then brought to the operating room in an urgent manner, where a large deltopectoral exposure is completed, crossing the antecubital fossa. The lacertus fibrosus is released, demonstrating pink and contractile muscles of the forearm. The brachial artery is identified, as is a traumatic complete laceration of the median nerve. The ulnar nerve is intact. The brachial artery is found transected and resected to healthy levels. Fogarty catheterization of the proximal and distal arterial stumps is performed, and brisk back bleeding from the distal artery is found. Non-traumatic vascular clamps are placed on the ends of the arterial defect, and definitive debridement and plating are completed (Case 2.2 – c, d). Local reversed cephalic vein graft is used to reconstruct this defect. His median nerve is grafted on postoperative day 3, with an 8 cm graft. Ten months later, the patient demonstrated 5/5 elbow flexion and 4/5 strength of his wrist and finger flexors and a palpable radial pulse.

These two cases demonstrate the varying degrees of ischemia, as they relate to the injured upper extremity. In the first (Case 2.1), the zone of injury is profound, as demonstrated by the plain X-ray revealing marked comminution and significant soft tissue injury, and collateral flow has been disrupted. This represents critical ischemia and the need for immediate return of arterial flow in order to salvage the arm and hand. In this case, shunting is recommended and compartment release mandatory, as the duration of absolute ischemia can be expected to incur reperfusion injury and resultant compartment syndrome.

In the latter case (Case 2.2), clinical markers such as dopplerable faint signals at the wrist, with preservation of some motor function of the extrinsic finger flexors, in addition to the operative findings of contractile forearm muscle and brisk back bleeding, confirm that perfusion, albeit at a reduced level, is occurring. Notably, the plain film demonstrates a relatively focal zone of injury compared to the first case. These findings allow the clinician to proceed with definitive debridement and plating, with no need for fasciotomy and local vein graft for reconstruction.

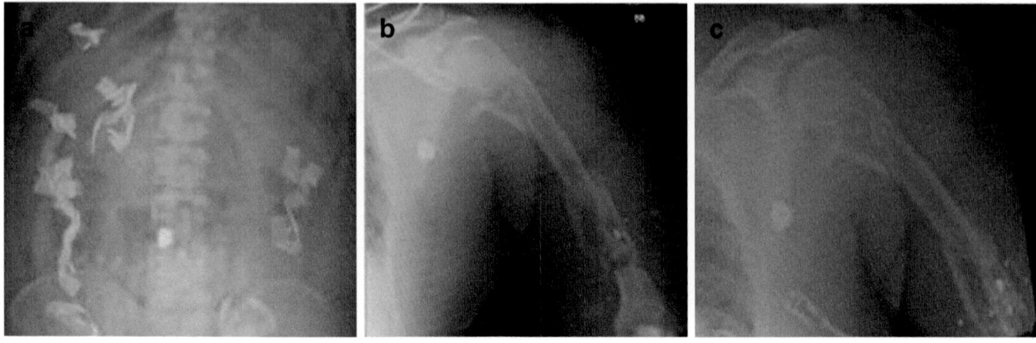

[**Case 2.3**]: A 36-year-old male is the victim of a multiple gunshot wounds to his left side, to include penetrating injuries to his (**a**) left chest, abdomen, and (**b**, **c**) left arm

[Case 2.3]: Upper Extremity Brachial Artery Injury with Associated Humeral Shaft Fracture: **Polytrauma Scenario**

The patient undergoes emergent thoracotomy, laparotomy, and resuscitation. Exploration of the left arm reveals partial transection of the left brachial artery, and intraoperative radiographs reveal a highly comminuted, segmental left humerus fracture (**Case 2.3 – b, c**).

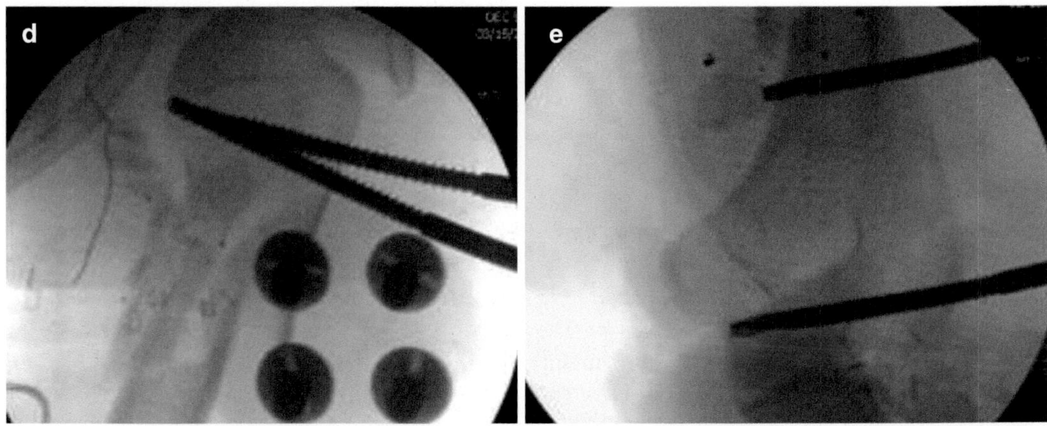

[Case 2.3]: (**d, e**) An external fixator is applied to the left arm in urgent fashion to protect the arterial repair

One week after his injury, his abdominal and chest wound has stabilized. Definitive fixation and alignment of his humerus are performed.

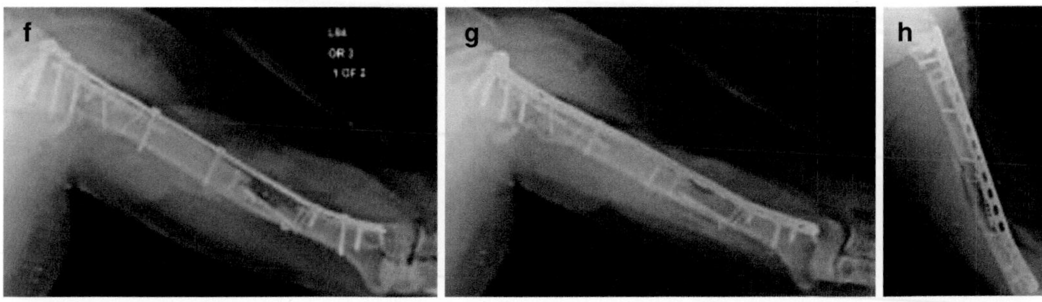

[Case 2.3]: (**f, g, h**) Different views showing the definitive fixation postoperatively of the humerus facture

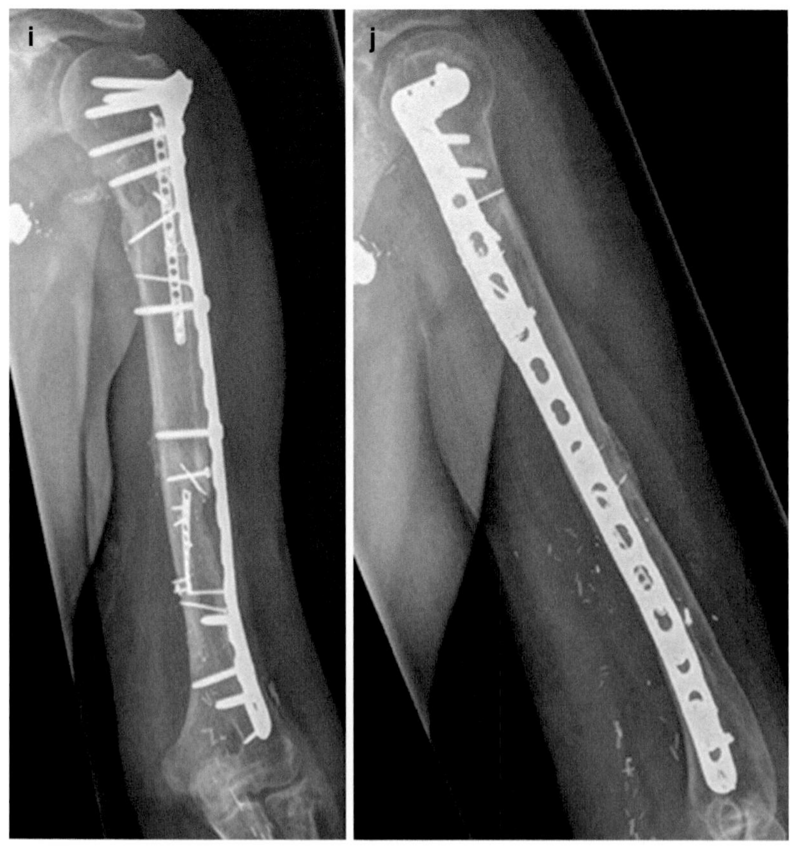

[**Case 2.3**]: (**i, j**) One year later, anteroposterior and lateral radiographs of the left humerus show adequate healing at the fracture sites

References

1. Song W, Zhou D, Dong J. Predictors of secondary amputation in patients with grade IIIC lower limb injuries: a retrospective analysis of 35 patients. Medicine (Baltimore). 2017;96(22):e7068.
2. Rutherford RB, Baker JD, Ernst C, et al. Recommended standards for reports dealing with lower extremity ischemia: revised version. J Vasc Surg. 1997;26(3):517–38.
3. Pederson WC. Replantation. Plast Reconstr Surg. 2001;107(3):823–41.
4. Haljamäe H, Enger E. Human skeletal muscle energy metabolism during and after complete tourniquet ischemia. Ann Surg. 1975;182(1):9–14.
5. Paradis S, Charles AL, Meyer A, et al. Chronology of mitochondrial and cellular events during skeletal muscle ischemia-reperfusion. Am J Physiol Cell Physiol. 2016;310(11):C968–82.
6. Better OS, Stein JH. Early management of shock and prophylaxis of acute renal failure in traumatic rhabdomyolysis. N Engl J Med. 1990;322(12):825–9.
7. Wolfe VM, Wang AA. Replantation of the upper extremity: current concepts. J Am Acad Orthop Surg. 2015;23(6):373–81.
8. Zeng X, Zhang L, Wu T, et al. Continuous renal replacement therapy (CRRT) for rhabdomyolysis. Cochrane Database Syst Rev. 2014;(6):CD008566.
9. Dennis JW, Frykberg ER, Veldenz HC, et al. Validation of nonoperative management of occult vascular injuries and accuracy of physical examination alone in penetrating extremity trauma: 5- to 10-year follow-up. J Trauma. 1998;44(2):243–52.
10. Feliciano DV. For the patient-evolution in the management of vascular trauma. J Trauma Acute Care Surg. 2017;83(6):1205–12.
11. deSouza IS, Benabbas R, McKee S, et al. Accuracy of physical examination, ankle-brachial index, and ultrasonography in the diagnosis of arterial injury

in patients with penetrating extremity trauma: a systematic review and meta-analysis. Acad Emerg Med. 2017;24(8):994–1017.

12. Frykberg ER, Dennis JW, Bishop K, et al. The reliability of physical examination in the evaluation of penetrating extremity trauma for vascular injury: results at one year. J Trauma. 1991;31(4):502–11.

13. Halvorson JJ, Anz A, Langfitt M, et al. Vascular injury associated with extremity trauma: initial diagnosis and management. J Am Acad Orthop Surg. 2011;19(8):495–504.

14. Zweifach SS, Hargens AR, Evans KL, et al. Skeletal muscle necrosis in pressurized compartments associated with hemorrhagic hypotension. J Trauma. 1980;20(11):941–7.

15. Mubarak SJ, Carroll NC. Volkmann's contracture in children: aetiology and prevention. J Bone Joint Surg Br. 1979;61-B(3):285–93.

16. Hafez HM, Woolgar J, Robbs JV. Lower extremity arterial injury: results of 550 cases and review of risk factors associated with limb loss. J Vasc Surg. 2001;33(6):1212–9.

17. Otto IA, Kon M, Schuurman AH, et al. Replantation versus prosthetic fitting in traumatic arm amputations: a systematic review. PLoS One. 2015;10(9):e0137729.

18. Levin PM, Rich NM, Hutton JE Jr. Collateral circulation in arterial injuries. Arch Surg. 1971;102(4):392–9.

19. Medina O, Arom GA, Yeranosian MG, et al. Vascular and nerve injury after knee dislocation: a systematic review. Clin Orthop Relat Res. 2014;472(9):2621–9.

20. Nagpal P, Maller V, Garg G, et al. Upper extremity runoff: pearls and pitfalls in computed tomography angiography and magnetic resonance angiography. Curr Probl Diagn Radiol. 2017;46(2):115–29.

21. Tan TW, Joglar FL, Hamburg NM, et al. Limb outcome and mortality in lower and upper extremity arterial injury: a comparison using the National Trauma Data Bank. Vasc Endovascular Surg. 2011;45(7):592–7.

22. Scerbo MH, Holcomb JB, Taub E, et al. The trauma center is too late: major limb trauma without a pre-hospital tourniquet has increased death from hemorrhagic shock. J Trauma Acute Care Surg. 2017;83(6):1165–72.

23. Tountas CP, Bergman RA. Tourniquet ischemia: ultrastructural and histochemical observations of ischemic human muscle and of monkey muscle and nerve. J Hand Surg Am. 1977;2(1):31–7.

24. Fields CE, Latifi R, Ivatury RR. Brachial and forearm vessels injuries. Surg Clin N Am. 2002;82(1):105.

25. Pederson WC. Acute ischemia of the upper extremity. Orthop Clin North Am. 2016;47(3):589–97.

26. Lebowitz C, Matzon JL. Arterial injury in the upper extremity: evaluation, strategies, and anticoagulation management. Hand Clin. 2018;34(1):85–95.

27. Gifford SM, Aidinian G, Clouse WD, et al. Effect of temporary shunting on extremity vascular injury: an outcome analysis from the Global War on Terror vascular injury initiative. J Vasc Surg. 2009;50(3):549–55.

28. Dragas M, Davidovic L, Kostic D, et al. Upper extremity arterial injuries: factors influencing treatment outcome. Injury. 2009;40(8):815–9.

Replantation of the Mangled Upper Extremity

6

John V. Ingari

First, it is necessary to be clear in the definition of replantation versus revascularization. Replantation in the upper extremity refers to the reattachment of a completely amputated limb, hand, or digit, whereas revascularization refers to the restoration of vascularity to an incompletely amputated limb, hand, or digit. The difference between complete amputation and near amputation can be crucial, because even a skin bridge may contain vital venous outflow in the case of incomplete amputation.

The first recorded successful replantation in the upper extremity was by Malt and McKann in Boston in 1962 [1]. Since then, microsurgical replantation has become reality in most trauma centers throughout the United States. In 2012, Peterson et al. surveyed 137 recognized level I trauma hospitals in the United States. Of the 117 level I hospitals who participated in the study, 64 (55%) reported on call microvascular replantation capability [2].

Additional 38 level II hospitals surveyed (29%) offered replantation capability, making replantation of severed digits, hands, and arms a very plausible and realistic event nationwide. With the advances in microsurgery, suture technology, and widely available microsurgical treatment, replantation of a mangled upper extremity may be preferable to revision amputation, when conditions allow. The condition of the amputated part must be considered, and the decision of replantation versus revision amputation should take into account more than the technical capabilities of an institution or surgeon. Only if the replanted part will add function, with minimal morbidity and pain, should replantation of a mangled extremity be considered. Some examples could include replantation of a thumb, a portion of a hand at the metacarpal level, through-wrist amputations, and more proximal level amputations in the forearm or brachium. An avulsion injury, a crush injury, or other tissue destroying mechanisms may preclude successful replantation, and each injury and each patient has to be considered individually. Use of the Mangled Extremity Severity Score (MESS) and Mangled Extremity Syndrome Index (MESI) has a place in evaluating the traumatized extremity, with a MESS score over 7 or a MESI over 18 being appropriate for amputation, while those limbs with lower scores are considered reasonable for limb salvage [3]. In the upper extremity, however, the MESS and MESI scores may be less reliable for several reasons [4, 5]. First, the muscle mass in the upper extremity is less than that of the lower extremity, and the physiologic burden of limb salvage may be less in the upper than lower extremity. Second, advanced lower extremity prostheses are quite functional, well tolerated, and can provide near-normal ambulation and

J. V. Ingari (✉)
Hand Surgery Division, Department of
Orthopaedic Surgery, Sinai Hospital of Baltimore,
Baltimore, MD, USA

© Springer Nature Switzerland AG 2021

R. A. Pensy, J. V. Ingari (eds.), *The Mangled Extremity*, https://doi.org/10.1007/978-3-319-56648-1_6

of the skin, nerves, and vessels and overall condition of the amputated part, allowing the surgeon to assess the possibility for replantation. Sometimes the decision whether to replant or amputate is best made only after intraoperative evaluation of the tissues, including magnified inspection of vascular, neural, and osseous injuries [16].

Initial Management

The initial patient management upon arrival at the emergency department should focus on life before limb. The "airway, breathing, circulation" (ABC) algorithm for initial care of the trauma victim should be followed. Special attention to expected blood loss and need for blood products should be anticipated [17]. Antibiotics should be administered, and tetanus immunization should be addressed. The cold (or warm) ischemia time, the mechanism of injury, the patient comorbidities, and the anticipation of needed blood products both preoperative and intraoperative should be factored into the initial evaluation. With a mangling upper extremity injury, concomitant injuries to organ systems, other bony injury, and head trauma are very possible and need to be assessed as well [16]. Initial radiographs of the pelvis, cervical spine, and chest are warranted. A complete blood count, electrolyte panel, serum glucose, and lactate levels should be drawn [18, 19]. Large-bore intravenous access should be initiated upon arrival. Hemorrhage remains the single most preventable cause of death on the battlefield, and with major limb amputations, blood loss management must be in the forefront of the treatment strategy as well [20].

A brief patient history to discern major medical comorbidities, allergies, time of injury, last meal, and medications is also warranted. Because ischemia time for the amputated part is critical, only the necessary history, physical examination, and laboratory data is gathered, with expedient transport to the operating room as a primary focus.

Assembling the Team

Once the patient is enroute to the trauma center, together with the amputated parts, and communication with the emergency personnel, both on the scene and in the emergency department of the trauma center, has occurred, the next step is to assemble a surgical team to address the potential replantation. Two teams are ideally required to optimize care of the patient and the part(s). One team should focus on evaluation of the patient and the residual limb, while one team is focused on the evaluation of the part or parts to assess the possibility of replantation. The team evaluating the amputated part(s) can proceed to the operating room (OR) with the parts to begin evaluation even prior to patient transport to the OR. The parts should be kept on ice, which can be facilitated by putting a sterile adherent plastic layer (i.e., Ioban) over a pan of ice. The part(s) should be cleansed with Hibiclens or betadine to optimize sterility. The surgical team can then assess the part under loupe or even microscopic magnification and make the necessary decision of whether replantation is an option or is primary amputation more suitable [21].

Once replantation is considered, expedient transport of the patient from the emergency department to the operating room is paramount. No extra time should be spent doing routine paperwork, focusing instead on only those emergent patient evaluations listed above. The operating room itself should be large enough to accommodate both surgical teams and the patient on the OR table with the amputated parts nearby. The teams then continue by dissecting out the vessels, nerves, tendons, muscles, and bony structures that will be reconnected during the multi-hour surgery.

Ischemia Time

Warm ischemia time of over 6–8 hours has been shown to be deleterious for replantation in ideal situations, but in the case of the mangled extremity, even more stringent restrictions should apply. Controversy, however, does exist in the literature. Lin et al. described a 64% success rate for replantation after 24 hours of cold ischemia time in 25 amputations in 14 patients [22]. Ten patients had multiple digital amputations, two had thumb amputations, and two had amputation at the wrist level, necessitating intensive care unit resuscitation leading to a 24-hour delay in surgery. Case reports of successful hand replantation after 54 hours of cold ischemia time, and even warm ischemia of up to 42 hours and up to 94 hours of cold ischemia time, have been described for digital replantation [23–25].

Additionally, new techniques in providing extracorporeal membrane oxygenation (ECMO) to perfuse limbs for up to 12 hours with subsequent successful replantation in a porcine model have been described [26]. This may provide a future method of reducing ischemia times, expanding time to replantation, and allowing successful replantation of amputated upper extremities despite unexpected delay in surgery. The concept of providing hypothermic oxygenated acellular fluids via an ECMO device to an amputated limb has potentially exciting ramifications not only in replantation surgery but also in transplant surgery as well [26].

With respect to replantation of the mangled upper extremity, ischemia time is also relative to the level of amputation. Amputations proximal to the hand, in the forearm, and especially at the transhumeral level all have muscle mass in the amputated part, unlike digital amputations, making ischemia time more critical to evaluate. For amputations proximal to the hand, warm ischemia of greater than 6–8 hours will lead to far more tissue damage including myonecrosis that can be both a problem in initial replant survival and to the patient in the early postoperative phase due to lactic acidosis, myoglobinemia, and myoglobinuria following major limb replantation. The routine use of intravenous fluids, Foley catheters, and monitoring urine and blood myoglobin levels cannot be overstated. Lactic acid levels should also be monitored in the more proximal level replantations.

In summary, with regard to ischemia times, although there are case reports of successful replants after prolonged ischemia up to 94 hours, the following guidelines from Wolfe and Wang's current concepts remain reasonable [27]. For digits, maximal warm ischemia of 12 hours and cold ischemia of 24 hours for consideration of replantation is recommended. For hand or more proximal amputations, 6-hour warm ischemia time or 12-hour cold ischemia time is the maximal time recommended for consideration of replantation [27]. It must be emphasized that these are guidelines only, and in the face of a mangled upper extremity amputation, ischemia times may be lessened regarding successful replantation attempts.

Appropriate Levels for Replanting Mangled Amputations

When considering replantation in a mangled upper extremity, the levels of amputation become even more important than when considering replantation under ideal, sharp amputation mechanisms. Individual mangled digits, with the possible exception of the thumb, for example, should not be replanted, as the function of a replanted mangled digit, even if technically achievable, would be less than that of a hand with a missing digit. Multiple digits can be considered for replantation after, but only if in the judgment of the surgeon or surgical team the less than perfect digits would enhance function versus the hand with completed revision amputations.

Through-hand amputations, wrist-level amputations, and more proximal forearm- or brachial-level amputations are those that warrant most careful consideration for replantation in the face of less than ideal mangled tissue and extended zone of injury mechanisms. The possibility of shortening the limb, with the ability to remove the most damaged zone of injured tissues, makes more proximal amputations a very reasonable consideration but must still take into account the most important principles of life before limb and thoughtful consideration of prosthetic options. The humerus tolerates five centimeters of shortening well, and that may allow primary repair of vessels and nerves while allowing appropriate tissue and muscle debridement as needed [28]. The forearm, similarly, can be shortened up to 4 cm without undue muscle tension disturbance [29]. The thumb has been shown to function adequately following replantation with a full centimeter of shortening [30]. Despite skeletal shortening, the possibility of intercalary vein grafting must remain foremost in the surgeons mind, despite potential for limb shortening, and a graft with two anastomoses is better than a primary single anastomosis done under tension or with damaged vessels. Toward this likely need for graft, taking the vein graft early in the case is recommended so that the surgeon has available graft(s) once the arterial and venous repairs are undertaken.

Surgical Techniques

The "Checklist"

Once the decision to attempt replantation has been made and the patient and the parts are in the operating suite, the actual surgical technique becomes the next and most important objective. The techniques differ for specific levels of replantation, and each level for replantation of a mangled upper extremity will be discussed individually. With that stated, one of the most helpful preparatory guidelines is to use a surgical "checklist," much like pilots use a checklist prior to leaving the ground in an aircraft. The most helpful checklist for replantation is an anatomic list of the mandatory structures to be repaired, reconnected, or otherwise reconstructed. The most useful one I have used is the following [31, 32]:

1. Bone(s)
2. Extensors
3. Flexors
4. Arteries
5. Nerves
6. Veins
7. Skin/closure

The acronym "B-E-F-A-N-V-S" is offered to help remember the seven categories in the replantation "checklist." The specific order of repair, anastomosis, or coaptation of the various structures may be altered depending on the level of amputation and the surgeon's experience, but the seven categories should be individually assessed and "checked off" once the replantation is underway.

The Equipment

The need for two surgical teams has already been mentioned, and the need for an operating suite of adequate size to accommodate both teams is clear. Next, the need to ensure the appropriate surgical equipment is ready and available cannot be overemphasized. Beginning with loupe magnification for initial dissection of the amputated part and the residual limb by individual teams, small hand instruments to include Adson forceps, smaller jeweler's forceps, or Bishop Harmon forceps, dissecting scissors such as tenotomy scissors or Littler tenotomy scissors will make initial exploration possible. Gerald and DeBakey forceps make handling of the vascular and neural tissues minimally traumatic in the initial dissection. Small retractors may be helpful, and using a suture like a 4-0 nylon to reflect and hold skin edges is also advantageous and minimally traumatizing. Small metallic clips, either from a disposable unit like a "Ligaclip" or Gem clip, are used to mark veins, arteries, and nerves as needed. Once these structures are identified and marked with small clips, valuable time is saved when the actual replantation is performed. Tendons can be individually identified as well, and a Tajima or Kessler suture can be placed with a steri-strip marked with sterile marker to make tendon repair expeditious during replantation (see Fig. 6.3).

The two surgical teams can identify and mark the structures in both the residual limb as well as the amputated part to make subsequent vascular anastomoses, nerve coaptations, and tendon repairs as straightforward as possible, saving

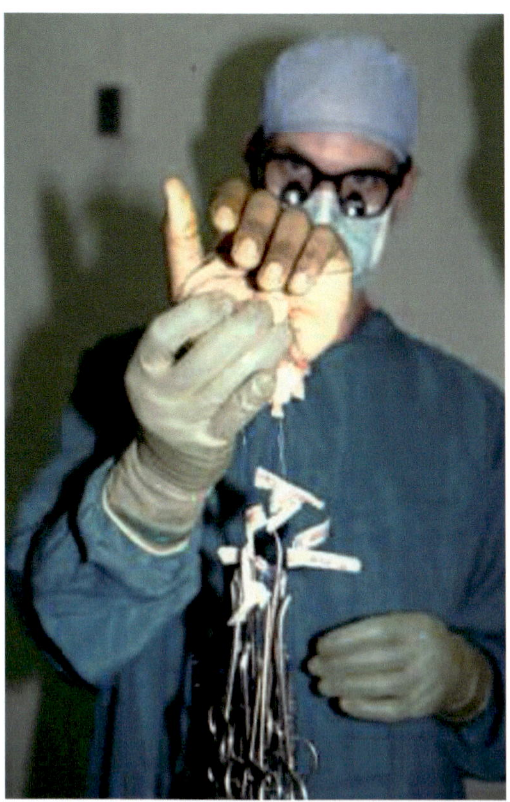

Fig. 6.3 Steri-strips marked with sterile marker attached to sutures to identify each tendon on the amputated part can facilitate expeditious tendon repair during subsequent replantation

valuable surgical time. The optimal hardware for bony osteosynthesis should also be included in the equipment list and may include K-wires, plates and screws, intramedullary fixation devices, or intraosseous wires.

Once the structures have been identified and marked on both the residual limb and the amputated part(s), the ensuing replantation requires microsurgical equipment, to include an appropriate two-headed microscope, capable of 20× magnification, microsuture (8-0 to 10-0 nylon) depending on the level of repair, and a complete set of micro-instruments. The micro-instruments are often based on surgeon's preference, but a basic list of needed instruments is fairly standard. Micro-instruments of stainless steel or titanium can be used, based on surgeon's preference. Titanium instruments avoid the distraction of magnetized instruments during the

procedure but are somewhat more fragile than stainless steel instruments. If stainless steel instruments are used, a commercial demagnetizer is useful to avoid magnetized instruments. Micro forceps, curved and straight, are necessary for handling vessels and nerves under the microscope. Microneedle drivers such as Castro-Villejo's, preferably non-locking are also needed. I prefer titanium, to avoid the distraction of magnetized instruments that can occur with the stainless steel instruments. Micro-scissors, both for dissection and suture cutting, are part of the basic list. A 30-gauge ophthalmology irrigating needle tip is useful to irrigate vessels prior to and during anastomoses. Vessel dilators are extremely helpful in optimizing vessel lumen dimensions prior to an anastomosis as well. When using a vessel dilator, care must be exercised to avoid intimal damage to the vessel. Vessel dilators should not be routinely used in place of forceps for handling tissue, as the small tips are easily bent, rendering the instrument unusable. Arterial and venous clamps, such as Acland clamps, are also needed once the vessels have been identified for anastomosis. Background material to place behind vessels for microanastomosis can be used based on surgeon's preference.

An operating microscope, with two viewing ports ("two-headed"), is an essential piece of equipment in any replant operation. While vessel anastomoses or nerve coaptations in the brachium may be achieved under loupe magnification, any replant below the elbow deserves the added advantage of enhanced visualization and precision offered by the operating microscope. 10–20× magnification is standard, and newer microscopes offer autofocus and zoom capabilities that make the surgical field optimally visualized. Surgeon preference dictates whether foot or hand controls are optimal, and both work well, allowing focus, zoom, as well as microscope head movements.

Specific Level Replantation: Thumb

The thumb is the most appropriate digit to consider replantation in the setting of a mangling injury if the resultant reconstruction will serve as a relatively pain-free post, which offers opposition and pinch capability. First, the part has to be evaluated for possible replantation, with special attention to vessels in the amputated part. Vessels that have been avulsed may have severe intimal damage that can preclude successful restoration of blood flow even if anastomosis can be done. If proximal avulsion of the flexor pollicis longus tendon precludes a primary tendon repair, transfer of brachioradialis to flexor pollicis longus can allow flexion through the interphalangeal joint in the face of irreparable flexor tendon avulsion. Thumb avulsions, while less than ideal, have been successfully replanted with reasonably functional results compared to amputation [33, 34]. When faced with thumb amputation, especially in the setting of somewhat mangled tissues, a vein graft from the thumb ulnar digital artery to the radial artery in the anatomic snuffbox is an ideal way to bypass injured vascular structures in the thumb and allow excellent inflow and has been shown to increase thumb replant survival rates [34, 35]. Bieber et al. reported on 28 avulsed thumbs, of which eight were successfully replanted (29%) using vein grafting [33]. The vein graft can be anastomosed to the amputated thumb vessels prior to bony fixation, making the surgical visualization and positioning somewhat easier for vascular repair [36]. If intimal damage is severe in the amputated thumb, the vein graft may be patent, but the likelihood of reestablishing blood supply to the part is low. If the a "ribbon" sign is visible on the skin, which is a red, somewhat squiggled line representing intimal and vessel injury as well as a tortuous remnant of digital artery, vascular repair is unlikely to be successful, despite a patent anastomosis. If replantation is to be attempted, resection of the injured arteries is required with intercalary vein grafting bridging the gap [34, 37].

If judged by the surgeon to be acceptable to attempt replantation, the surgical "checklist" as delineated above should be followed.

The bony reconstruction depends on whether the amputation is through a joint or periarticular or conversely through the shaft of the bone. In the case of articular or periarticular amputation in the thumb, fusion of the involved joint is a suitable way to begin osteosynthesis. This can be done with K-wires or modular plates and screws designed for phalangeal fixation. Alternatively, one or more headless compression screws can be used to fuse a joint, either at the metacarpalphalangeal level or more proximally at the carpometacarpal level. The surgeons experience with each of the above methods as well as equipment availability should dictate which of the methods of arthrodesis is selected.

If the amputation is through diaphyseal bone, then the surgeon can use the method of osteosynthesis that is most stable, is expeditious, and allows minimal soft tissue disruption. This may be K-wires, 90-90 wiring, modular hand plates, or combinations thereof. Again, the surgeon's comfort and familiarity should dictate which method of bony fixation is chosen.

Once the bone fixation is complete, the checklist continues with repair of extensors, which, for the thumb, is primarily the extensor pollicis longus, although at more proximal levels it may include extensor pollicis brevis as well. I prefer prolene sutures, 3-0 or 4-0 for tendon repair, using a grasping suture such as a Kessler or Tajima. The Tajima modification of the Kessler suture is particularly attractive in replants as both the proximal and distal tendon stumps can be independently sutured, joining the sutures and tying them once the bone fixation is complete.

Next on the checklist are flexors, which, for the thumb the flexor pollicis longus and possibly flexor pollicis brevis in a more proximal amputation, can be considered for repair. As noted above, an avulsed tendon or tendons do not preclude successful replantation but may involve either primary or staged tendon transfer. Alternatively, arthrodesis can be used to stabilize a joint, if tendon repair or transfer is deemed unacceptable. 3-0 or 4-0 prolene in a tendon-grasping configuration is recommended. An epitenon suture is advised if achievable given the tissue condition. The extensors tendons can be next repaired under loupe magnification, prior to beginning the microscopic portions of the replantation.

Once the tendons have been addressed, the microscope is brought in to allow vessel and nerve repair under optimal visualization. Vein grafts, which ideally have already been harvested, can be used as needed for vascular repair. 9-0 or 10-0 nylon suture on a BV75 or BV100 needle works well for vascular repair. The necessary microscopic instruments are listed earlier in the chapter. I prefer to begin with arterial repair prior to venous repair to allow the earliest inflow of blood to the amputated part as possible. Although some prefer to do vein anastomoses first, I find that it is easier to find the ideal veins to anastomose once blood is flowing through them. In addition if arterial repair is deemed unsuitable or flow cannot be reestablished due to the injury severity, then precious time has not been wasted in prior vein anastomoses. In general, one artery and two veins are the minimum required for optimal restoration of vascular flow and patency. As mentioned earlier, arterial anastomosis in the thumb with vein grafting can be made easier if the vascular work actually precedes bony fixation, as described by Caffee [36].

In the same microscopic field as the artery is the digital nerve(s), and those can be repaired primarily if bony shortening allows or with allograft nerve grafts. Allograft nerve for sensory nerve gaps of 5–50 mm has proven superior to nerve conduits, making nerve tubes or conduits less than ideal for nerve coaptations [38–40].

Finally, on the dorsal aspect of the thumb, veins can be anastomosed, preferably at least two veins for optimal outflow. Vein grafting remains an option, as does primary anastomosis when bony shortening allows.

Transmetacarpal-Level Amputation

A hand amputation through a level proximal to the metacarpal heads may be amenable to replantation in a mangled hand case if the resultant reconstructed hand can be expected to offer digital function with minimal pain and stiffness. This is perhaps one of the most difficult decisions as it may seem advantageous to replant the multiple digits affected by a transmetacarpal-level amputation, but stiff, painful fingers with no intrinsic function may be more deleterious to

function than a well-done amputation at this level. In a sharply cut, guillotine style mechanism of injury, a transmetacarpal-level amputation is indicated for replantation, but with crushing, avulsing, or tearing mechanisms, the likeliness of stiffness, tendon adhesions, and loss of intrinsic function is quite high and may best served by amputation, especially in a hand with an intact thumb. Recognizing the ultimate goal of not merely to preserve all living tissue through nonselective replantation, but rather to preserve one's quality of life by improving their function and appearance, is critically important [41]. The objective remains to care for the patient with the intent to optimize function as well as appearance and should be an important guide to decision-making [41].

If, in the mind of the surgeon, replantation of a mangled transmetacarpal-level amputation is feasible and reasonable, the surgical "checklist" as outlined in the above sections should be followed. In addition to bony shortening, vein grafts should be anticipated as well as the possible need for soft tissue coverage.

Wrist-Level Amputation

Amputation through the carpus is a severely debilitating loss, and if possible, replantation at this level may be advantageous even in the setting of avulsion, sawing, tearing, or otherwise mangling injury, especially if the zone of injury does not extend to the digits (see Figs. 6.4 and 6.5).

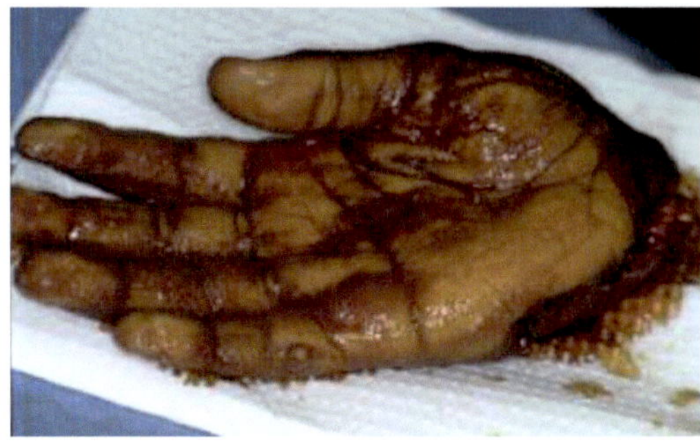

Fig. 6.4 A transcarpal disarticulation from a sawing mechanism in an industrial accident. Notice the amputated hand has been initially cleansed with betadine scrub

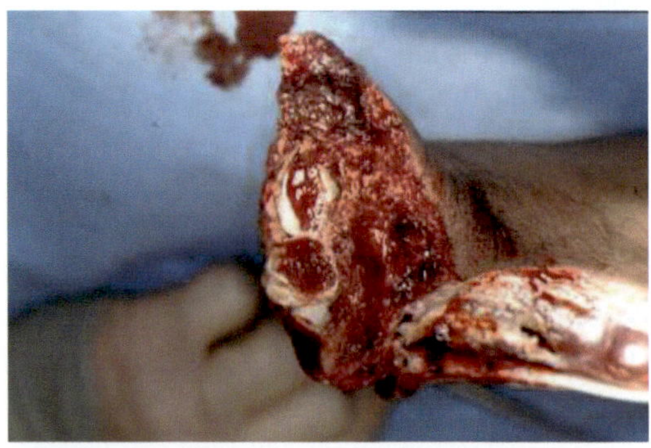

Fig. 6.5 The proximal residual limb was judged to be in reasonable condition to allow replantation despite injury to the carpus

Shortening of bone can be accomplished via proximal row carpectomy and subtotal or even total wrist fusion (see Fig. 6.6). The surgical "checklist" is much the same as for more distal amputations, with bones, extensors, and flexors being addressed initially. As with more distal amputations, plans for vein grafting and soft tissue coverage are needed. When addressing the arterial repair, either the radial or ulnar artery can be reanastomosed, if a complete arch is present distally. If an incomplete arch is present, both arteries will need to be anastomosed to reestablish flow to all digits. Intraoperative evaluation with Doppler signal to

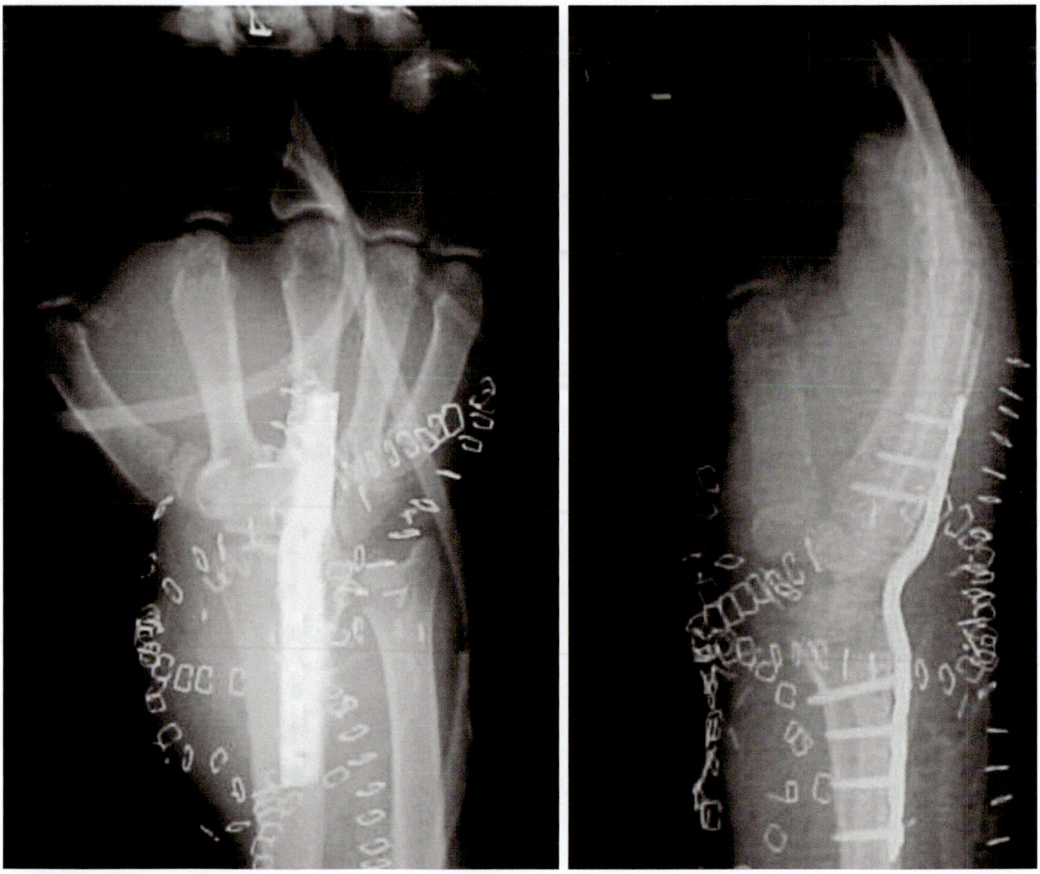

Fig. 6.6 Arthrodesis of the wrist in this case with a proximal row carpectomy achieved stout bony fixation, with enough skeletal shortening to allow primary nerve and arterial repair

the digits is an ideal way to assess distal flow following anastomosis of the radial and/or ulnar artery. If Doppler flow is audible in all digits, then a single arterial repair is acceptable. Conversely, if inadequate digital flow is achieved following single artery repair, then proceeding with repair of the second artery is indicated.

Repair of the artery may need to precede completion of the flexor repairs, as the flexor carpi radialis overlies the radial artery and the flexor carpi ulnaris overlies the ulnar neurovascular bundle. Specifically, the radial artery anastomosis should be completed prior to repair of the flexor carpi radialis, and the ulnar artery and nerve should be repaired prior to flexor carpi ulnaris repair. Although this does not follow the "checklist" exactly, accommodation for specific anatomy is warranted.

If a wrist arthrodesis is chosen for bony fixation, the tendons for wrist flexion and extension do not require specific repair, making those tendons available as transfers or even source for primary tendon graft material. Finally, after vessel anastomoses are complete, nerve coaptations are done, and fasciotomy as needed should be considered, including release of the carpal tunnel following a wrist-level replantation. Soft tissue coverage needs may include skin graft or skin graft substitutes, such as acellular dermal matrix (see Fig. 6.7).

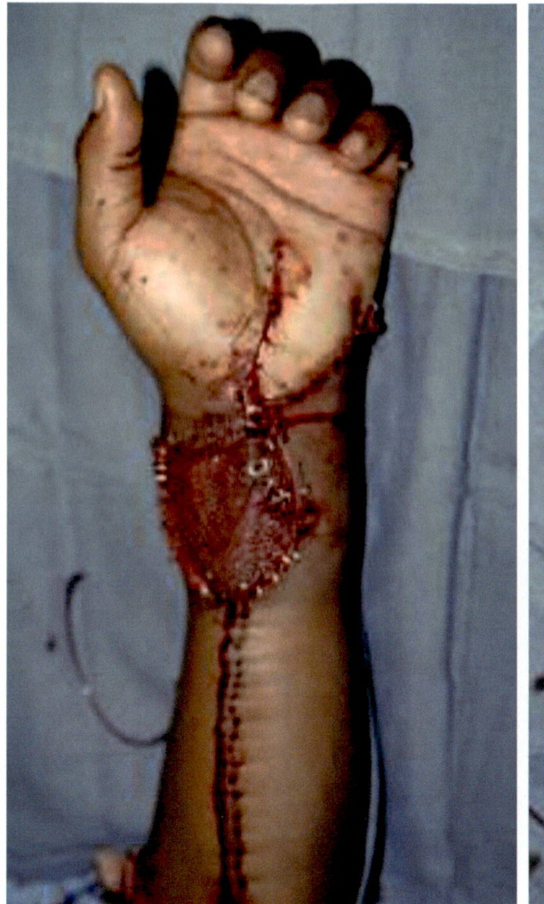
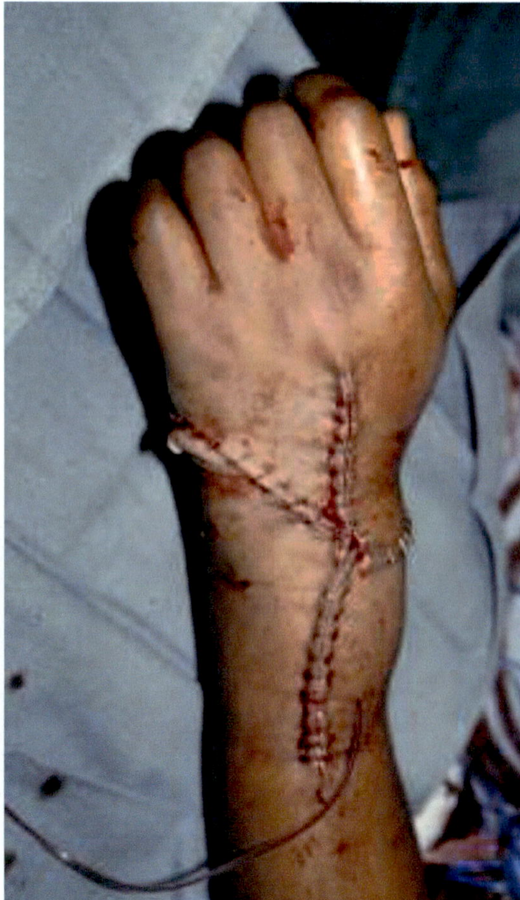

Fig. 6.7 Successful replantation with reestablished blood flow 4 hours post-injury. Notice the skin graft required for soft tissue coverage in the face of acute swelling

Forearm-Level Amputation

In forearm-level amputation, if replantation is considered a viable option, the bony fixation is much like that for fixation of a both bone forearm fracture with standard plating options for the radius and ulna [42] (see Figs. 6.8 and 6.9). Bone shortening up to four centimeters is well tolerated in the forearm and may make vascular anastomoses and nerve coaptations more amenable to direct end-to-end repair [43]. The level of amputation will dictate whether tendon repair is feasible or, if more proximal in the forearm, muscle tendon junction repair strategies need to be used. The more proximal level amputations include muscle tissue in the amputated part, and close attention to myoglobin levels in the blood and urine needs to be given in the early postoperative phase. Reperfusion fasciotomy to include carpal tunnel release distally should be included. The order of fixation in the surgical checklist may be modified in more proximal injuries to include ini-

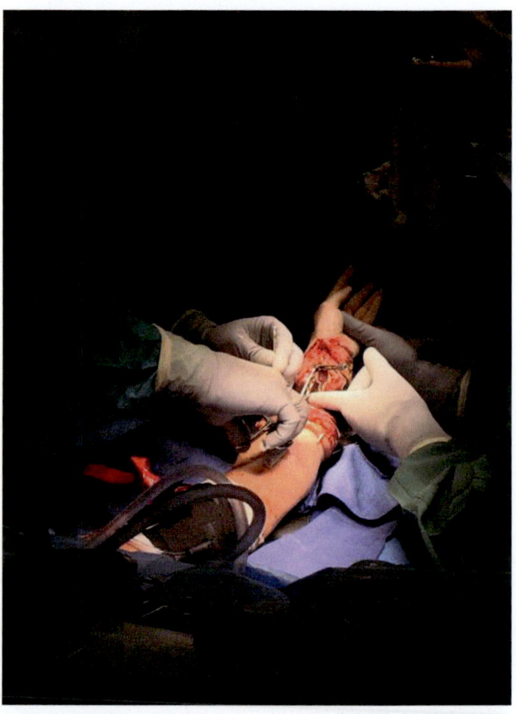

Fig. 6.9 Replantation at the forearm level begins with plate fixation of the radius and ulna. (Photo courtesy of Dr. Ray Pensy)

tial use of temporary vascular shunts even prior to bony fixation to minimize ischemia times and allow more detailed fixation of nerves, tendons, and bone [44]. Despite the mangling mechanism of injury, replantation of through forearm-level amputations can lead to acceptable patient functional and cosmetic outcomes in the majority of cases [45].

Transhumeral Amputations

Transhumeral-level mangling amputations are among the most difficult decisions clinically. With advanced prosthetics, myoelectric hands, wrist, and elbows are available for the transhumeral amputee, and with minimal sensation expected in replant patients at this level, serious consideration to revision amputation rather than attempted replantation with limited motor and sensory return distally is warranted. Conversely, with the relatively large vessel and

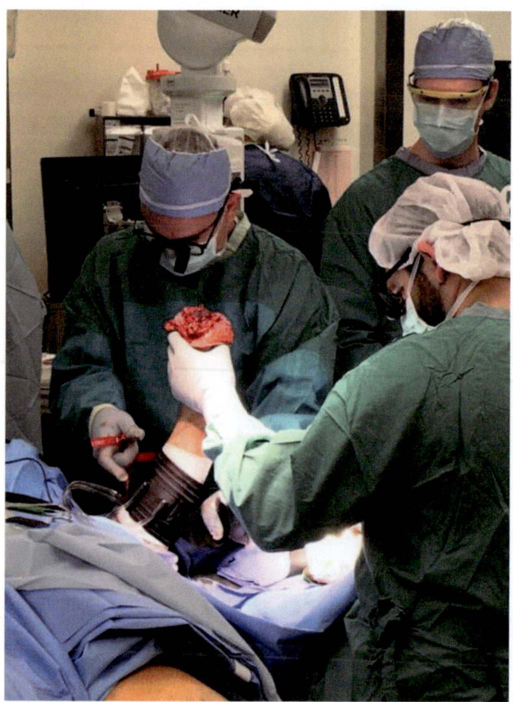

Fig. 6.8 Avulsion amputation at the forearm level can be a reasonable choice for replantation. (Photo courtesy of Dr. Ray Pensy)

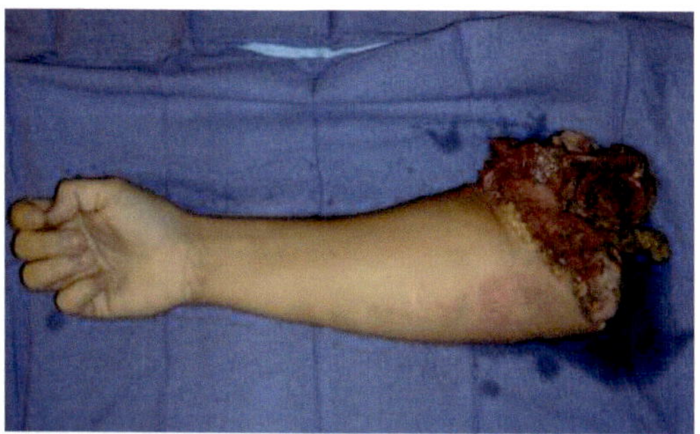

Fig. 6.10 A distal transhumeral amputation should be considered for replantation if the patient has a functional shoulder. (Photo courtesy of Dr. Jaimie Shores)

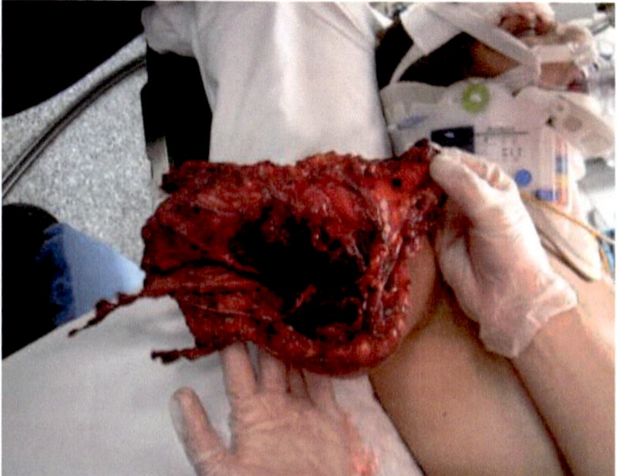

Fig. 6.11 A mangled transhumeral amputation, judged to be an acceptable situation for replantation. (Photo courtesy of Dr. Jaimie Shores)

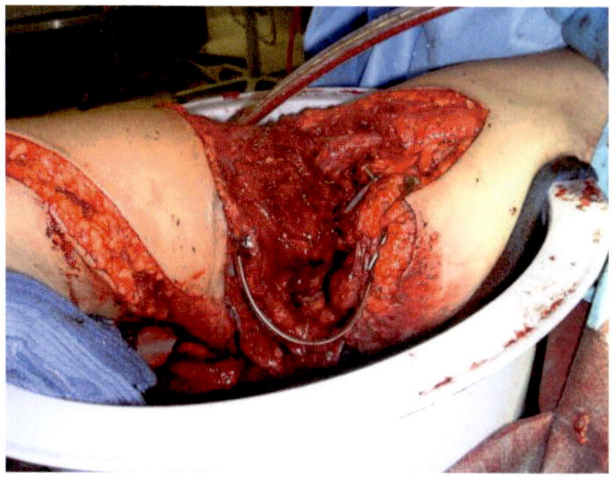

Fig. 6.12 Arterial and venous vascular shunts provided early inflow, prior to formal vessel anastomosis

nerve caliber and fewer muscle/tendon units to repair and stout bony fixation for the humerus, replantation is technically feasible in many cases and does remain an option (see Figs. 6.10 and 6.11). In a highly motivated patient with realistic expectation, an intact functioning shoulder should be considered an indication for attempted replantation [46]. A "helper" arm can still be achieved even in an avulsion-type amputation [46].

If replantation is considered, several technical points are worth mentioning here. Even prior to bony fixation, a temporary vascular shunt can provide early revascularization to the amputated limb, allowing a less rushed bone, muscle, and nerve repair (see Fig. 6.12). Plating of the humerus is recommended, with consideration of up to five centimeters of bone shortening to help

with subsequent definitive vascular anastomosis and neural coaptations. With successful muscle repair, functional elbow flexion and extension can be expected (see Figs. 6.13 and 6.14). At the level of the brachium, deep veins including the brachial veins can be anastomosed, along with the more superficial cephalic and basilic veins. Anastomosis of at least two major veins is recommended. With a brachial-level replantation, significant physiologic burden of injured muscle mass must be expected as noted previously, and increase in serum and urinary myoglobin should be anticipated. Reperfusion fasciotomy of the entire limb to include the carpal tunnel should also be included.

Postoperative Care

Initial admission to a surgical intensive care unit is mandatory. Maintaining the room at a warmed temperature is standard. Maintaining high level of IV hydration with normal saline or equivalent will help "flush" out myoglobin from the blood and urine. Anticoagulation with aspirin is effective, but if significant difficulty was encountered during vessel repair, consideration of heparin drips has also been found to be effective. Intravenous antibiotics should be routinely administered both preoperatively and in the early postoperative phase of recovery. Tetanus prophylaxis should be administered, if not already done pre-op.

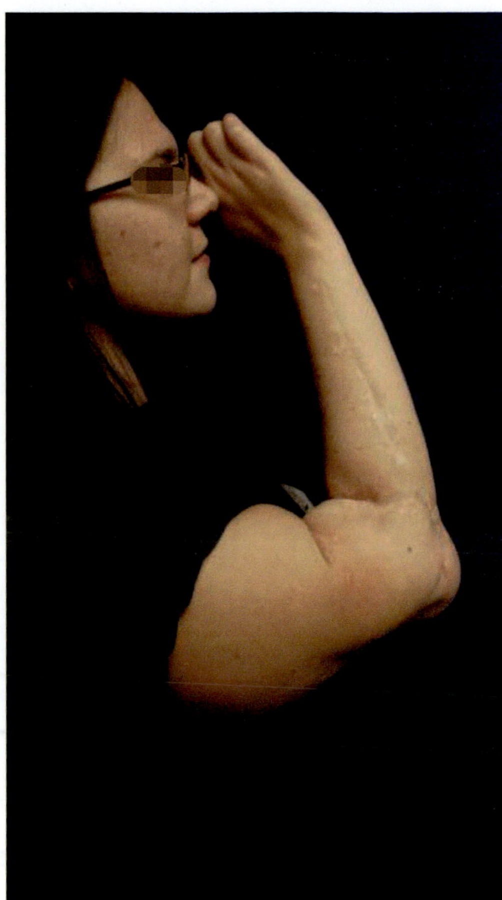

Fig. 6.13 Successful transhumeral replantation allows elbow flexion. (Photo courtesy of Dr. Jaimie Shores)

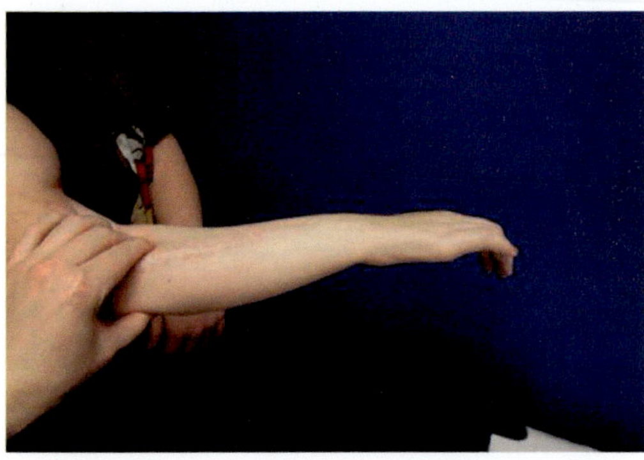

Fig. 6.14 Elbow and digital extension in the same patient from Figs. 6.10, 6.11, 6.12, and 6.13. (Photo courtesy of Dr. Jaimie Shores)

Pain management for the replanted limb should include an indwelling catheter, both for optimal pain control and for the chemical sympa-thectomy that the regional anesthetic affords. This can help in avoiding vessel spasm in the area of arterial anastomosis. The reader is urged to refer to the chapter on pain management for more detailed strategies.

Summary

When faced with a mangling amputation in the upper extremity, the surgeon is challenged with much more than the technical challenges of the microscopic and macroscopic surgical proce-dure. Evaluating the patient as a whole, for medi-cal comorbidities, psychological factors, and often polytraumatic injury patterns is the first order of business in assessing the possibility of replantation. Saving life before limb, while sounding trite, must be strictly in the forefront of the surgeon's mind in these cases.

The evaluation of the amputated part must be thorough yet expeditious, and if tissue con-dition is unacceptable for replantation, or if ischemia time precludes, a revision amputation is the better choice. Long-term function must be considered as a primary goal, rather than focusing on just the technical ability to perform a replantation. Yet despite these misgivings, successful replantation of a mangling upper extremity amputation, with the proper consid-erations noted throughout this chapter, can be accomplished and may offer patient function and satisfaction greater than that of an ampu-tated limb.

References

1. Malt RA, McKhann C. Replantation of severed arms. JAMA. 1964;189:716–22.
2. Peterson BC, Mangiapani D, Kellogg R, Leversedge FJ. Hand and microvascular replantation call avail-ability study: a national real-time survey of level-I and level-II trauma centers. J Bone Joint Surg Am. 2012;94(24):e185.
3. Slauterbeck JR, Britton C, Moneim MS, Clevenger FW. Mangled extremity severity score: an accu-rate guide to treatment of the severely injured upper extremity. J Orthop Trauma. 1994;8(4):282–5.
4. Kumar RS, Singhi PK, Chidambaram M. Are we jus-tified doing salvage or amputation procedure based on

mangled extremity severity score in mangled upper extremity injury. J Orthop Case Rep. 2017;7(1):3–8.

5. Togawa S, Yamami N, Nakayama H, Mano Y, Ikegami K, Ozeki S. The validity of the mangled extremity severity score in the assessment of upper limb injuries. J Bone Joint Surg Br. 2005;87(11):1516–9.

6. Pet MA, Morrison SD, Mack JS, Sears ED, Wright T, Lussiez AD, et al. Comparison of patient-reported outcomes after traumatic upper extremity amputation: replantation versus prosthetic rehabilitation. Injury. 2016;47(12):2783–8.

7. Shores JT, Malek V, Lee WPA, Brandacher G. Outcomes after hand and upper extremity transplantation. J Mater Sci Mater Med. 2017;28(5):72.

8. Shores JT, Brandacher G, Lee WP. Hand and upper extremity transplantation: an update of outcomes in the worldwide experience. Plast Reconstr Surg. 2015;135(2):351e–60e.

9. Shores JT, Imbriglia JE, Lee WP. The current state of hand transplantation. J Hand Surg Am. 2011;36(11):1862–7.

10. Boulas HJ. Amputations of the fingers and hand: indications for replantation. J Am Acad Orthop Surg. 1998;6(2):100–5.

11. Ahmadi A, Hirschberg E. Indications for replantation in psychiatric patients exemplified by hand replantation in a patient with schizophrenia. Handchir Mikrochir Plast Chir. 1990;22(1):46–8.

12. Hustedt JW, Chung A, Bohl DD, Olmscheid N, Edwards S. Evaluating the effect of comorbidities on the success, risk, and cost of digital replantation. J Hand Surg Am. 2016;41(12):1145–52.e1.

13. Kwon GD, Ahn BM, Lee JS, Park YG, Chang GW, Ha YC. The effect of patient age on the success rate of digital replantation. Plast Reconstr Surg. 2017;139(2):420–6.

14. Bumbasirevic M, Stevanovic M, Lesic A, Atkinson HD. Current management of the mangled upper extremity. Int Orthop. 2012;36(11):2189–95.

15. VanGiesen PJ, Seaber AV, Urbaniak JR. Storage of amputated parts prior to replantation--an experimental study with rabbit ears. J Hand Surg Am. 1983;8(1):60–5.

16. Russell RC, O'Brien BM, Morrison WA, Pamamull G, MacLeod A. The late functional results of upper limb revascularization and replantation. J Hand Surg Am. 1984;9(5):623–33.

17. Mardian S, Krapohl BD, Roffeis J, Disch AC, Schaser KD, Schwabe P. Complete major amputation of the upper extremity: early results and initial treatment algorithm. J Trauma Acute Care Surg. 2015;78(3):586–93.

18. Parsikia A, Bones K, Kaplan M, Strain J, Leung PS, Ortiz J, et al. The predictive value of initial serum lactate in trauma patients. Shock. 2014;42(3):199–204.

19. Okello M, Makobore P, Wangoda R, Upoki A, Galukande M. Serum lactate as a predictor of early outcomes among trauma patients in Uganda. Int J Emerg Med. 2014;7:20.

20. Koo A, Walsh R. A brief history on the evolution of amputation hemorrhage control and surgical technique. Am Surg. 2016;82(6):118–9.

21. Goldner RD, Urbaniak JR. Indications for replantation in the adult upper extremity. Occup Med. 1989;4(3):525–38.

22. Lin CH, Aydyn N, Lin YT, Hsu CT, Lin CH, Yeh JT. Hand and finger replantation after protracted ischemia (more than 24 hours). Ann Plast Surg. 2010;64(3):286–90.

23. Molski M. Thumb replantation after 22 hours of ischemia: a case report and review of literature. Chir Narzadow Ruchu Ortop Pol. 1999;64(4):457–62.

24. VanderWilde RS, Wood MB, Zu ZG. Hand replantation after 54 hours of cold ischemia: a case report. J Hand Surg Am. 1992;17(2):217–20.

25. Baek SM, Kim SS. Successful digital replantation after 42 hours of warm ischemia. J Reconstr Microsurg. 1992;8(6):455–8; discussion 9.

26. Kueckelhaus M, Dermietzel A, Alhefzi M, Aycart MA, Fischer S, Krezdorn N, et al. Acellular hypothermic extracorporeal perfusion extends allowable ischemia time in a porcine whole limb replantation model. Plast Reconstr Surg. 2017;139(4):922e–32e.

27. Wolfe VM, Wang AA. Replantation of the upper extremity: current concepts. J Am Acad Orthop Surg. 2015;23(6):373–81.

28. Khan MS, Sahibzada AS, Khan MA, Sultan S, Younas M, Khan AZ. Outcome of plating, bone grafting and shortening of non-union humeral diaphyseal fracture. J Ayub Med Coll Abbottabad. 2005;17(2):44–6.

29. Wolfe S, editor. Green's operative hand surgery. 6th ed. Philadelphia: Elsevier; 2011.

30. Goldner RD, Howson MP, Nunley JA, Fitch RD, Belding NR, Urbaniak JR. One hundred eleven thumb amputations: replantation vs revision. Microsurgery. 1990;11(3):243–50.

31. Barbary S, Dap F, Dautel G. Finger replantation: surgical technique and indications. Chir Main. 2013;32(6):363–72.

32. Wood MB. Finger and hand replantation. Surgical technique. Hand Clin. 1992;8(3):397–408.

33. Bieber EJ, Wood MB, Cooney WP, Amadio PC. Thumb avulsion: results of replantation/revascularization. J Hand Surg Am. 1987;12(5 Pt 1):786–90.

34. Nystrom A, Backman C. Replantation of the completely avulsed thumb using long arterial and venous grafts. J Hand Surg Br. 1991;16(4):389–91.

35. Hamilton RB, O'Brien BM, Morrison A, MacLeod AM. Survival factors in replantation and revascularization of the amputated thumb--10 years experience. Scand J Plast Reconstr Surg. 1984;18(2):163–73.

36. Caffee HH. Improved exposure for arterial repair in thumb replantation. J Hand Surg Am. 1985;10(3):416.

37. Van Beek AL, Kutz JE, Zook EG. Importance of the ribbon sign, indicating unsuitability of the vessel, in replanting a finger. Plast Reconstr Surg. 1978;61(1):32–5.

38. Cho MS, Rinker BD, Weber RV, Chao JD, Ingari JV, Brooks D, et al. Functional outcome following nerve repair in the upper extremity using processed nerve allograft. J Hand Surg Am. 2012;37(11):2340–9.

39. Brooks DN, Weber RV, Chao JD, Rinker BD, Zoldos J, Robichaux MR, et al. Processed nerve allografts for peripheral nerve reconstruction: a multicenter study of utilization and outcomes in sensory, mixed, and motor nerve reconstructions. Microsurgery. 2012;32(1):1–14.

40. Rinker BD, Ingari JV, Greenberg JA, Thayer WP, Safa B, Buncke GM. Outcomes of short-gap sensory nerve injuries reconstructed with processed nerve allografts from a multicenter registry study. J Reconstr Microsurg. 2015;31(5):384–90.

41. Wilhelmi BJ, Lee WP, Pagenstert GI, May JW Jr. Replantation in the mutilated hand. Hand Clin. 2003;19(1):89–120.

42. The Hoang N, Hai LH, Staudenmaier R, Hoehnke C. Complete middle forearm amputations after avulsion injuries--microsurgical replantation results in Vietnamese patients. J Trauma. 2009;66(4):1167–72.

43. Kusnezov N, Dunn JC, Stewart J, Mitchell JS, Pirela-Cruz M. Acute limb shortening for major near and complete upper extremity amputations with associated neurovascular injury: a review of the literature. Orthop Surg. 2015;7(4):306–16.

44. Hornez E, Boddaert G, Ngabou UD, Aguir S, Baudoin Y, Mocellin N, et al. Temporary vascular shunt for damage control of extremity vascular injury: a toolbox for trauma surgeons. J Visc Surg. 2015;152(6):363–8.

45. Assouline U, Feuvrier D, Lepage D, Tropet Y, Obert L, Pauchot J. Functional assessment and quality of life in patients following replantation of the distal half of the forearm (except fingers): a review of 11 cases. Hand Surg Rehabil. 2017;36(4):261–7.

46. Dagum AB, Slesarenko Y, Winston L, Tottenham V. Long-term outcome of replantation of proximal-third amputated arm: a worthwhile endeavor. Tech Hand Up Extrem Surg. 2007;11(4):231–5.

Non-microsurgical Soft Tissue Coverage of the Mangled Limb

Alexander Hahn and Ebrahim Paryavi

Introduction

The destructive forces that lead to a mangled extremity can create complex fractures and strip and devitalize the soft tissue envelope. Salvaging the limb often requires osseous reconstruction and soft tissue coverage to provide an environment conducive to fracture healing while preserving or restoring function. Fortunately, there is a spectrum of soft tissue coverage options that vary in complexity and utility.

The "reconstructive ladder" describes tiers, or rungs, of increasingly complex soft tissue coverage options from local wound care, primary closure, skin graft, to local flaps, pedicled flaps, free flaps, or complex allotransplantation [1, 2]. The principle behind the ladder is to use the most simple, clinically appropriate option to provide soft tissue coverage while optimizing function, whether it is simple primary closure or complex microsurgical free flaps. The reconstructive ladder has been modified and revisited several times as technologic advances and new products such as negative pressure wound therapy and dermal matrices are applied to soft tissue management [2, 3].

There is some criticism to using the ladder concept dogmatically and strictly using the simplest technique for wound coverage in every case. Gottlieb coined the term "reconstructive elevator" to describe a more individualized treatment algorithm for a wound [4]. He argues that the surgeon should consider optimal form and function postoperatively for the wound rather than defaulting to the "simplest" technique. This may mean using a flap instead of a split-thickness skin graft to improve function. The hand in particular is an example of where wound coverage is only part of the goal, as mobility, function, sensation are equally important goals of treatment [5].

Whether climbing the "ladder" or taking the "elevator," the treating team must take into account the anatomy of the injury, patient-specific personal factors, and the complexity of the procedure versus risk to the patient [6]. This chapter will focus on the non-microsurgical soft tissue coverage options such as local and regional flaps, fasciocutaneous, muscle, and myocutaneous flaps, which are powerful tools a non-microsurgical trained surgeon can use to provide coverage of a mangled extremity. The lower tiers of wound coverage options such as skin and skin substitute products will not be covered in this chapter, nor will the higher tiers of microsurgical options that require specialized training. The techniques described below are considered "workhorse" flaps for upper and lower extremity

A. Hahn
Orthopaedics, University of Maryland Medical Center, Baltimore, MD, USA

E. Paryavi (✉)
Orthopaedic Surgery, Alaska Native Medical Center, Anchorage, AK, USA

© Springer Nature Switzerland AG 2021
R. A. Pensy, J. V. Ingari (eds.), *The Mangled Extremity*, https://doi.org/10.1007/978-3-319-56648-1_7

coverage, but there are several other options that are beyond the scope of this chapter.

Indications

Non-microsurgical soft tissue coverage techniques are useful for wounds that need more than a split-thickness skin graft, but may not necessarily need a free flap. These techniques are generally indicated for wounds that are unable to close primarily, as well as wounds unlikely to heal by secondary intention. Primary or delayed primary closure works well for clean, easily approximated wound edges that are not under much tension. In the mangled extremity, this scenario is rare as most wounds require multiple procedures to debride and resect devitalized tissue, and the swelling that has occurred by the time of closure usually precludes tension-free closure. Healing by secondary intention is also not an ideal option when tendons, vessels, and/or nerves are exposed. Unfortunately, mangled extremities are subject to wound breakdown leading to exposed internal fixation implants, vasculature, or tendons, which would also be an indication for local or rotational flap coverage.

Patients with mangled extremities are often polytrauma victims that have other injuries that do not allow for a prolonged operative procedure, and in some cases, they may lack healthy donor sites to provide free-flap coverage. In this scenario, non-microsurgical soft tissue coverage can be used to provide a protective environment for large defects or exposed tendons or neurovascular structures to promote healing and reduce the risk of continued infection while sparing the patient from a physiologically demanding and extensive procedure.

Preoperative Workup

A thorough history to obtain the mechanism, timing, and location of injuries is important for appropriately managing a mangled extremity. For example, if the patient is a polytrauma patient requiring other life-saving procedures, communication with the trauma team is important to discuss timing and tolerance of limb surgery [11]. The degree of contamination and mechanism of injury help anticipate the likelihood of salvage versus amputation, as well as provide clues as to how much healthy soft tissue will be available after multiple debridements. The patient's nutrition, smoking, and psychological status are also important factors to consider when planning soft tissue coverage. For example, patients who are poor hosts due to smoking or malnutrition may not be the best candidates for flaps, and psychiatric conditions or social barriers to adequate participation with postoperative restrictions or wound care will impact inpatient as well as outpatient disposition [6]. Physical exam findings with regard to vascular and neurologic status, degree of soft tissue damage, and bone or joint exposure will help dictate type of coverage needed as well as what soft tissue will be available.

Initial radiographs to determine bony injuries should be obtained. Advanced diagnostic imaging studies such as angiography, CT angiography, or ultrasound are useful if the vessels to the planned soft tissue coverage are in question, but these studies are usually optional.

Several objective measures have been described to predict outcomes of attempted limb salvage versus amputation. For example, the Mangled Extremity Severity Score (MESS) was described by Johansen et al. in 1990 to rate lower extremity trauma based on measures of skeletal or soft tissue injury, limb ischemia, shock, and age [12]. They set a cutoff score of 7 as predictive of amputation. However, later studies including LEAP (Lower Extremity Assessment Project) study group data and PROOVIT (PROspective Observational Vascular Injury Treatment) registry data were unable to establish a predictive value of MESS for functional status nor need for amputation [13, 14]. While objective scoring systems are helpful to generally categorize injury severity, the ultimate decision to attempt limb salvage versus amputation should be a team approach that incorporates the input from orthopedic, plastic, and trauma surgical teams as well as patient factors. As the time for operative management of the mangled extremity approaches, backup plans for coverage should be discussed beforehand with all teams, so that the necessary equipment and staff are available.

Wound, Patient, and Timing Considerations

When managing a wound that requires soft tissue coverage, the treating surgeon should consider several factors to decide on the appropriate coverage method and timing. Elevating rotational skin and muscle flaps requires available, non-traumatized local donor options. Ideally, this would be supple, non-edematous tissue in the desired area of flap elevation. Adequate debridement and the treatment of any preexisting infection are mandatory prior to flap coverage. In some situations, the wound dimensions or location may preclude local coverage options. These wounds may be better suited to distant free tissue transfer options.

Patients with significant comorbid conditions who are poor candidates for limb salvage could be a contraindication to soft tissue reconstruction. Furthermore, the patient's financial, social, and emotional circumstances should be taken into consideration when determining coverage options [6]. In a scenario where the patient's injury or their ability to be a good steward of their wounds are compromised, the surgeon should pause and consider other options before moving forward with using complex techniques requiring significant resources.

With regard to the timing of soft tissue coverage, factors such as amount of contamination, amount of swelling, and availability of a microsurgical team are all part of determining when to cover a wound. Repeating debridements until a wound was culture negative before definitive coverage in open tibia fractures was shown to have low rates of deep infection [7]. Even with institution of an ortho-specific microsurgery team, coverage of open fractures can be delayed by several days, although no statistically significant difference was seen between early (<7 days) and late coverage [8]. Delaying coverage and elevating the traumatized limb until swelling is reduced and tissue equilibrium is achieved decreases the technical difficulty of dissecting

tissue planes and also reduces vessel friability. A German study showed a low rate of flap complications in retrospectively reviewed cases of delayed (>3 days) soft tissue reconstruction of open extremity fractures [9]. However, there is also opinion that exposed structures, especially in the upper extremity, should be covered as soon as possible, or less than 72 hours, if feasible [10].

Non-microsurgical Soft Tissue Coverage Options

Local Flaps

Local skin flaps provide subcutaneous fat and skin coverage of wound defects. This option can provide sensate tissue over the wound, but local flaps depend on available nearby lax soft tissue. If the local manipulation of skin and fat causes too much tension, it may necessitate skin grafting the donor site. Options such as Z-plasty or rhomboid (Limberg) flap are commonly used methods to cover small wounds [15, 16]. In general, mangled extremities have defects too large to be adequately covered using these methods, but if the wound is appropriate, local, random pattern transposition flaps are straightforward and useful coverage options.

Case: A 38-year-old male with a history of right brachial artery pseudoaneurysm and forearm abscess treated with brachial artery reconstruction, irrigation, and debridement who presented with a non-healing wound at initial follow-up. The non-healing portion was excised, and a local flap was raised to cover the defect (Fig. 7.1). Split-thickness skin grafting was applied to the donor site.

Fascial and Fasciocutaneous

Local skin flaps with underlying fascia attached are helpful in staged reconstructions. Compared to myocutaneous flaps, they are less scarred and fibrotic when they heal, providing functional and cosmetic benefits. Theoretically, decreased scarring allows structures such as tendons and neurovascular structures to glide underneath the flap.

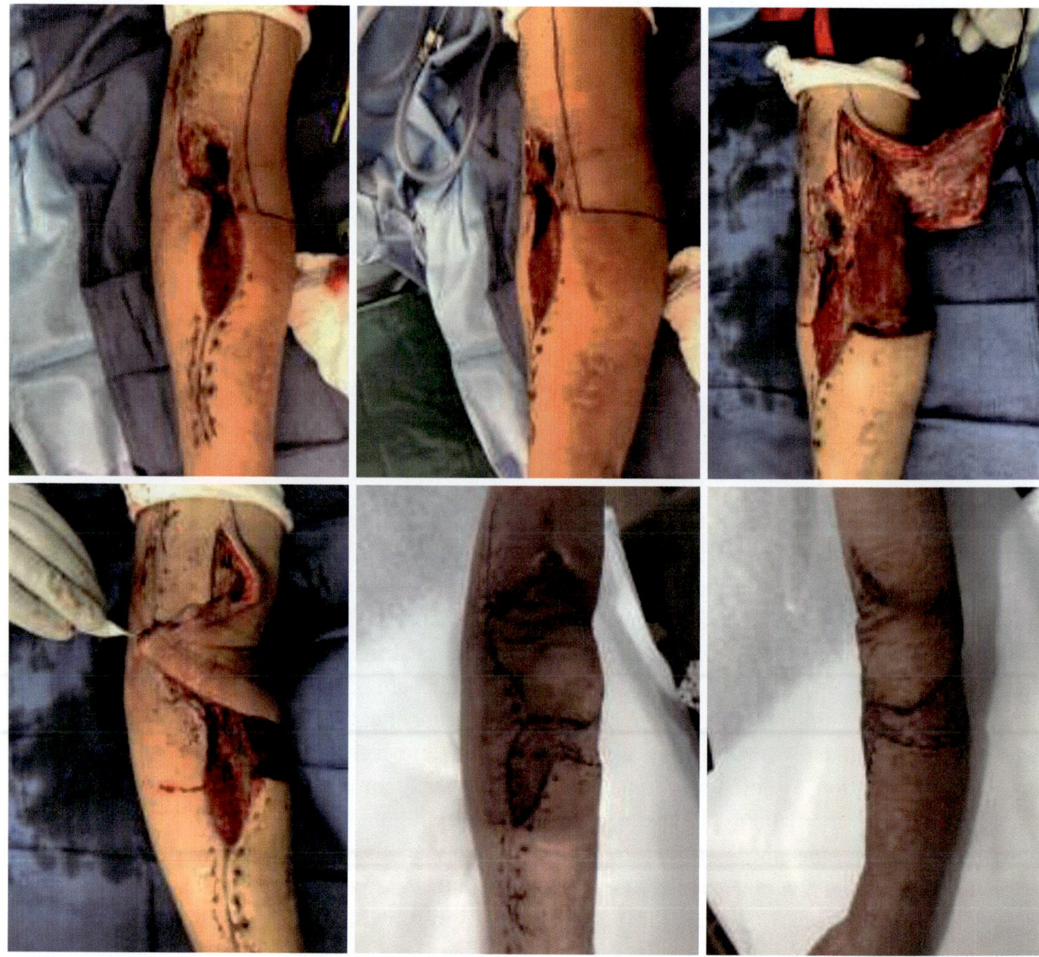

Fig. 7.1 Non-healing over antecubital fossa covered with local flap intraoperatively and at 2-week follow-up

These flaps also tend to have better cosmetic outcomes than myocutaneous flaps due to their decreased relative bulk if they are transferred as fascia-only flaps. Wound healing is thought to be promoted by restoration of venous and lymphatic circulation.

Radial Forearm

The radial forearm flap is a versatile option for covering defects of the distal upper extremity given that it can be used both as a free and pedicled flap. It is a radial artery-based flap with sensation provided through the medial and lateral antebrachial cutaneous nerves. It can be used as an antegrade or reversed flow flap depending on the location of the defect to be covered.

Preoperatively, an Allen test is mandatory to assess for any pathologic results to avoid ischemia to the hand. The radial artery course is marked out and the amount of coverage needed is templated out, centered over the radial artery. This should be planned with consideration of the axis around which the flap will pivot.

The flap should be harvested from distal and ulnar to proximal and radial. The dissection can be carried out in either a sub- or supra-fascial manner, depending on the need. During dissection, the paratenon of the flexor carpi radialis tendon should be preserved. Once the intermuscular septum is encountered, perforators to the bone are carefully taken down, while perforators to the skin are preserved. The artery should be separated from the surrounding tissue until the flap is free enough to either rotate or tunnel. The donor site can be closed primarily if the defect is small; however, this site often requires a separate full- or split-thickness skin graft [17].

Lateral Arm Flap

The lateral arm flap is taken from the lower lateral aspect of the arm above the epicondyle. This flap is based on the posterior radial collateral artery with sensation from the lateral brachial cutaneous nerve and can provide a fairly substantial amount of tissue when elevated as an extended flap [18–20]. The extended lateral arm flap is useful as an axial transposition flap for posterior elbow and olecranon wound coverage [21].

The desired flap is outlined, the anterior incision is made first, the fascia of the brachialis and brachioradialis muscles is elevated, and the radial nerve is identified in the interval and can be protected. The posterior incision can then be made, elevating triceps fascia, and the flap is then elevated from a distal to proximal direction, essentially subperiosteally off of the lateral humeral ridge in order to include the pedicle that runs with the lateral intermuscular septum. There are several perforators within the septum that are preserved by elevating in this manner, ensuring perfusion of the skin island. Once the flap is raised, it can be rotated, or tunneled as an island flap [22].

Case: A 76-year-old female with history of open reduction internal fixation of right distal humerus fracture with a wound dehiscence about her elbow. A lateral arm flap was used to cover the bony prominence, with split-thickness skin grafting of the donor site (Fig. 7.2). She went on to healing at follow-up.

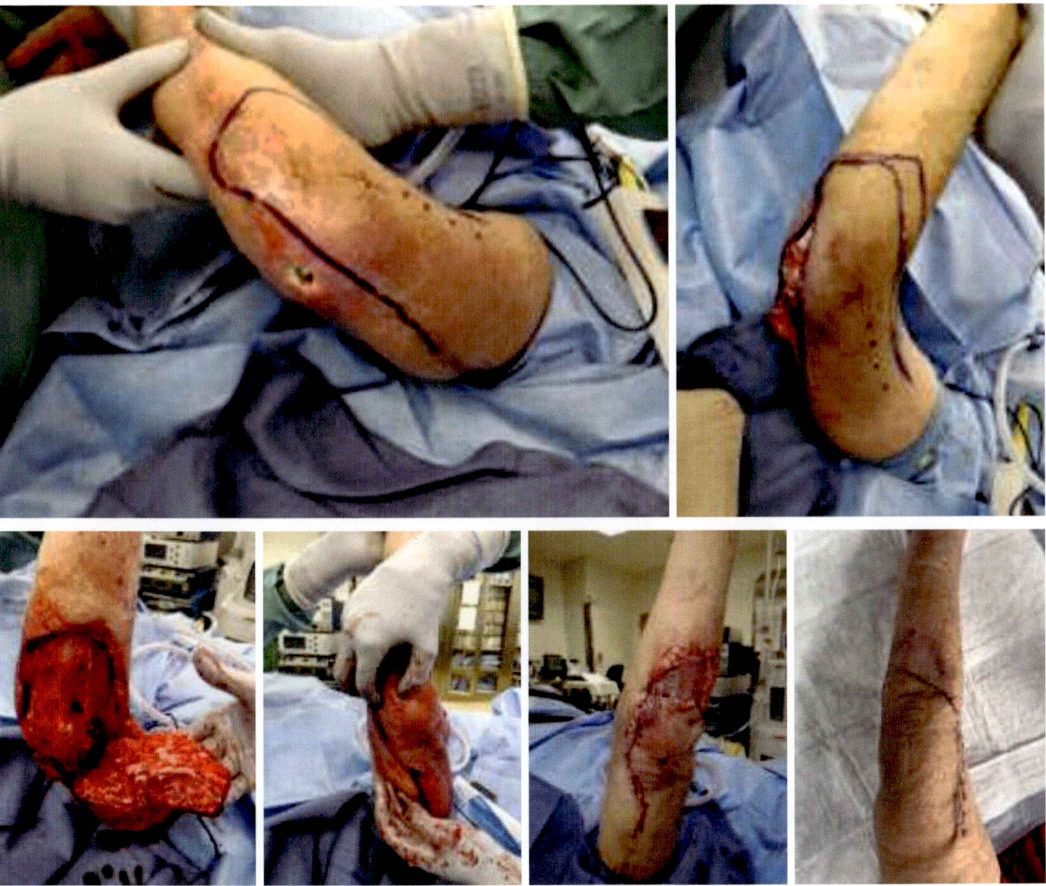

Fig. 7.2 Lateral arm flap used to cover exposed hardware as well as the bony prominence of the olecranon

Groin Flap

The groin flap is a technique described in 1972 by McGregor and Jackson to provide coverage of upper extremity traumatic soft tissue defects [23]. This flap is based on the superficial circumflex artery and provides a large surface area to work with. The flap is raised starting from lateral to medial including the fascia lata medial to the anterior superior iliac spine terminating at the medial border of the sartorius muscle [24]. When planning the outline of the flap, an additional 2–3 cm can be added to the length for some mobility [25]. Once the flap is mobilized, coverage is obtained, and the unused portion is tubed. Although this method provides reliable soft tissue coverage, patients treated with this technique are subjected to a period of bed rest, and the grafted limb is immobilized until the second stage of detachment. In a polytrauma patient that remains intubated or sedated, this may not be of much consequence. However, the patient with an isolated mangled extremity may experience some discomfort with their positional and activity restrictions.

Case: A 26-year-old male sustained a ballistic injury to his hand during a home invasion. He required acute internal fixation as well as a groin flap (Fig. 7.3). After detachment, he went on to full healing and retained some intrinsic hand motion.

Propeller Flap

The pedicled propeller flap can be useful in the lower extremity, especially in the distal third of the limb where the thin soft tissue envelope can leave bone, tendon, and neurovascular structures exposed after trauma [26]. Proximally, there is a thicker soft tissue envelope, and perforator vessels arise from the posterior tibial artery, anterior tibial artery, and the peroneal artery. Flaps can be raised from any of these vessels, and a single perforator can perfuse a fairly large surface area [27].

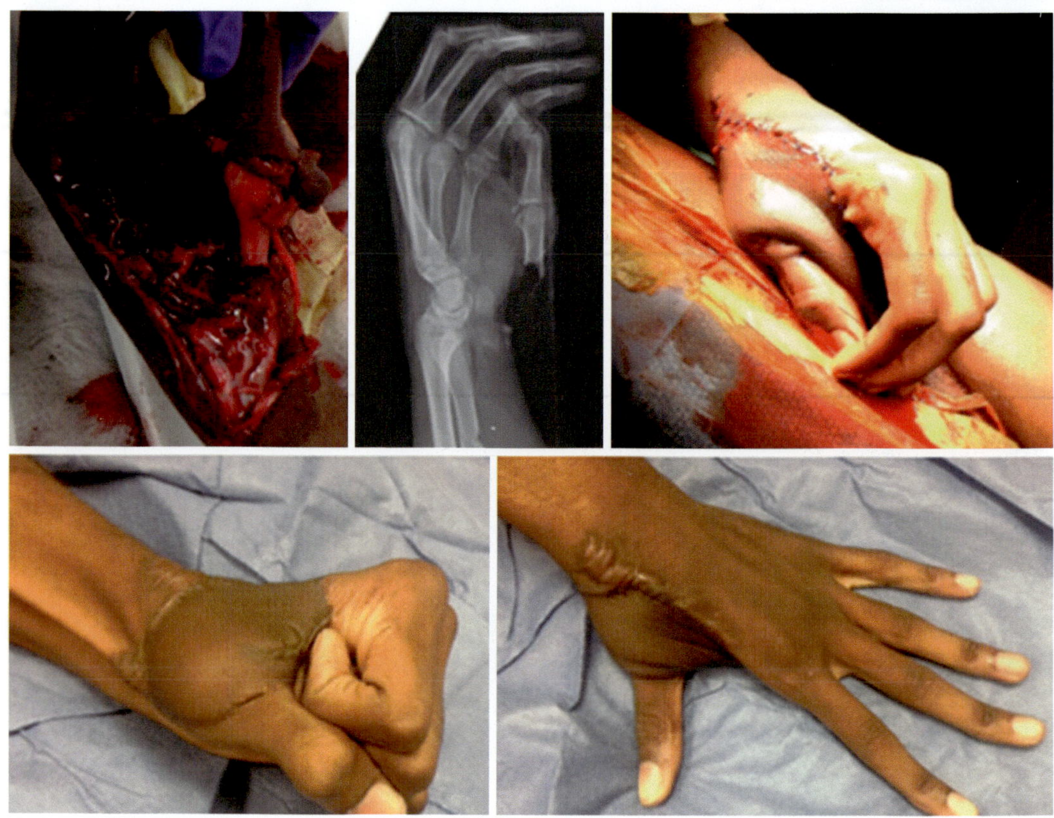

Fig. 7.3 Ballistic injury to hand requiring internal fixation and soft tissue coverage with a groin flap acutely. (Pictures courtesy of Raymond Pensy, MD)

Perforator arteries are first detected using a handheld ultrasound Doppler and marked out. The outline of the flap is then planned to provide adequate length and coverage. Subfascial dissection is carried out to directly visualize the perforator vessel around which the flap will rotate. The perforator branch is then isolated and dissected free to allow for appropriate rotation. Once the flap is mobilized to cover the defect, perfusion is carefully checked and verified before the flap is closed over drains [26–28].

Case: A 40-year-old male with open distal tibia fracture requiring open reduction internal fixation with a soft tissue defect that required a propeller flap for coverage (Fig. 7.4).

Reverse Sural Artery Pedicle Flap

Reverse sural artery pedicle flap is a peroneal artery-based flap that can be used for fasciocutaneous coverage of the lower leg and foot. It is a useful flap due to its reliable blood supply that does not need to be sacrificed, as well as its fairly straightforward dissection with generally low blood loss. It is extremely useful for distal lower extremity coverage with demonstrated success in blast victims [29]. It does have a reputation for high rate of venous congestion, but a wide pedicle width can enhance venous drainage and reduce this risk [30].

The patient is placed in a prone or lateral decubitus position. After the flap is traced out, the incision is made distal to proximal. The sural nerve and the short saphenous vein should be kept together and preserved with the flap. Perforators are identified 5–10 cm proximal to the tip of the lateral malleolus. The sural nerve can be transected and ligated proximally to mobilize the flap. The flap should be attached with minimal tension with anchoring sutures. The donor sites may be able to be closed primarily depending on the size, but some may require split-thickness skin grafts [29, 31].

Case: A 53-year-old male with wound breakdown after Achilles tendon repair. After multiple debridements, the wound was ready for coverage (Fig. 7.5). After measuring and planning, a reverse sural artery flap was raised and rotated to

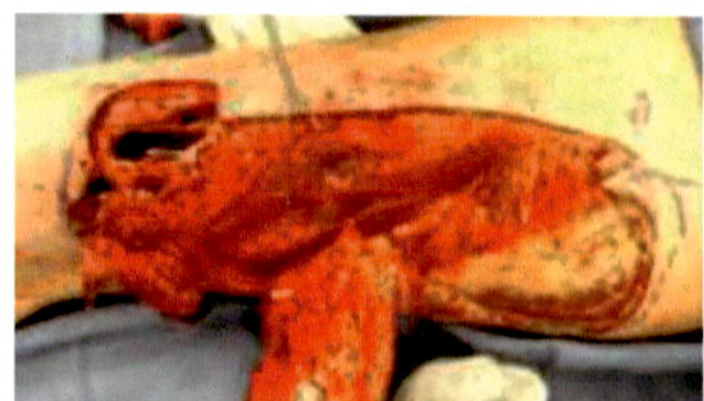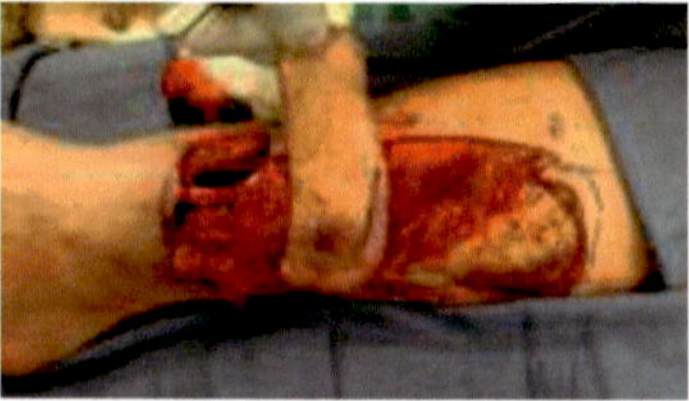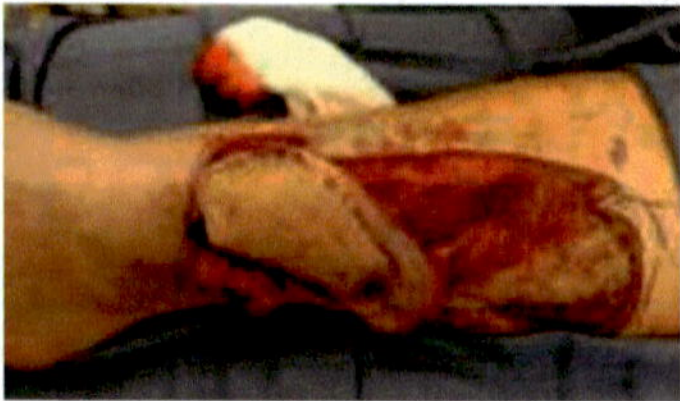

Fig. 7.4 Exposed hardware and soft tissue defect in distal lower extremity requiring a propeller flap with demonstration of rotation of the flap. (Pictures courtesy of Raymond Pensy, MD)

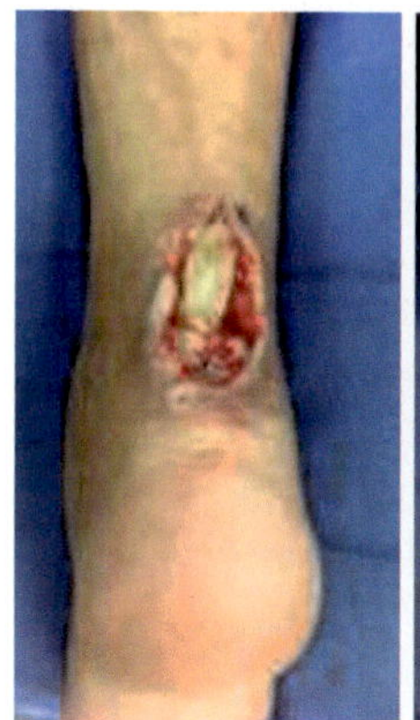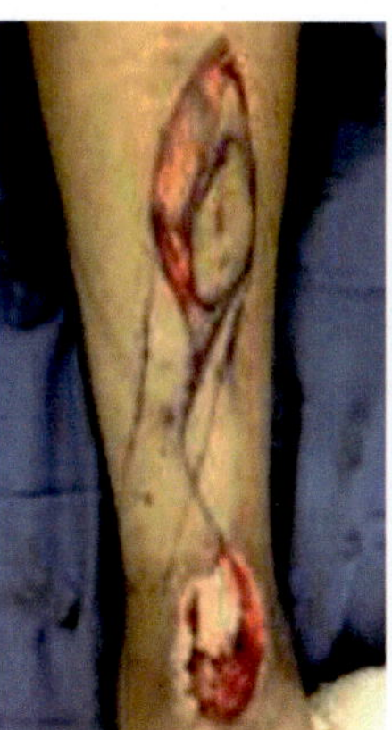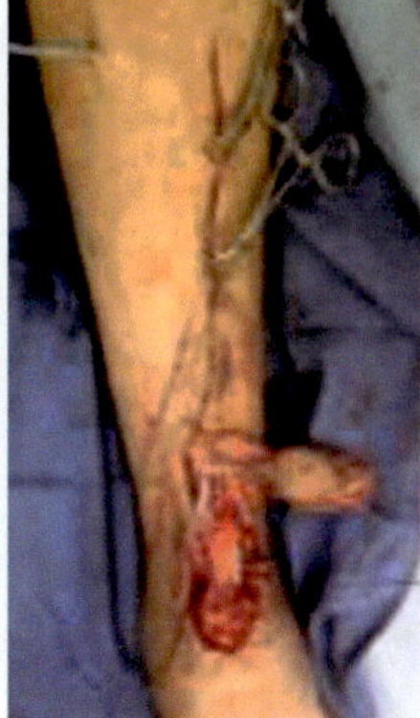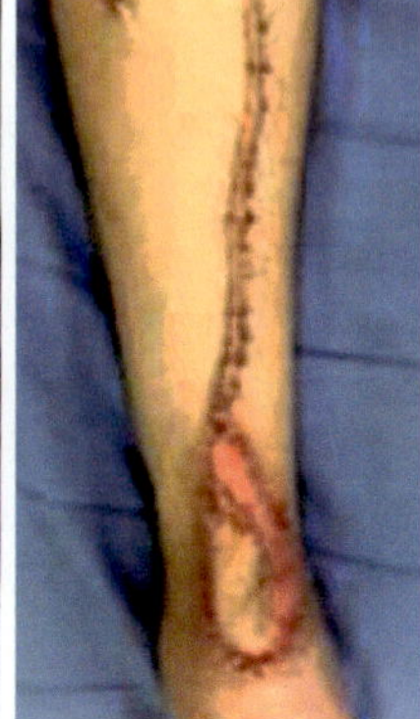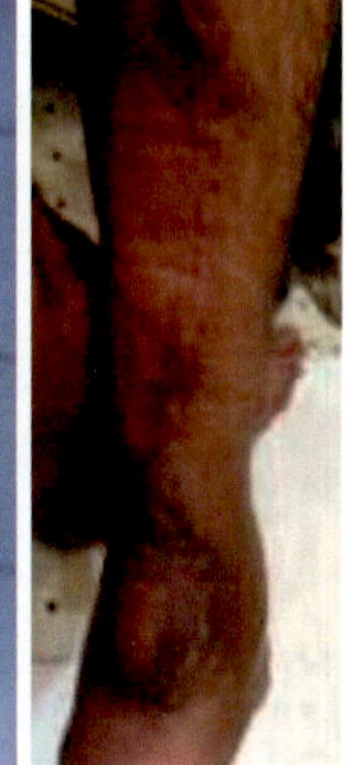

Fig. 7.5 Posterior lower leg wound breakdown with exposed tendon treated with reverse sural artery flap and split-thickness skin graft that went on to subsequent healing. (Pictures courtesy of Sam Fuller, MD)

cover the defect. The donor site was closed primarily, and the remaining exposed skin was covered with split-thickness skin graft. (Case and pictures courtesy of Dr. Sam Fuller)

Muscular and Myocutaneous

Myocutaneous or pedicled muscular flaps can be used in cases of underlying osteomyelitis, areas where there are large defects from debridement, or in wounds that were grossly contaminated. The increased bulk of muscle flaps may be cosmetically displeasing in areas with previously thin soft tissue coverage; however, in regions with deeper, larger defects, the increased bulk of the flap can help fill these spaces in. These flaps do incur a fairly large donor site morbidity and may result in compromised function in the donor region.

Flexor Carpi Ulnaris (FCU) Flap

The FCU flap is a useful and reliable option for posterior elbow coverage where lack of muscle and other subcutaneous tissue predisposes this area to coverage issues [32]. The FCU muscle belly receives its blood supply from the ulnar artery and the posterior ulnar recurrent artery, with ulnar nerve innervation. The flap provides approximately 4 cm of coverage [32–34]. The FCU is also bipennate, which can reduce donor morbidity if it is split rather than taken in whole, although this is rarely indicated in our practice. This muscle can also be harvested as a myocutaneous flap with an overlying skin paddle centered over the muscle belly at the junction between the distal two thirds of the forearm. The dominant perforators enter the muscle at this level and do not need to be visualized or specifically isolated.

The flap is raised from distal to proximal along the posterior ulnar border from the pisiform. The FCU muscle is then elevated similarly from distal to proximal with ligation of minor perforators. The dominant pedicle enters approx-imately 6 cm distal from the olecranon tip and should be isolated with careful dissection to allow for mobilization. Flap stabilization and wound closure should be done with the elbow at 90° to assess the tension on the flap with elbow flexion [33].

Case: A 50-year-old female with history of open reduction internal fixation of the ulna with a wound dehiscence. A FCU flap was used to cover the defect, and healing was seen upon follow-up (Fig. 7.6).

Gastrocnemius Flap

The gastrocnemius flap is a pedicled muscular soft tissue coverage option for the upper third of the leg that has been used frequently for defects about the knee (Fig. 7.7). This rotational flap provides a good bulk of tissue with excursion that can be used to cover defects after a mangled extremity or in the sequelae thereafter if there is chronic osteomyelitis or exposed hardware. The medial and lateral heads of the gastrocnemius are supplied, respectively, by the medial sural and lateral sural artery branches of the popliteal artery [35].

For a medial gastrocnemius flap, the incision is made on the medial aspect of the leg from the medial tibia posterior to the pes anserine tendons proximally to about 10 cm above the ankle [35]. The superficial posterior compartment fascia is released, and the medial gastrocnemius is isolated from the lateral head and from the soleus. The muscle is transected distally. Dissection can then proceed proximally to free the attachment to the medial femoral condyle. The muscle flap can then be tunneled or rotated over to cover the defect. The skin is closed over drains. The defect covered by the gastrocnemius will require a split-thickness skin graft or synthetic equivalent.

The lateral gastrocnemius flap is harvested with an incision on the lateral aspect of the leg about 2 cm posterior to the fibular head and parallel with the shaft [35]. Neurovascular structures are carefully dissected, and the small saphenous

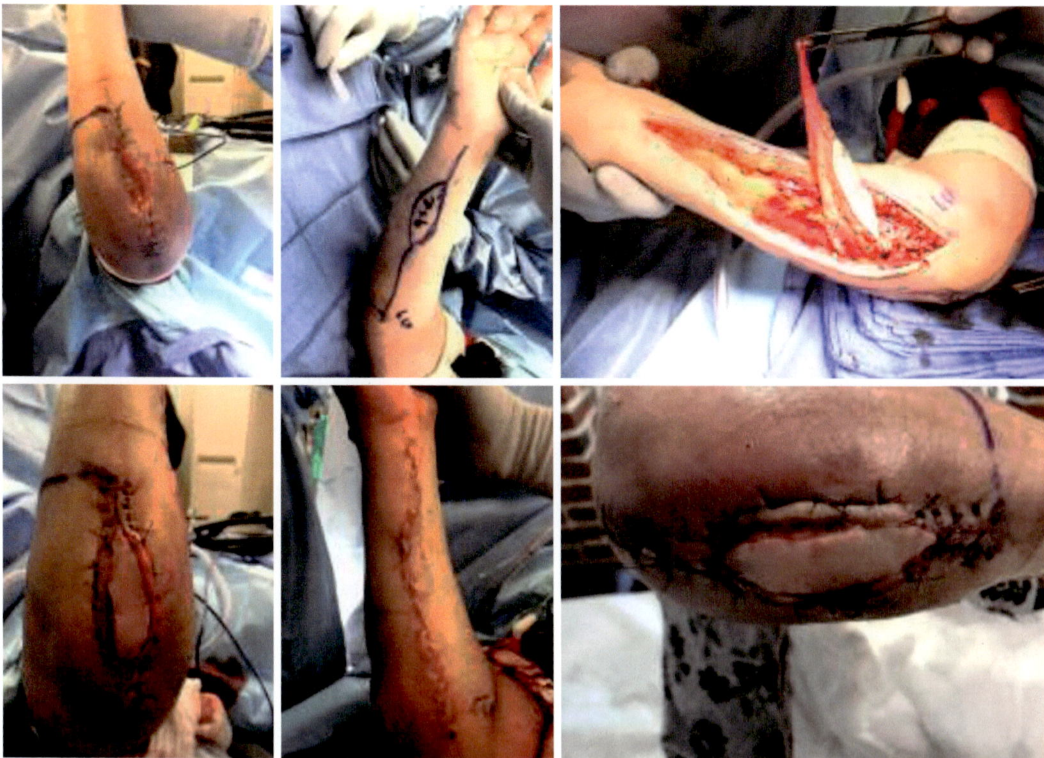

Fig. 7.6 Wound dehiscence with FCU flap planned, raised, and tunneled to the defect with primary closure of the donor site. (Pictures courtesy of Ebrahim Paryavi, MD)

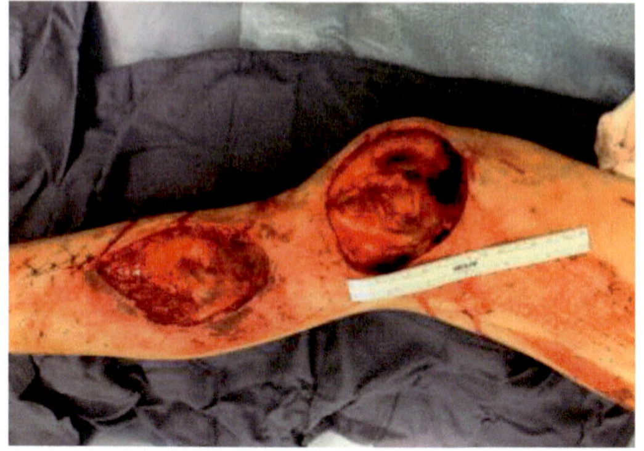

Fig. 7.7 A 25-year-old male with significant road rash and soft tissue defects after motorcycle accident, amenable to a lateral gastrocnemius flap. (Picture courtesy of Ebrahim Paryavi, MD)

vein and sural nerve can be used to identify the median raphe [36]. The muscle belly should be bluntly dissected as in the medial flap away from the soleus and transected distally once freed. The flap can be tunneled and rotated as needed.

Latissimus Dorsi Flap

The latissimus dorsi flap is a pedicled muscular or myocutaneous flap that can provide a large area of soft tissue coverage for the upper extremity. Its primary blood supply is the thoracodorsal artery, but it also has secondary blood supply from perforators [37]. The muscle is innervated by the thoracodorsal nerve, and if necessary, the flap can be used as a functional muscle tendon transfer. If soft tissue coverage is the only need, the muscle can be denervated to allow for atrophy and less bulk.

Graft harvest is done with the patient in the lateral decubitus position with a wide area prepped out. If the flap is to be used as a myocutaneous flap, this should be incorporated into the planned incision. The flap should be raised from distal to proximal to approach the pedicle, which should be 10–12 cm from the axilla [37]. The pedicle is isolated, and the muscle is elevated before tunneling or rotating to the defect.

Case: A 23-year-old landscaper status post lawn mower rollover accident sustained heavily contaminated open scapular acromion and glenoid fractures (Fig. 7.8a, b). He was treated with debridement and open reduction internal fixation (Fig. 7.8c, d) and underwent a flap on the first postoperative day with a good outcome (Fig. 7.8e–g).

Conclusion

Each mangled extremity case will provide unique challenges and opportunities for management. There is no one-technique or one-flap-fits-all when managing open wounds. The condition of the wound as well as the condition of the patient will help guide coverage options. In situations where primary closure or microsurgical techniques are not possible, there are several flap options that do not require microsurgical training. When used appropriately, these non-microsurgical flaps are valuable tools for any surgeon that manages mangled extremities. However, they should be planned out carefully and used appropriately to achieve the goal of reliable coverage and optimal function postoperatively.

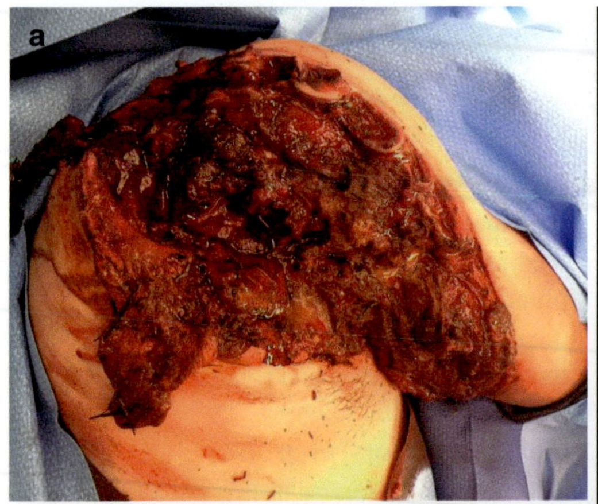
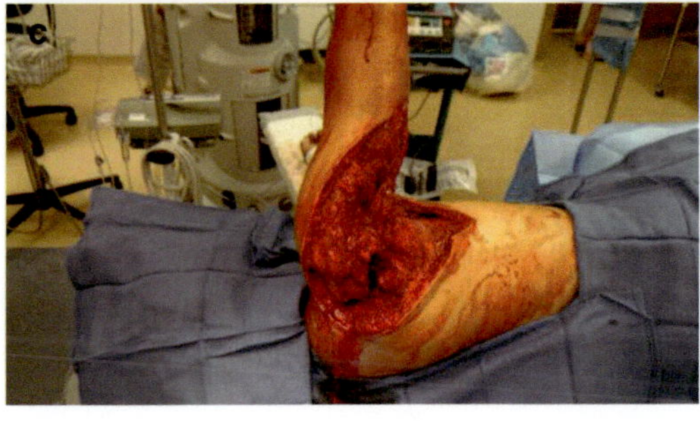
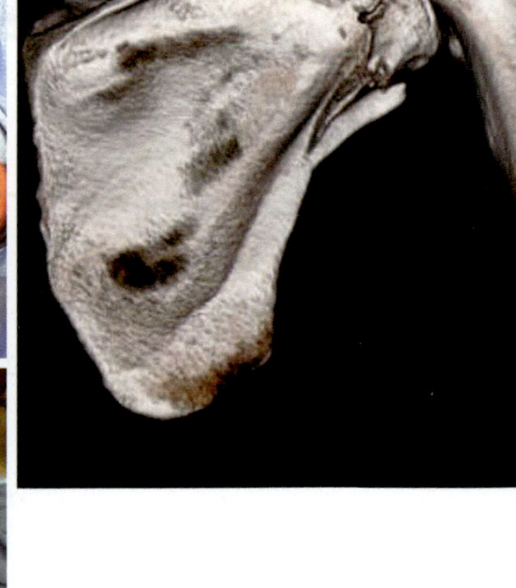

Fig. 7.8 (**a**) Clinical photograph on presentation demonstrating significant contamination and devitalized tissue. (**b**) 3D CT reconstruction. (**c**, **d**) Debridement followed by fixation (same day). Debridement was completed followed by re-prep, re-drape, new back table and fresh instruments, and new gowns for all operative staff prior to fixation at same setting. (**e**) Pedicled latissimus flap POD#1 to achieve soft tissue coverage, anchoring latissimus to scapula and remnants of supra- and infraspinatus tendons for additional abduction/external rotation strength. (**f**, **g**) Final follow-up clinical photos. (**a–g** Courtesy of Raymond Pensy, MD)

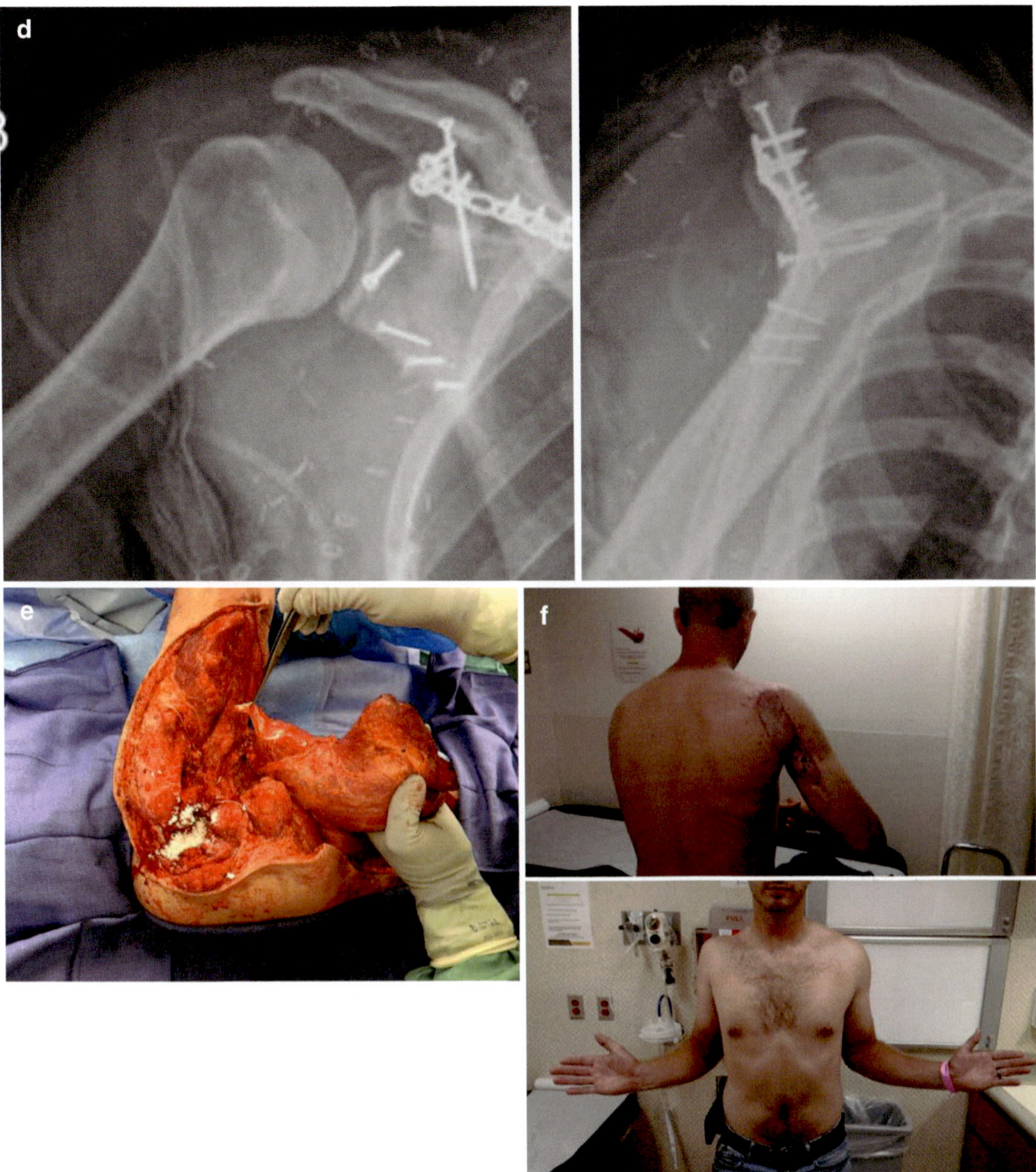

Fig. 7.8 (continued)

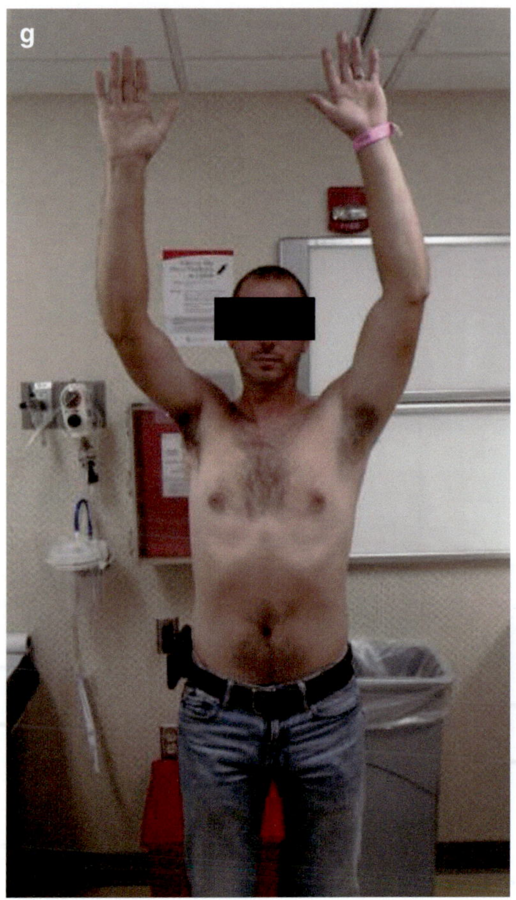

Fig. 7.8 (continued)

References

1. Tintle SM, Levin LS. The reconstructive micro-surgery ladder in orthopaedics. Injury [Internet]. 2013;44(3):376–385. Available from: https://doi.org/10.1016/j.injury.2013.01.006.
2. Fleming ME, O'Daniel A, Bharmal H, et al. Application of the orthoplastic reconstructive ladder to preserve lower extremity amputation length. Ann Plast Surg. 2014;73(2):183–9.
3. Janis JE, Kwon RK, Attinger CE. The new reconstructive ladder: modifications to the traditional model. Plast Reconstr Surg. 2011;127((Suppl 1 S):205–12.
4. Gottlieb LJ, Krieger LM. From the reconstructive ladder to the reconstructive elevator. Plast Reconstr Surg [Internet]. 1994;93(7):1503–4, [cited 11 Aug 2018]. Available from: http://www.ncbi.nlm.nih.gov/pubmed/7661898.
5. Miller EA, Friedrich J. Soft tissue coverage of the hand and upper extremity: the reconstructive elevator. J Hand Surg Am [Internet]. 2016;41(7):782–92. Available from: https://doi.org/10.1016/j.jhsa.2016.04.020.
6. Sandberg LJM. The plastic surgery compass. Plast Reconstr Surg – Glob Open [Internet]. 2016;4(9):e1035. Available from: http://insights.ovid.com/crossref?an=01720096-201609000-00025.
7. Lenarz CJ, Watson JT, Moed BR, et al. Timing of wound closure in open fractures based on cultures obtained after debridement. J Bone Jt Surg A. 2010;92(10):1921–6.
8. Vandenberg J, Osei D, Boyer MI, et al. Open tibia shaft fractures and soft-tissue coverage: The effects of management by an orthopaedic microsurgical team. J Orthop Trauma. 2017;31(6):339–44.
9. Steiert AE, Gohritz A, Schreiber TC, et al. Delayed flap coverage of open extremity fractures after previous vacuum-assisted closure (VAC®) therapy – worse or worth? J Plast Reconstr Aesthetic Surg [Internet]. 2009;62(5):675–83. Available from: https://doi.org/10.1016/j.bjps.2007.09.041.
10. Bumbasirevic M, Stevanovic M, Lesic A, et al. Current management of the mangled upper extremity. Int Orthop. 2012;36(11):2189–95.
11. Prasarn ML, Helfet DL, Kloen P. Management of the mangled extremity. Strategies Trauma Limb Reconstr. 2012;7:57.
12. Johansen K, Daines M, Howey T, Helfet DHSJ. Objective criteria accurately predict amputation following lower extremity trauma. J Trauma. 1990;30(5):568–72.
13. Loja MN, Sammann A, DuBose J, et al. The mangled extremity score and amputation: time for a revision. J Trauma Acute Care Surg. 2017;82(3):518–23.
14. Ly TV, Travison TG, Castillo RC, et al. Ability of lower-extremity injury severity scores to predict functional outcome after limb salvage. J Bone Jt Surgery Am [Internet]. 2008;90(8):1738–43. Available from: http://content.wkhealth.com/linkback/openurl?sid=WKPTLP:landingpage&an=00004623-200808000-00017
15. Hudson DA. Some thoughts on choosing a Z-plasty: the Z made simple. Plast Reconstr Surg [Internet]. 2000;106(3):665–71. Available from: http://content.wkhealth.com/linkback/openurl?sid=WKPTLP:landingpage%7B&%7Dan=00006534-200009030-00024
16. Chasmar LR. The versatile rhomboid (Limberg) flap. Can J Plast Surg [Internet]. 2007;15(2):67–71. Available from: http://www.ncbi.nlm.nih.gov/pubmed/19554188, http://www.pubmedcentral.nih.gov/articlerender.fcgi?artid=PMC2698804
17. Megerle K, Sauerbier M, Germann G. The evolution of the pedicled radial forearm flap. Hand. 2010;5(1):37–42.
18. Lanzetta M, Bernier M, Chollet A, et al. The lateral forearm flap: an anatomic study. Plast Reconstr Surg [Internet]. 1997;99(2):460–4, [cited 24 Mar 2018]. Available from: http://www.ncbi.nlm.nih.gov/pubmed/9030155.
19. Wettstein R, Helmy N, Kalbermatten DF. Defect reconstruction over the olecranon with the distally

extended lateral arm flap. J Plast Reconstr Aesthetic Surg [Internet]. 2014;(8):67, 1125–1128. Available from: https://doi.org/10.1016/j.bjps.2014.04.036.

20. Kelley BP, Chung KC. Soft-tissue coverage for elbow trauma. Hand Clin [Internet]. 2015;31(4):693–703, [cited 2018 Mar 24]. Available from: http://www.ncbi.nlm.nih.gov/pubmed/26498556.

21. Mears SC, Zadnik MB, Eglseder WA. Salvage of functional elbow range of motion in complex open injuries using a sensate transposition lateral arm flap. Plast Reconstr Surg [Internet]. 2004;113(2):531–5, [cited 20 May 2018]. Available from: https://insights.ovid.com/crossref?an=00006534-200402000-00009.

22. Prantl L, Schreml S, Schwarze H, et al. A safe and simple technique using the distal pedicled reversed upper arm flap to cover large elbow defects. J Plast Reconstr Aesthetic Surg. 2008;61(5):546–51.

23. McGregor IA, Jackson IT. The groin flap. Br J Plast Surg [Internet]. 1972;25(1):3–16, [cited 24 Mar 2018]. Available from: http://www.ncbi.nlm.nih.gov/pubmed/4550433.

24. Knutson GH. The groin flap: a new technique to repair traumatic tissue defects. Can Med Assoc J [Internet]. 1977;116(6):623–5. Available from: http://www.pubmedcentral.nih.gov/articlerender.fcgi?artid=1879168&tool=pmcentrez&rendertype=abstract.

25. Bajantri B, Latheef L, Sabapathy SR. Tips to orient pedicled groin flap for hand defects. Tech Hand Up Extrem Surg. 2013;17(2):68–71.

26. Jakubietz RG, Jakubietz MG, Gruenert JG, et al. The 180-degree perforator-based propeller flap for soft tissue coverage of the distal, lower extremity: a new method to achieve reliable coverage of the distal lower extremity with a local, fasciocutaneous perforator flap. Ann Plast Surg. 2007;59(6):667–71.

27. Tos P, Innocenti M, Artiaco S, et al. Perforator-based propeller flaps treating loss of substance in the lower limb. J Orthop Traumatol. 2011;12(2):93–9.

28. Pignatti M, Pasqualini M, Governa M, et al. Propeller flaps for leg reconstruction. J Plast Reconstr Aesthetic Surg. 2008;61(7):777–83.

29. Orr J, Kirk KL, Antunez V, et al. Reverse sural artery flap for reconstruction of blast injuries of the foot and ankle. Foot Ankle Int [Internet]. 2010;31(1):59–64. Available from: https://doi.org/10.3113/FAI.2010.0059.

30. Sugg KB, Schaub TA, Concannon MJ, et al. The reverse superficial sural artery flap revisited for complex lower extremity and foot reconstruction. Plast Reconstr Surg – Glob Open [Internet]. 2015;3(9):e519. Available from: http://content.wkhealth.com/linkback/openurl?sid=WKPTLP:landingpage&an=01720096-201509000-00009.

31. Finkemeier CG, Neiman R. Reverse sural artery pedicle flap. J Orthop Trauma [Internet]. 2016;30(Suppl 2):S41–2, [cited 24 Mar 2018]. Available from: http://content.wkhealth.com/linkback/openurl?sid=WKPTLP:landingpage&an=00005131-201608001-00020.

32. Wysocki RW, Gray RL, Fernandez JJ, et al. Posterior elbow coverage using whole and split flexor carpi ulnaris flaps: a cadaveric study. J Hand Surg Am [Internet]. 2008;33(10):1807–12. Available from: https://doi.org/10.1016/j.jhsa.2008.08.019.

33. Bayne CO, Slikker W, Ma J, et al. Clinical outcomes of the flexor carpi ulnaris turnover flap for posterior elbow soft tissue defects. J Hand Surg Am [Internet]. 2015;40(12):2358–63. Available from: https://doi.org/10.1016/j.jhsa.2015.09.004.

34. Andre A, Bonnevialle N, Grolleau J-L, et al. Soft-tissue coverage of olecranon with musculocutaneous flexor carpi ulnaris flap. Orthop Traumatol Surg Res [Internet]. 2014;100(8):963–6. Available from: http://www.ncbi.nlm.nih.gov/pubmed/25459453.

35. Walton Z, Armstrong M, Traven S, et al. Pedicled rotational medial and lateral gastrocnemius flaps: surgical technique. J Am Acad Orthop Surg. 2017;25(11):744–51.

36. Boopalan PRJVC, Nithyananth M, Jepegnanam TS. Lateral gastrocnemius flap cover for distal thigh soft tissue loss. J Trauma [Internet]. 2010;69(5):E38–41, [cited 2018 May 2018]. Available from: https://insights.ovid.com/crossref?an=00005373-201011000-00053.

37. Pierce TD, Tomaino MM. Use of the pedicled latissimus muscle flap for upper-extremity reconstruction. J Am Acad Orthop Surg. 2000;8(5):324–31.

ing teams for microsurgical reconstruction of the mangled upper or lower limb.

By definition the mangled limb results in major trauma to three of the four tissue types (skin, bone, arteries, and nerves). Open fractures and soft tissue defects necessitate coordinated care to achieve bony union, guard against infection, and maximize functional outcome. In the late 1950s, the Arbeitsgemeinschaft für Osteosynthesefragen group (AO) developed four basic principles for surgical treatment of fractures. These include:

1. Anatomic reduction
2. Stable internal fixation
3. Preservation of blood supply with careful attention to soft tissue handling
4. Functional rehabilitation of the injured limb

The development of these principles emphasized the importance of soft tissue and has led to the awareness that successful management of major orthopedic trauma is inseparable from successful management of the soft tissue envelope. It is imperative that both the orthopedic surgeon and the reconstructive plastic surgeon be familiar with the needs and approaches of the other to optimize a functional outcome for the patient. In the senior author's (L.S.L.) opinion, the two disciplines are so critically intertwined in the management of the mangled extremity that an "orthoplastic" approach is paramount for functional limb salvage [14–16]. Valuing the respective roles of the orthopedic and plastic surgeon in mangled limb reconstruction is crucial for successful management of these complex cases [14–16].

An orthoplastic approach to limb salvage is a modernization of the century-old concept of the reconstructive "ladder" in assessing wounds and selecting appropriate closure. During World War I, with the influx of battlefield extremity trauma in Europe, Sir Harold Gillies introduced the concept of replacing "like with like." The reconstructive ladder for wound closure ranges from simple procedures at the bottom rungs (primary closure, secondary closure, skin grafts) to more complex procedures (local flaps, regional flaps, and free tissue transfer) depending on the soft tissue coverage needs of the patient [17]. This principle has

been used as a framework for wound coverage by plastic surgeons for decades. However, with the advances in microsurgery, this framework can be modernized to describe a "microsurgery reconstructive ladder" for the mangled limb (Fig. 8.1a) [15]. At the lowest rung of this ladder, basic microsurgical techniques apply, progressing to the most complex microsurgical reconstructions at the top rung. The ladder progresses, therefore, from simple direct microvascular and neural repairs to interpositional nerve and vein grafts, nerve transfers, replantation, free tissue transfer, composite tissue transfer, functioning muscle transfers, toe to hand transfers, perforator flaps, prefabricated flaps, pre-expanded flaps, and finally vascularized composite allotransplantation (Fig. 8.1). All of these techniques are available to the modern reconstructive surgeon and have taken their place in the management of mangled limb reconstruction over the past few decades [14–16, 18]. Since the lower rungs on this ladder do not necessarily have to be utilized to ascend to higher rungs, perhaps the concept of a "microsurgical reconstructive elevator" is more appropriate (Fig. 8.1b).

In this chapter, we review the multifaceted requirements for successful microsurgical soft tissue reconstruction of the mangled limb—from the trauma center facilities and staff, patient factors, principles of free flap selection, and pre- and postoperative management. Adequate microsurgery facilities, an experienced multidisciplinary surgical team, a clear preoperative strategy, postoperative monitoring protocols, and a rehabilitation plan are all paramount for success.

Indications for Microsurgical Reconstruction

Using the microsurgical reconstructive ladder or elevator as a framework, the indications for local versus free flap coverage in the upper or lower mangled extremity can be defined. The definitive reconstructive plan will depend on the zone of injury, the blood supply to the extremity, the surgeon's capability and resources, and the patient's underlying clinical status. A local flap is preferred

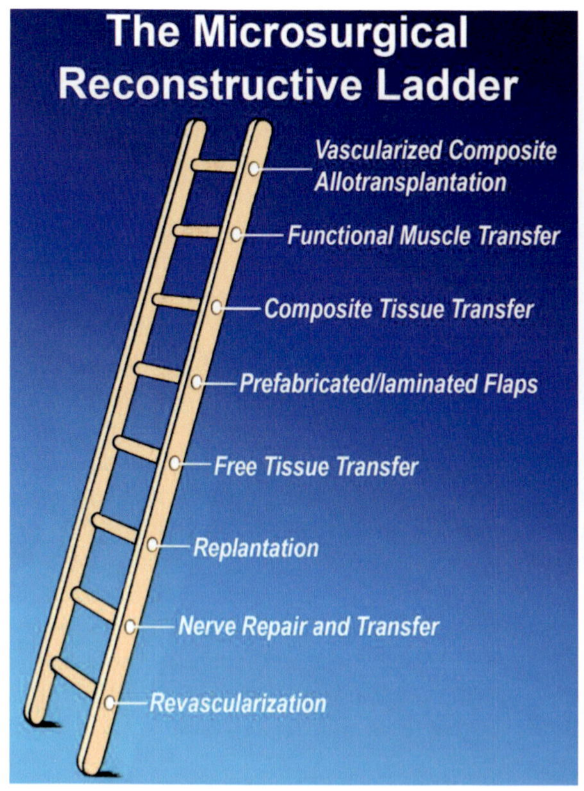

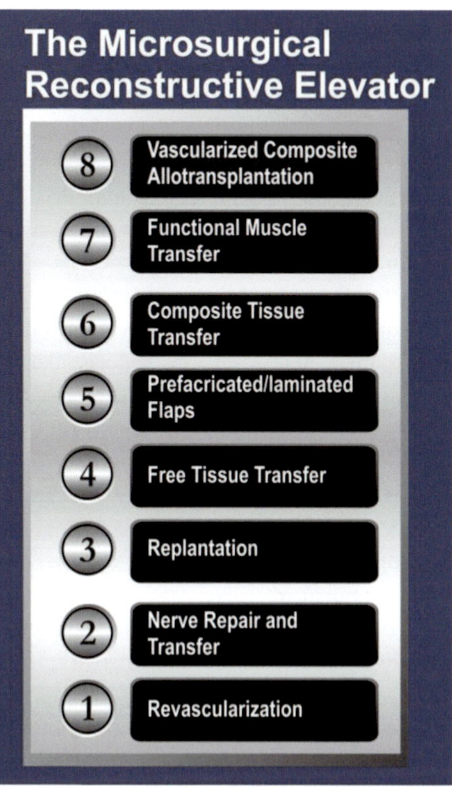

Fig. 8.1 The microsurgical reconstructive ladder demonstrating microsurgical techniques going from relatively simple at the bottom rung to more complex at the top rung (left). (Adapted with permission from Wolf et al. [52]). The concept of a reconstructive "elevator" is likely more appropriate in reconstructive surgery since at times complex problems require more complex microsurgical solutions without utilizing simpler solutions first (right)

if it is out of the zone of injury, has an adequate pedicle length, and has a large enough surface area for a viable, stable coverage of a defect following transfer. In a mangled limb, local flap options are often not available. Therefore, microsurgical soft tissue reconstruction is indicated in the salvageable limb when the wound has:

1. An extensive zone of injury
2. Local or regional flaps within the zone of injury are insufficient for coverage or must be preserved for remaining viable tissue
3. Exposed vital structures (bone, arteries, nerves) that do not have a local coverage option
4. Severe combined tissue injuries (skin, bone, arteries, nerve)
5. Previous failure with local or regional flaps

A common mistake to avoid is to underestimate an extensive wound and select local tissue for reconstruction when a microsurgical reconstruction is indicated. This can occur when facility resources, the surgical team, or the postoperative care are not equipped for microsurgical techniques and a local option is selected because it appears easier. This often leads to additional procedures, prolonged morbidity, increased hospitalizations, patient transfers, and often ultimately a salvage free tissue transfer. This scenario is avoided by assessing a wound appropriately and selecting more complex rungs of the reconstructive ladder, or taking the reconstructive "elevator" directly to an appropriate microsurgical reconstruction [19–21] (Fig 8.1).

Facility and Patient Requirements

Facility and Staff Requirements

The trauma center should be equipped to manage a critically ill patient with a mangled limb. A well-equipped emergency room and resuscitation resources are crucial, as is an experienced trauma team to triage life-threatening injuries and stabilize the patient. Subspecialty consultants in orthopedics, plastic surgery, and vascular surgery are all essential. Once a mangled limb is stable for microsurgical reconstruction, an operating room with an operating microscope, microsurgery instruments, microsurgery needles/venous couplers, on-table fluoroscopy and angiography, intraoperative Doppler, 2 Fr. Fogarty catheters, and a surgical intensive care unit for postoperative care are all required. The surgical team should be comfortable with microsurgical techniques and the nursing and anesthesia staff experienced in the intraoperative needs of a free tissue transfer patient. An operating room pharmacy with availability of free tissue transfer intraoperative medications is desirable (i.e., intravenous heparin, intraoperative vasodilating agents such as papaverine, lidocaine, or nitroglycerin), and streptokinase or tissue plasminogen activator (TPA) in the event of a "take back" for thrombosis. The availability of the operating room and nursing staff 24 hours a day is a necessity in the event that a free flap must be emergently re-explored.

Patient Requirements and Contraindications

The main contraindications for microsurgical soft tissue reconstruction can be described in terms of either the wound or patient factors. A microsurgical reconstruction is contraindicated in a poorly debrided wound, or in a wound that has been determined to have a poor long-term functional outcome by the entire reconstructive team. Patient factors can also influence candidacy for microsurgical soft tissue reconstruction. A critically ill patient who may be hemodynamically unstable (e.g., on vasopressors), be requiring blood products, have a bleeding coagulopathy, be malnourished, have multisystem organ failure, or have an evolving life-threatening condition is not an appropriate candidate for free tissue transfer. Relative contraindications include chronic conditions such as renal failure, severe diabetes, diminished mental capacity, or psychiatric illness that could prolong healing or compliance with postoperative care. In these cases, the reconstructive surgeon must make a determination if these complex pathophysiologic states can be controlled enough for the risk-benefit analysis to favor proceeding with free tissue transfer. Of note, smoking has been shown to affect blood flow and wound healing, although it may not affect the overall rate of anastomotic patency or flap survival. It is generally preferable to recommend a patient to be nicotine-free before surgery [22]. Patient age, interestingly, does not appear to be a major factor in patient selection for free tissue transfer [23, 24].

Preoperative Imaging

A mangled limb requiring microsurgical reconstruction usually has an extensive zone of injury. The trauma team, following ACLS protocols, is the initial team that may obtain imaging in suspected major vessel injury. These imaging studies (CT scans with angiography) are usually a baseline assessment of inflow and possible microsurgery vessel targets for reconstruction. However, the full extent of the zone of injury is only verified after surgical debridement is complete, often after second- or third-look debridement [13, 15, 25–28]. Soft tissue reconstruction follows definite debridement. Imaging studies can be completed prior to reconstruction if needed.

For preoperative planning, a detailed history and physical examination of the patient and examination of pulses of the upper and lower extremity is the standard of care. If physical examination and the trauma survey imaging studies are inadequate, high-resolution CT angiography or formal percutaneous angiography following patient stabilization is desirable.

Bedside Doppler probe examination can assist in detecting arterial inflow and distal perfusion following debridement. Formal preoperative imaging is not necessary in all cases and is up to the judgment of the reconstructive surgeon on a case-by-case basis. However, in the mangled lower extremity, vessel anatomy can be unpredictable, the reconstructive team should be prepared for variability intraoperatively, and preoperative imaging is helpful [29, 30]. Venous anatomy can be defined by preoperative ultrasound vein mapping if concerns exist regarding outflow or vein grafts will be needed, especially if saphenous vein grafts have already been utilized for revascularization. Coordinating the preoperative studies needed by all specialists in an orthoplastic approach can streamline the preoperative assessment and minimize patient radiation exposure.

Flap Selection and Options for Small, Medium, and Large Defects

Presently, there are a variety of free flap options for coverage of the mangled upper or lower extremity that are of different sizes and tissue types. There is no free flap that can provide a solution to all problems, but there are commonly used flaps that are well described that have reliable anatomy, large cutaneous or muscular territories, vascular pedicles of good caliber, and acceptable donor site morbidity. Flap selection depends on the size of defect and the need for skin, fascia, muscle, bone, or combined tissues. Characteristics of commonly used free flaps are summarized in Table 8.1 and are organized below by defect size.

Small Defects (up to 10 cm)

- Radial forearm flap
- Lateral arm flap
- Gracilis flap
- Serratus anterior flap
- Groin flap
- Dorsalis pedis flap

For smaller defects in need of free tissue transfer, the radial forearm flap has a long history of being a workhorse flap with large diameter vessels but is somewhat limited by forearm donor site morbidity. When raising the flap, care must be taken to leave paratenon on the flexor carpi radialis and digital flexor tendons to prevent poor skin graft take on the donor site. Careful imbrication of soft tissue over the tendons during closure can help with this issue. Creation of a one vessel hand by taking the radial artery can cause some hesitation in selecting this flap, so one must document ulnar artery dominance with an Allen's test preoperatively. Other options for small defects include the lateral arm flap, gracilis muscle flap, and the serratus anterior flap. Less commonly used flaps that remain viable options are the groin flap that is limited by its short pedicle and the dorsalis pedis flap that is limited by poor skin graft take over the extensor tendons of the foot and donor site morbidity.

Medium Defects (10–20 cm)

- Anterolateral thigh flap
- Scapular and parascapular flaps
- Rectus abdominus flap
- Gracilis (long narrow defects)

The workhorse of medium-sized defect reconstruction has become the anterolateral thigh (ALT) flap, commonly with primary closure of the donor site possible when used for defects up to 8 cm wide. This flap does have the limitation of being quite thick in more overweight or obese patients of the Western world. Scapular/parascapular flaps offer a reliable pedicle with the versatility of using fasciocutaneous, bone, and muscle components (Fig. 8.2). The rectus abdominus and gracilis flaps have proven to be straightforward and reliable muscle flaps for many years and remain a good option reconstruction of small-, medium-, and occasionally large-sized defects. The limitation of the rectus flap is the donor site with hernia a possibility and the gracilis flap is the narrow nature of the flap, although it can be folded side to side to cover medium-sized defects or stretched out for long narrow defects (Fig. 8.3).

Table 8.1 Flap options for microsurgical reconstruction of the mangled extremity

Tissue type	Donor site	Maximum size of flap (cm)	Comments	Disadvantages
Skin	Radial forearm flap (RFF)	10 × 30 cm	Workhorse flap	Donor site; compromises arterial inflow to hand
	Groin	10 × 25 cm	Easily disguised	Short pedicle, complex vascular anatomy
	Anterolateral thigh (ALT)	18 × 25 cm	Large skin and fascia territory	Aesthetics; less reliable pedicle; thick adipose layer
	Lateral arm	8 × 15 cm	Can be innervated; osteocutaneous variant with portion of humerus	Very small pedicle
	Scapular and parascapular flaps	7 × 20 cm	Simple, reliable pedicle; osteocutaneous variant with strip of scapula	Spreading scar common; thick; not innervated
	Dorsalis pedis	12 × 14 cm	Can harvest with tendons; thin, pliable	Requires skin graft to donor site, often poor take on foot
	Deep inferior epigastric artery perforator (DIEP)	17 × 50 cm	Favorable donor site, large skin paddle	Usually thick, requires secondary debulking/liposuction
Muscle	Latissimus dorsi	25 × 40 cm	Workhorse flap; largest muscle flap	Seroma formation from donor site common
	Gracilis	6 × 24 cm	Easily disguised donor site; no deficit	Distal skin paddle unreliable
	Serratus anterior	10 × 15 cm	Small defects, thin pliable muscle	Winging of scapula if more than four strips removed
	Rectus abdominis	6 × 25 cm	Easily harvested	Hernia possible
Fascia	Radial forearm	8 × 20 cm	Fascia alone improves donor site	Loss of radial artery
	Temporoparietal	8 × 15 cm	Thin, pliable	Possible frontal branch of facial nerve injury; alopecia
	Serratus fascia (lateral thoracic fascia)	12 × 18 cm	Thin, scar hidden in axilla/lateral thorax	Possible winging of scapula if long thoracic nerve injured
Bone	Fibula	25 cm	Long bony strut	Peroneal nerve palsy; flexor hallucis longus contracture, short pedicle length
	Radius	10 × 11.5 cm	Distal radius can be harvested with RFF	Radius fracture, can be prevented by prophylactic plating of radius
	Scapula	3 × 11 cm	Harvested with scapular/parascapular flap	Bone thin, not easily worked
	Humerus	1 × 10 cm	Harvested with lateral arm flap	Bone thin, not easily worked
	Iliac crest	4 × 12 cm	Curved bone for curved defects	Inguinal hernia possible
	Medial femoral condyle	3 × 3 cm	Long pedicle, ease of harvest	Small pedicle diameter, variable anatomy

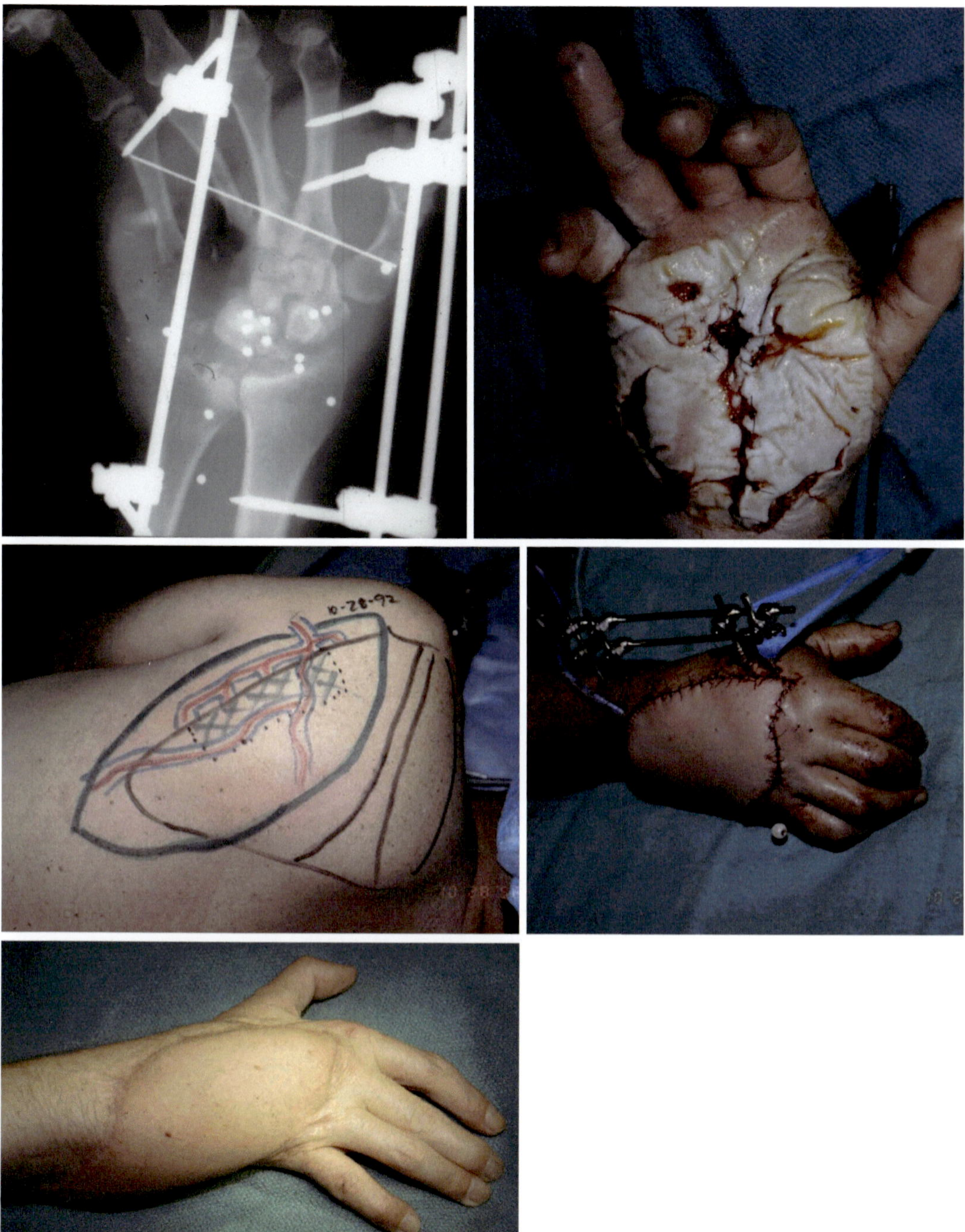

Fig. 8.2 Shotgun blast to the hand with bone and soft tissue loss. The defect was reconstructed with an osteocutaneous scapular flap

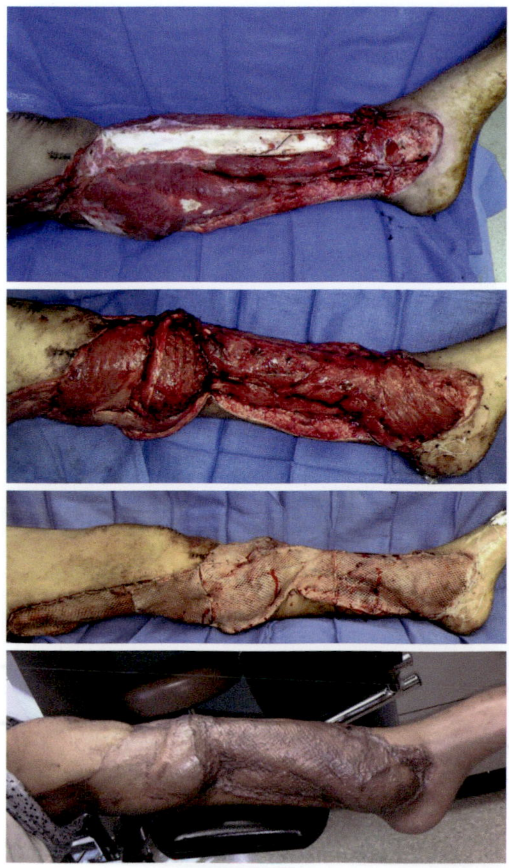

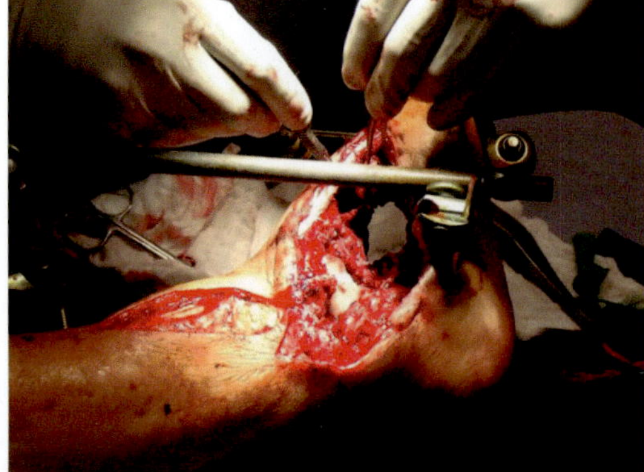

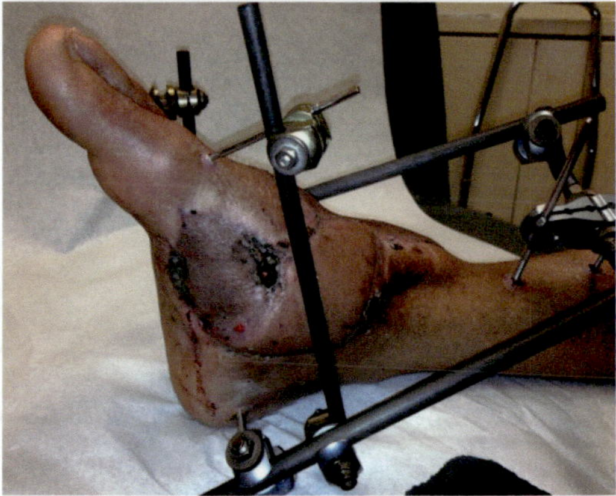

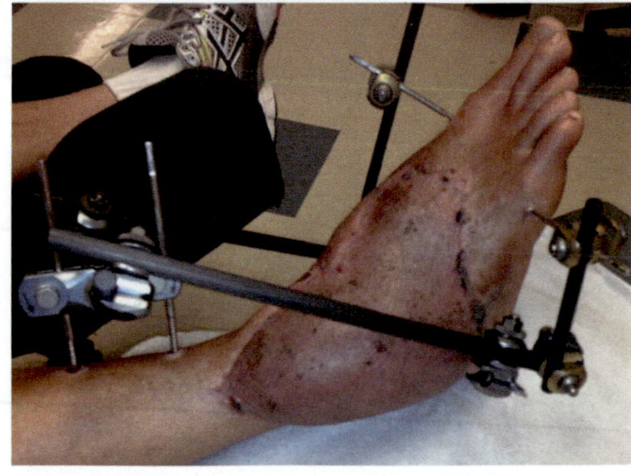

Fig. 8.3 Mutilating lower extremity injury that started as a gunshot wound which was complicated by necrotizing fasciitis after placement of tibial intramedullary nail. Reconstruction of the large defect was accomplished with a combination of local muscle flaps (medial gastrocnemius and medial hemi-soleus) and a free gracilis muscle flap. (Photos courtesy of Nada Berry MD)

Large Defects (>20 cm)

- Anterolateral thigh flap (with skin grafting of donor site)
- Latissimus dorsi flap
- Deep inferior epigastric perforator artery flap
- Pre-expanded scapular/parascapular flap

The latissimus dorsi (LD) flap is the largest muscle flap (25 × 40 cm) and has long been a workhorse flap for covering extensive defects with exposed vital structures and bone (Fig. 8.4). The downside to this flap remains donor site seroma formation, but this is often treatable with drains and compression. The ALT flap offers a good fasciocutaneous alternative to the LD flap with a potential size of 18 × 25 cm

Fig. 8.4 Gunshot wound through the forefoot with a large through-and-through defect. This was reconstructed with a latissimus myocutaneous flap that was pulled through the defect and used to close both sides, demonstrating the ability of this flap to fill dead space and cover large wounds

when the donor site is skin grafted. The ALT donor site, when skin grafted, can be problematic as healing is sometimes impeded by the dynamic rectus femoris and vastus lateralis muscles underlying the graft. The deep inferior epigastric artery perforator flap (DIEP) is most commonly used for breast reconstruction but can be used for extremity reconstruction. This flap provides a large cutaneous paddle for reconstruction of extensive defects and has the advantage over the LD flap of supine positioning of the patient during harvest [31]. Another advantage is a favorable donor site especially in the female patient. The downside to the flap is that it can be quite thick and require contouring procedures/liposuction in the future. Pre-expanded scapular/parascapular flaps can also be useful for large extremity defects [32], but in the setting of mutilating injuries, this is not an option.

Considerations for Skin, Fascia, or Muscle Flaps Depending on Future Reconstructive Needs

Skin or Fasciocutaneous Flaps

Skin or fasciocutaneous flaps contain skin and underlying fascia with a named vascular pedicle. Fasciocutaneous flaps are advantageous for staged reconstructions where elevation of the flap is predicted such as in the need for removal of antibiotic spacers and subsequent bone grafting (i.e., the Masquelet technique) [33], because they are easier for secondary procedures [34]. They also provide very good gliding surface for underlying tendons and can be elevated later for tenolysis procedures. These flaps are often thin and pliable and can result in acceptable cosmesis. Common flaps in this category are the radial forearm flap, anterolateral thigh flap, parascapular/scapular flap, and lateral arm flap [18, 21, 26]. Some of these flaps can be harvested as sensate flaps or as composite flaps with underlying bone for functional reconstruction. Relative advantages and disadvantages are summarized in Table 8.1.

Fascial Flaps

Fascial flaps are indicated in superficial defects requiring very thin coverage (e.g., dorsum of the hand or fingers). They are advantageous from donor site viewpoint, but the flap must be covered with a skin graft, which can produce further contractures.

Fascial flaps, similar to fasciocutaneous flaps, can be elevated later for tenolysis, but not as easily since the overlying skin grafts can cause scarring/fibrosis of the flap. Relative advantages and disadvantages of fascia flaps are summarized in Table 8.1.

Muscle Flaps

Free muscle flaps have been widely utilized in extremity reconstruction. Despite the advantages of fasciocutaneous flaps that offer effective coverage of large wounds, there are still indications for free muscle flaps. These include the presence of osteomyelitis or in highly contaminated wounds that leave large areas of dead space following definitive debridement. Such scenarios take advantage of muscle bulk to obliterate dead space and provide highly vascular tissue for underlying bone and hardware (Fig. 8.4). Muscle flaps also tend to do better on the plantar surface of the foot where they become more fibrotic to the underlying bone and are good for walking compared to fasciocutaneous flaps that shear more and are less stable for ambulating. A muscle flap can be harvested with overlying skin (e.g., myocutaneous flap) to serve as a source of skin for coverage and for monitoring of perfusion. In addition, muscle flaps can be harvested as functioning muscle transfers when incorporating the motor nerve to the muscle in addition to the vascular pedicle. The motor nerve is sutured to a recipient nerve with the goal of achieving reinnervation and voluntary control of the muscle. The most commonly used muscle flaps are the latissimus dorsi, gracilis, serratus anterior, and rectus abdominis, which all have well-described anatomy [18, 28, 34, 35]. Relative advantages and disadvantages of these muscle flaps are summarized in Table 8.1.

Bone Flap Options

Microsurgery has revolutionized the treatment of large segmental bone defects through the use of vascularized bone transfer. Since its description by Taylor et al. in 1975, the vascularized fibula has been used extensively due to its size, acceptable donor site morbidity, and predictable dissection [29, 30]. Free fibular vascularized grafts have been utilized for segmental defects of the upper and lower extremity and have a pivotal role in traumatic reconstruction (Fig. 8.5). The bone can be harvested in isolation or can be harvested as an osteocutaneous flap due to the consistent anatomy of the peroneal artery perforators. The vascular supply of to the fibula is based on the peroneal artery, though there is reported variability in the takeoff of the peroneal artery from the posterior tibioperoneal trunk [30]. Other large vascularized bone grafts described include the partial radius, scapula, humerus, and iliac crest [26]. Relative advantages and disadvantages of these bone flaps are summarized in Table 8.1.

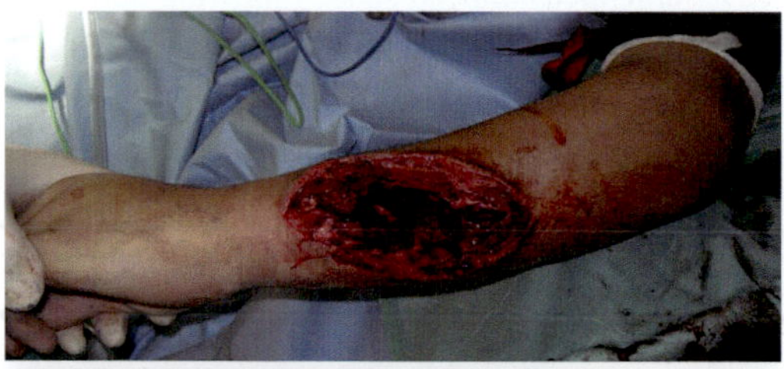

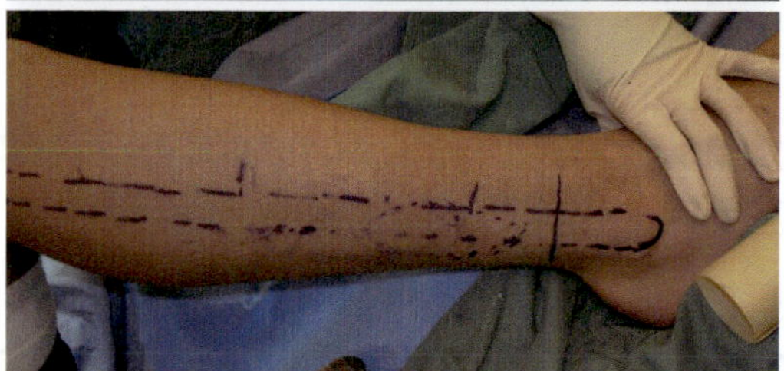

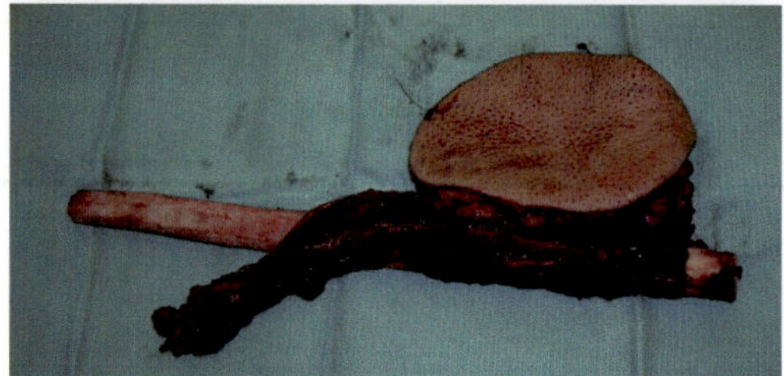

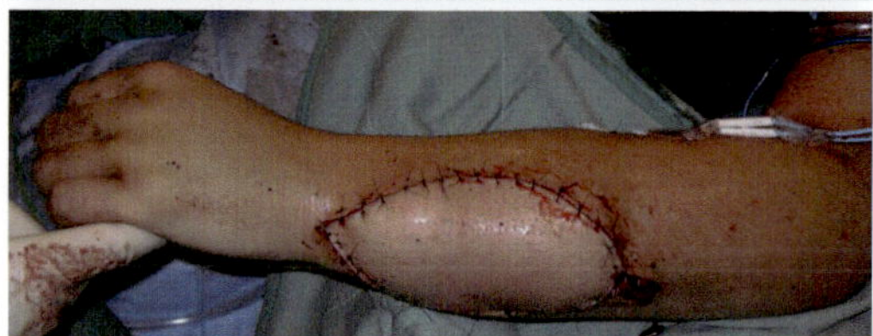

Fig. 8.5 Gunshot wound of the forearm with soft tissue and bone loss. Reconstruction consisted of a free fibula osteocutaneous flap, which offers ample bone and a long pedicle for reconstruction of significant composite defects

Free vascularized bone grafts from the medial femoral condyle are increasing in versatility and popularity. The medial femoral condyle flap or medial genicular artery flap as a source of vascularized bone transfer has had a surge in use in a variety of bony reconstructions. It has been utilized with increased frequency for larger bone grafting procedures and has become a reliable alternative to free fibular grafts for intermediate to large osseous defects [36–40]. The flap has more recently been described as a method of supplying well-vascularized cortico-periosteum as a method of treating recalcitrant nonunions all including the foot/ankle, tibia, femur, scaphoid, radius, ulna, humerus, and clavicle [41]. The vascular anatomy has been well described by Yamamoto et al. [42]. The nutrient vessels of the medial femoral condyle were consistently supplied by the descending genicular artery, the superomedial genicular artery, or both. The descending genicular artery is a branch off the superficial femoral artery just proximal to the adductor hiatus and often divides into two or three branches: (1) the osteoarticular branch, (2) muscular branch, and (3) the saphenous branch. The descending genicular artery was found in 89% of specimens and branches off the superficial femoral artery approximately 13.7 cm above the knee joint. The superomedial genicular artery was present 100% of the time and serves as a backup. The main challenges to this flap are the relatively small vessel diameter of the pedicle (1–1.5 mm) and the amount of bone available for reconstruction so as to not disrupt the knee joint (usually 3 cm × 3 cm × 1 cm). Nevertheless, it is a versatile flap used routinely by the senior author (L.S.L.) in a variety of reconstructions, including segmental bony free flap reconstructions of the foot and ankle (see case example and Fig. 8.6) [43].

Special Considerations for Skeletal Stabilization Methods Around Time of Free Tissue Transfer

Mutilating extremity injuries often involve significant bony comminution and contamination which require temporary external fixation and repeat irrigation and debridements. If the bone

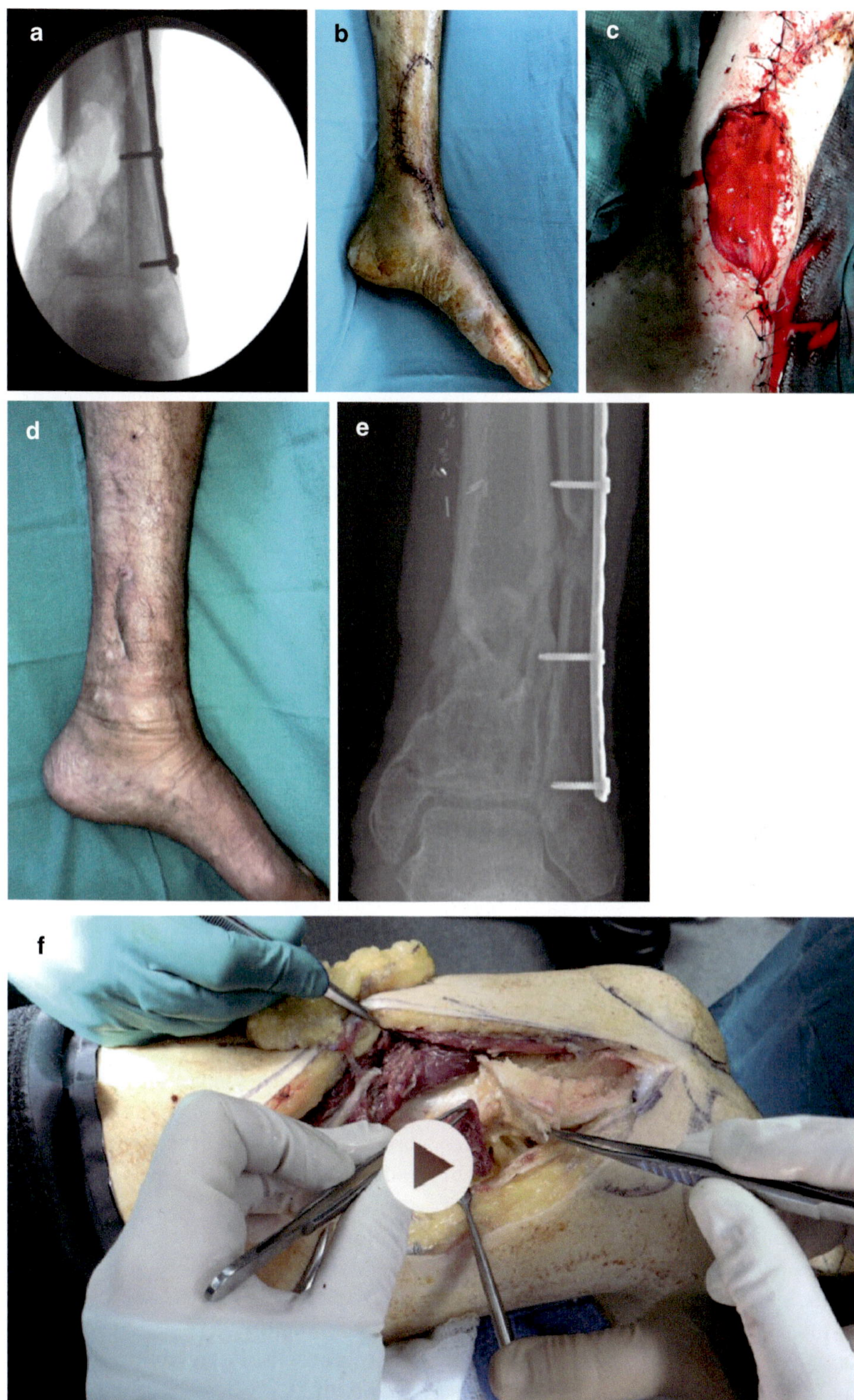

Fig. 8.6 Case example of tibial osteomyelitis and fibular nonunion after motor vehicle crash. Fluoroscopic view of the bony defect (**a**) and the tenuous soft tissue envelope (**b**) following first stage debridement and antibiotic bead placement. This was reconstructed with a myo-osseous medial femoral condyle flap. Panel (**c**) shows the inset muscle component of the flap prior to skin grafting; panels (**d** and **e**) show the healed muscle and bone flaps, respectively. A video is available online (**f**) demonstrating the flap in situ prior to dividing the pedicle

contamination is significant or there is concern for ongoing infection, fractures require external fixation as the definitive treatment until bone healing. Important soft tissue reconstruction principles must be considered with placement of external fixation pins and bars as follows:

- Pins should be as far from the wound as possible while maintaining fracture stability.
- Bars should not obstruct the soft tissue window around the zone of injury.
- In the leg, mid anterior pins are better than medial or lateral pins to allow for vascular access for free flaps and rotational muscle and perforator flaps.
- The frame must be easily loosened for adjustments needed during reconstruction.

Conversion from external fixation to plates or intramedullary nails in open fractures that have been thoroughly debrided in combination with immediate soft tissue coverage has proven effective in the treatment of severe extremity trauma [44, 45]. This approach is ideal when possible and allows for reconstruction to proceed without interference of external fixator devices.

Intraoperative Care

Following careful preoperative planning and choice of reconstruction, the patient is taken to the operating room under general anesthesia. Central and arterial lines may be desirable for close monitoring of central venous pressure and mean arterial pressure. Foley catheterization is essential. Proper positioning and padding of pressure points for the desired procedure is critical to prevent iatrogenic nerve palsies or pressure ulcer formation. A two-team approach is often used to maximize efficiency and minimize fatigue, with one team raising the tissue to be transferred while the other team preparing the recipient sites. Even the most accomplished surgeon will have a failure rate of 2% to 5%, and part of the definitive reconstructive plan is to have alternatives to the initial procedure should complications arise.

Perioperative strategies are directed toward maximizing flap perfusion. In the mangled limb scenario, inpatient stabilization of the patient should ensure proper resuscitation and confirm homeostasis in hydration, normothermic conditions, and adequate urine output. Once in the operating room, the patient should be maintained normothermic with the application of hot air blankets, padding, and warmed intravenous fluids. The optimal hematocrit level is 30, which is good for appropriate oxygenation while maintaining relatively low blood viscosity and blood flow. The mean arterial pressure desirable for free flap perfusion is 70 mmHg, maintaining blood pressure in normal ranges with the use of fluid volume rather than vasopressors (which can complicate microvascular flow in free flap physiology). A urine output of 1 mL/Kg/hr. is desirable. An indicator of appropriate hemodynamic parameters is flow through the pedicle once isolated. Poor flow through the pedicle can be related to low blood pressure state or hypothermia which can be investigated intraoperatively and corrected to improve flap circulation.

The use of agents to alter clotting or viscosity is controversial and surgeon dependent. There is a lack of high-quality scientific data to support their agent both intraoperatively or perioperatively. Aspirin, heparin, and dextran are used often in microsurgery [46]. The senior author's (L.S.L.) usual free flap regimen is the use of 2500 units of intravenous heparin intraoperatively prior to harvesting the free flap pedicle for transfer, heparinized saline flushes during the microsurgery, use of local papaverine on the pedicle and around the anastomosis as needed, followed postoperatively with PO aspirin 325 mg daily for 10–14 days. The use of an implantable venous Doppler can monitor flow through the flap, versus external Doppler probe monitoring on the flap itself, confirmed intraoperatively and marked for the nursing staff postoperatively.

Postoperative Care

Postoperative Patient and Flap Monitoring

The patient is usually admitted to a surgical intensive care unit (ICU) following free flap reconstruction unless there are very well-trained personnel on a regular floor unit. For uncomplicated procedures, the patient is extubated and provided with adequate parenteral pain control. In complicated cases due to patient comorbidities or polytrauma, there may be a benefit in keeping the patient intubated and sedated to minimize fluctuations in blood pressure. Adequate perfusion of the free flap is monitored with clinical observation (skin color, temperature, capillary refill, turgor, and external Doppler probe). At the discretion of the surgeon, other techniques for monitoring may be employed such as temperature differential probes, laser or implantable Doppler probes, real-time pulse oximetry, or external real-time tissue oximetry devices. An experienced nursing staff is critical as they are the first caregivers to detect any compromise in the flap. Perfusion checks are up to the judgment of the surgeon. At our institution, perfusion checks are every 1 hour while in the ICU and are progressively spaced to every 2 hours or every 4 hours when transferring to step-down units or the ward.

Clinical exam is still the standard of care for detecting a compromised flap. Arterial insufficiency is indicated in a pale, cool flap with delayed capillary refill and failure to bleed upon a pinprick. Venous insufficiency leads to a blue, mottled color with immediate capillary refill and swelling of a flap (i.e., a "congested"-appearing flap). On occasion, a signal loss is related to patient positioning or a technical issue with the Doppler. Furthermore, free flap congestion can be occasionally relieved by removal of selected sutures, changes in position, or loosening constricting bandages. However, if bedside maneuvers are exhausted and arterial or venous compromise is suspected, the surgical team should be alerted immediately. Both conditions are indications for immediate return to the operating room.

Free Flap Complications and Management

The most common complication is an acute problem with flap circulation for a variety of reasons. In an acute arterial or venous compromise of a fresh free flap, immediate return to the operating room is mandatory. Early return to the operating room allows the salvage of >50% of compromised flaps [24]. The pedicle is inspected for kinking, torsion, or compression, and any bleeding is stopped. Hematomas are evacuated. Patency of the pedicle is inspected visually, tested with the strip test across the anastomosis, and evaluated with sterile Doppler probe. When there is no obvious problem, the anastomosis may need to be redone. Intraoperative thrombolytic agents, such as urostreptokinase or more commonly tissue plasminogen activator (TPA), may be used if thrombus within the flap is suspected. The venous outflow of the flap must be disconnected from the outflow vein to avoid systemic administration, and thrombolytic can be injected into the arterial pedicle to break down thrombi within the flap. 2 Fr. Fogarty catheters can also be used to help extract thrombi from flap vessels. Postoperative anticoagulation is an option to minimize clotting following these salvage maneuvers and is surgeon dependent. Two retrospective analyses of free flap take-backs for flap compromise identified surgeon experience and preoperative thrombocytosis as independent risk factors for intraoperative and perioperative thrombosis [47, 48]. If detected preoperatively, thrombocytosis can be managed expectantly or with the aid of hematology consult recommendations prior to free flap reconstruction. Intraoperative heparin anticoagulation and complete thrombectomy were essential in these cases for flap salvage [47, 48].

Besides problems with the anastomosis, the most serious complications of free tissue transfer are partial or complete failure of the flap (i.e., partial or complete ischemic necrosis of tissue). Flap failure occurs more frequently early in the reconstructive surgeon's experience. Different tissue types have different tolerance of ischemia insults. Muscle flaps are the least tolerant, while skin, fascia, and bone have a greater tolerance to ischemia. Partial flap loss can be salvaged with debridement and local wound care and secondary procedures. Interestingly, experimental data and anecdotal evidence suggest hyperbaric oxygen treatment may be used as an adjunct to support ischemic grafts and flaps, although more clinical trials are needed [49–51].

Complete flap loss is the most serious complication and requires definitive debridement and planned, staged secondary reconstruction. Failure of the original flap should be exhaustively investigated to prevent further complications on redo free flap procedures.

Rehabilitation (Elevation, Edema Control, Dangling, and Therapy)

Rehabilitation should proceed in stages: from early-protective, intermediate-mobilization, to late-strengthening. Rehabilitation of microsurgical soft tissue reconstruction begins in the operating room following free tissue transfer with appropriate splinting of the injured extremity, but allowing movement of uninvolved limbs. Peripheral nerve blocks, epidural anesthesia, and brachial plexus indwelling catheters decrease narcotic requirements and are useful. Tight circumferential casts or wraps are avoided, and superficial dressings are cut along the axis of the injured extremity to prevent constriction from bandaging. Edema is a major consideration and should be controlled with extremity elevation on two pillows while an inpatient and during the rehabilitation period. A patient-specific approach should be adopted depending on the defect location, free flap choice, and the stability of the skeletal fixation. Dangle protocols for lower extremity free flap reconstructions vary, but typically the senior author's (L.S.L) preference is a conservative approach with no dependent ambulation for 2 weeks following surgery with progressive dangling thereafter under the direct supervision of the reconstructive surgery team and physical therapists versed in free flap rehabilitation. Weight-bearing should proceed based on the stability of the bony reconstruction. Patients should also be offered referrals for psychological support and social assistance to guard against post-traumatic stress disorder (PTSD) and depression following catastrophic injuries. Follow-up is critical in first 6 months to a year and can be yearly thereafter to assess need for secondary procedures such as free flap debulking, contouring, and contracture releases as needed.

Case Example

Patient Presentation

A 49-year-old police dispatcher suffered a comminuted fracture of distal tibia and fibula from a motor vehicle accident, originally managed by open reduction and internal fixation and complicated by fibular nonunion, hardware failure, and chronic osteomyelitis of the tibia with an open draining sinus. He had multiple debridements and revision procedures and presented with suspected chronic hardware colonization of spanning plates of both the tibia and fibula over antibiotic beads. The patient's post-debridement fluoroscopic x-rays and tenuous soft tissue envelope are shown in Fig. 8.6a, b. The surgical plan was staged reconstruction with removal of tibial hardware and antibiotic beads (previously placed), wide debridement of sinus tract, bony nonunion, and new antibiotic bead placement. Interval IV antibiotic treatment for osteomyelitis was planned, followed subsequently by free vascularized MFC bone flap reconstruction of distal tibial defect.

Surgical Technique

Preparation of the Recipient Site
After multiple debridements and removal of the colonized hardware, the patient was taken to the operating room and placed under general anesthesia with regional block. The original incisions were opened and subcutaneous tissues were divided. The pretibial defect was identified and the antibiotic beads were removed without difficulty. Dissection was then carried down beyond the tibialis posterior tendon and muscle belly to the posterior tibial neurovascular bundle. The posterior tibial artery and vena comitantes were identified and isolated proximal to the zone of injury.

Raising the Medial Femoral Condyle and Vastus Medialis Chimeric Flap
The free medial femoral condyle flap was then raised by making longitudinal incision over the left knee. The fascia of the vastus medialis was

incised and the muscle was retracted anteriorly. The medial geniculate artery system was identified distally as it approached the medial face of the diaphysis of the medial femoral condyle. Retrograde dissection was carried out and muscle perforators to the vastus medialis were identified and preserved for possible harvest of a composite flap. There were no direct perforators coming off the medial geniculate that could be used for a skin paddle, so muscle was chosen as the composite/chimeric flap. The pedicle measured approximately 1.5 mm as it came off the SFA. The bone flap was then designed on the medial femoral condyle. The periosteum was incised with a Bovie, protecting the pedicle proximally. A periosteal elevator was used to elevate the pedicle and periosteum proximal to the osteotomy sites. An oscillating saw was then used to harvest a 1 × 3 × 3.5 cm bone block from medial femoral cortex which included cortex, cancellous bone, and periosteum. A portion of the vastus medialis was then taken based on the muscle perforator proximally and the pedicle was divided (see Video 8.1). The bone flap was trimmed and impacted into the medial tibial defect, osteotomizing the undersurface of the flap so that a gentle curve could exist from the medial native tibia to the cortico-cancellous graft. Anastomosis was performed end-to-end on the posterior tibial artery to the medial geniculate artery with excellent flow. Outflow was obtained through multiple veins that were coalesced into one outflow vein. A 3 mm venous coupler was then used to couple the veins with excellent inflow and outflow and strong Doppler signals. The muscle was advanced and placed over the chronic wound area above the periosteum of the bone component of the composite flap. A 3-0 nylon was used to close the remainder of the skin without tension over the pedicle. A split-thickness skin graft was applied over the muscle flap. An intraoperative photo of the inset muscle flap is shown in Fig. 8.6c.

Follow-Up

At 6 months, his intercalary defect of his tibia was bridged with the medial femoral condyle flap with a good lateral column of bone without any evidence of lucency by CT scan. He was able to plantar flex to 60 degrees. Mild lower extremity edema is managed by compression stocking and he is full weight-bearing. The well-healed flap and a follow-up radiograph of his bony bridging are shown in Fig. 8.6d, e.

Clinical Pearls and Pitfalls

Pearls

- Microsurgery indications include a large zone of injury, exposed vital structures, and severe combined injuries (e.g., segmental bony defects) with no local coverage options.
- Principles of flap selection follow the tissue types requiring reconstruction using the microsurgical reconstructive ladder.
- Ideally free tissue transfer should be timed within 7 days of the injury to maximize outcomes.

Pitfalls

- Contraindications to microsurgery include inadequate wound debridement, unstable patient, and chronic uncontrolled medical comorbidities.
- Inadequate facilities, staff capabilities, and postoperative care will affect outcomes.
- Negative pressure wound therapy and dermal substitutes should not replace the need for microsurgical soft tissue reconstruction when indicated.

Conclusion

Free tissue transfer can provide stable, durable coverage of mangled extremity wounds when indicated. Indications include an extensive zone of injury, exposed vital structures, or severe combined injuries of different tissue types. The microsurgical reconstructive ladder is a conceptually useful framework for proper free flap selection. Pitfalls arise when the facility, staff

Growing Bone: Lengthening and Grafting

Jessica C. Rivera, Janet D. Conway,
Michael J. Assayag, and John E. Herzenberg

Introduction

Segmental bone loss occurs in patients with a variety post-traumatic, infectious, and malignant pathologies. In the setting of the mangled extremity, large segmental bone losses can be treated with bone grafting or gradual distraction to grow new bone. The use of bone grafts has a long history in orthopedic and maxillocraniofacial applications such that it is difficult to pinpoint the pioneering surgeons. Wolff and Ollier both made early observations that transplanted bone could regenerate new bone [1, 2]. Duhamel credited periosteum as the source of osteogenic elements, coining the term "cambium layer" of periosteum [2]. Dobrotworski is credited with successful autogenous rib grafting for cranial defects, and Albee is credited with an early series of hundreds of successful graftings in the lower extremities [1]. Bone grafting is now the second most common type of tissue transfer performed after skin grafting.

Similarly, surgical limb lengthening has been attempted since the late nineteenth century start-ing with the first applications of first-generation external fixation [3]. Diagnoses treated in this period by external fixation included post-traumatic malunions and post-poliomyelitis deformities via various combinations of osteotomies, acute distractions, and/or gradual traction. Codivilla gave the first English literature report to describe the concept of "continuous extension" using a calcaneal transfixion pin and traction, a precursor to gradual lengthening [3]. Bosworth was credited with the first use of the term "bone distraction," and other pioneers including Bost, Larsen, and Wagner performed work that supported gradual distraction [3, 4]. Professor Gavriil Ilizarov solidified the concept of bone distraction as a means to grow new bone in treating post-traumatic pathologies by observing new bone formation spanning a gradually widening gap. He termed this phenomenon "distraction osteogenesis," and the term "distraction histogenesis" can be applied as soft tissue also expands with this technique. Ilizarov distraction principles include periosteal and blood supply sparing corticotomy and placement of stable, ring external fixators applied to the limb via tensioned wires followed by a latency period and a specific rate and rhythm of distraction [5, 6]. Distraction osteogenesis principles first elucidated by Ilizarov are the basis for bone transport procedures used to fill segmental bone defects.

J. C. Rivera · J. D. Conway · M. J. Assayag
J. E. Herzenberg (✉)
International Center for Limb Lengthening, Rubin Institute for Advanced Orthopaedics, Sinai Hospital of Baltimore, Baltimore, MD, USA
e-mail: jherzenberg@lifebridgehealth.org

© Springer Nature Switzerland AG 2021
R. A. Pensy, J. V. Ingari (eds.), *The Mangled Extremity*, https://doi.org/10.1007/978-3-319-56648-1_9

Approach to Patients with Bone Loss

The clinical need for bone grafting or other biologic treatment for segmental bone loss is assumed if the bone defect is not expected to heal despite appropriate stabilization [7]. The threshold of bone loss, or critical defect, is not clearly defined in the orthopedic literature. Traditionally, a long bone defect of 1–2 cm and/or loss of greater than 50% of the cortical circumference of bone is accepted as a critical defect [8]. However, this size-based definition is not necessarily accepted by the orthopedic trauma community as local and systemic biology of the limb will affect healing regardless of the defect size [9]. Young children in particular are known to be able to spontaneously heal seemingly critical defects assuming an intact periosteum. Despite no consensus on what constitutes a critical defect, recommendations for bone loss reconstruction have been published based on defect size vis-à-vis what defects are amendable to bone grafting. In addition to dogma related to what defects can be grafted, additional dogma exists which suggests there is a limit to what percentage of a bone can be lengthened or transported. *For the purpose of this chapter, the authors suggest that proper assessment of the patient's physiology, proper stabilization of the mangled extremity including meticulous regard for the soft tissue, and proper understanding of the surgeon's skill set, institutional support, and patient's psychosocial support are cumulatively more important than any specific rule related to size of segmental bone loss.*

Regardless of defect size, reconstruction requires a physiologically amenable tissue bed and host [10]. Locally, vascularity must be adequate to sustain viability of the injured limb and healing tissue. Soft tissue coverage is essential as the muscle – bone interface is critical for bone healing [11]. The remaining bone after debridement must be viable and optimally should be infection-free or have infection adequately suppressed. Achieving this local environment may require peripheral vascular work-up and treatment, multiple procedures for local debridement, and/or multiple modalities geared toward soft tissue reconstruction before, during, and after the bony reconstruction.

The patient with a mangled extremity will undergo multiple surgeries whether bone grafting or bone transport methods are used to achieve limb reconstruction [12, 13]. As a result, the patient must be optimized for multiple anesthetics and prolonged physiologic stress of limb salvage. Advanced Trauma Life Support (ATLS) and damage control orthopedics principles apply. Comorbid conditions which are modifiable should also be optimized such as cardiac conditions, blood glucose control, nutritional optimization with adequate protein intake and replacement as needed for healthy bone metabolism (e.g., vitamin D replacement), nicotine cessation, and establishment of psychosocial support [10]. The Lower Extremity Assessment Project (LEAP) study found that patient-reported outcomes following severe lower extremity trauma were affected by the patient's self-efficacy, or the patient's belief that he or she could achieve the desired goal of being well [14]. As such, psychosocial optimization toward improving the patient's self-efficacy should be addressed alongside medial/physiological optimization.

The wound bed itself should be optimized. Antibiotics should be administered as soon as possible following open limb injury [15, 16]. The limb should have adequate vascularity. All necrotic and devitalized tissue should be debrided including bone edges to healthy, bleeding margins [17]. This bleeding margin of bone is indicated by a "paprika sign" which describes the appearance of the healthy, bleeding bone edge. There is some support for retention of osteochondral bone fragments since composite tissues are not yet able to be regenerated or reconstructed, while devitalized diaphyseal bone should be debrided [18]. Soft tissue, particularly in a trauma and infection setting, should be stabilized by way of bony stabilization, including provisional stabilization and/or immobilization. Open wounds which cannot be closed can be treated with local wound care. The use of negative pressure wound dressings are now common and associated with lower infection rates, improved edema control, and reduction in soft tissue reconstruction complexity [19–21]. However, use of negative pressure wound dressings should not delay or replace soft tissue flap coverage if clearly indicated as a delay in definitive soft tissue coverage beyond 7 days has been associated with increased risk of infection [22, 23]. Surgeons must have a plan for the management of soft tissue injury which requires one's own technical ability to perform rotational or local flap coverage of the bony reconstruction or adequate support from a microvascular or plastic surgery-trained colleague.

Principles of Bone Grafting

Autograft

Autograft bone is considered the gold standard graft material due to the inherent osteoconductive, osteoinductive, and osteogenic properties of the patient's own bone tissue and no risk of rejection [24]. Autograft may be obtained from various anatomic sites. The iliac crest is a common area for harvest because it is an ample source of both cancellous and cortical autograft and may be easily accessed with the patient in a supine position [25]. Other sites of cancellous autograft harvest include the posterior superior iliac spine, distal radius, distal femur, proximal tibia, and calcaneus. At each of these sites, a direct surgical approach may be made and small oscillating saw or osteotome used to make a cortical window. Curettes are then used to extract chunks of cancellous bone. In the case of the iliac crest and from the long bones, the harvest can be directed through a relatively small cortical window and curettes directed proximally and distally to optimize the volume of cancellous bone extracted. Disadvantages of this type of autograft harvest include morbidity associated with an additional surgical incision, particularly at the iliac crest. For large bone defects, this type of autograft harvest may also fail to yield adequate graft volumes [24].

An additional source of graft material from the femur or tibia is intramedullary reaming debris which contains viable cellular and growth factor components [26]. The Reamer-Irrigator-Aspirator (RIA) reamer (DePuy Synthes) was initially designed to reduce intramedullary pressure and risk of fat embolism, but its use has expanded to harvest cancellous graft from the intramedullary space using standard reaming techniques [27, 28]. The proprietary reamer and associated components have an effluent trap and filter to capture aspirated cancellous graft while the reamer is being passed into the intramedullary canal. For this system, the reamer heads start at 12 mm diameter and are thus suited for appropriately sized long bones. The surgical approach to pass the RIA reamer is the same as any other intramedullary approach to the long bone, and the RIA may be passed in the femur (antegrade or retrograde) and the tibia. In the femur, the antegrade approach preferred is the trochanteric start point as the large-diameter reaming via the piriformis start point risks creating a stress rise in the femoral neck. Several studies have demonstrated that cancellous graft harvested by RIA contains ample cells and growth factors comparable to iliac crest bone graft while yielding a greater volume of graft material and with fewer complications [29–31]. The disadvantage to the RIA system is the risk of cortical breach and/or fracture of the harvest bone. To reduce this risk, the reamer should be passed in the central canal and monitored along the bone length using fluoroscopic guidance.

Cancellous autograft contains osteoconductive scaffold required for vascular in-growth and cell migration, osteoinductive growth factors, and osteogenic cells but does not offer structural support [24]. Cortical autograft can also be harvested from the iliac crest, fibula, or rib. Vascularized cortical graft (e.g., cortical pedicle at the distal radius, free vascularized fibula) requires significant technical skill and may not be practical for all surgeons. Cortical graft harvest, whether avascular or vascular, increases donor site morbidity compared to cancellous graft harvest. Vascularized fibular graft specifically is associated with donor site complications and fracture complications in as high as 32% of procedures [32].

Allograft

Cortical allograft bone graft is useful for structural support in the setting of fracture-related bone loss as strut to support fixation or to fill in segmental bone loss. Intramembranous bone formation and creeping substitution at the allograft borders results in some incorporation of the graft into the host bone; however this is limited by the size of the allograft and the host bone ability to vascularize large allograft segments [33, 34]. As a result, extreme bone loss that is treated with cortical graft is recommended for vascularized autograft to avoid failure at persistently nonvascular segments of long cortical allografts. However, there is no evidence for what amounts to a critical length defect which requires vascularized graft [35]. Non-structural allografts including cancellous bone chips and demineralized bone matrix provide osteoconductive substrate. Depending on the product processing and sterilization methods, these products also retain some osteoinductive factors, more so with demineralized bone matrix [24]. Non-structural allografts are particularly useful to expand the volume to be used in conjunction with autograft in cases where the amount of autograft harvested is insufficient to fill the required void.

Bone Graft Substitutes

Several synthetic bone graft substitutes are now marketed, most commonly composed of calcium phosphate or calcium sulfate [24, 36]. Bone graft substitutes are useful for their osteoconductive properties rather than structural properties and can be helpful adjuncts to dead space management [24]. Calcium phosphate ceramics and cements are available in preparations that closely resemble the porosity of cancellous bone. Calcium phosphate bone graft substitutes also demonstrate some axial stability which is advantageous while the patient's bone heals. Calcium sulfate preparations are attractive in settings where fully resorbable substitute is desired. Both calcium phosphate and calcium sulfate bone graft substitutes have been used to deliver antibiotics, demonstrating superior elution properties compared to polymethylmethacrylate (PMMA) cement [36–38]. Bone graft substitutes are regulated by the Food and Drug Administration (FDA) as devices and are labeled as indicated for use in bone segments in which structural stability is not required (and thus not indicated as substitutes in the setting of segmental bone loss).

Biologic Adjuncts to Bone Grafting

Various autogenous and recombinant adjuncts have been used to augment healing or supplement grafting. This discussion is beyond the scope of this chapter. However, recombinant human bone morphogenetic protein (rhBMP)-2 is FDA approved for treatment of acute tibia fractures within 14 days of injury and after intramedullary nail stabilization and soft tissue management [39, 40]. Studies on BMP uses in segmental and critical size defect models are plentiful in the basic science literature though conclusive clinical studies on segmental bone loss in humans are lacking. What randomized or pooled results are available is inconclusive though the single randomized trial exploring segmental bone loss specifically concluded that autogenous bone graft and rhBMP-2 plus allograft were equivocal [41–43].

Another source of biological adjunct for bone grafting is aspiration of autologous bone marrow, so-called bone marrow aspirate concentrate (BMAC). BMAC is a reliable source of mesenchymal stem cells and growth factors, yielding some of the biological advantage of autogenous bone graft without the donor site morbidity [44]. BMAC requires a point of care centrifuge which isolates the stem cell layer of an aspirate or which there are several marketed. The concentrate can then be mixed with bone graft (auto- or allograft) or bone graft substitute. Theoretical benefits of BMAC are the ease of obtaining the graft without substantially prolonging surgery time and without donor site morbidity [45]. Two studies have been published supporting the use of BMAC added to a scaffold for repair of segmental bone loss, though multiple animal studies have demonstrated benefit in radiographic healing, bone histologic assessment, and torsional stiffness [46–48].

Principles of Induced Membrane Techniques

Described by AC Masquelet in the 1970s, the induced membrane technique is a two-stage procedure for the treatment of segmental bone defects [49]. Assuming prerequisite procedures for thorough debridement and infection eradication are completed, the initial procedure involves placing a PMMA cement spacer into the segmental defect. The cement spacer allows for length retention and dead space management while the patient's body forms a tissue layer, or induced membrane, around the spacer as a foreign body reaction. The spacer is shaped to fill as much space as possible and must be extended to wrap around the host bone ends for 2–3 cm [50]. The second stage utilizes this induced membrane by careful removal of the spacer and placing bone graft inside the space surrounded by membrane. Masquelet recommends a period of 6–10 weeks separate the two stages and strongly advised against using this technique in the setting of active infection [50].

Multiple basic science investigations have explored the biological activity of the induced membrane [51]. These indicate that the induced membrane is vascular, with maximum vascularity forming between 2 and 4 weeks. Mesenchymal stem cells capable of osteogenic differentiation are inherent to the membrane and/or effectively recruited by the membrane. Growth factors including bone morphogenetic protein-2 (BMP-2), vascular endothelial growth factor (VEGF), and transforming growth factor-β (TGF-β) have been identified in induced membranes, generally with maximal levels by 6 weeks. While these properties may lead to in situ osteogenesis, Masquelet reports that the induced membrane is most critical to contain autogenous bone graft placed into the biologically active membrane at the second procedure [50]. Extending the time between stages is not beneficial, and various investigations on varying the spacer material, composition, or texture have not shown benefit in bone healing beyond the original description using PMMA cement.

This technique has the advantage of greater accessibility to a wide spectrum of surgeons who may not have training or experience with circular external fixation/distraction osteogenesis. Avoiding an external fixator is also considered advantageous and is also not dependent on patient compliance with a distraction program. The disadvantages include the requirement for infection eradication, stable and contained soft tissue envelope, and need for stable fixation proximal and distal to the induced membrane site. The Masquelet technique was originally described for the treatment of bone loss associated with lower extremity infected nonunions but theoretically can be applied at any skeletal site where bone loss is present. However, it is most successful in contained, partial defects which may limit its effectiveness toward larger, segmental bone loss. Furthermore, regardless of bone grafting technique chosen, soft tissue management and proper boney stabilization is critical.

Principles of Distraction Osteogenesis

The technique used to restore lost bone using gradual bone distraction is called distraction osteogenesis. Classically described, distraction osteogenesis is achieved following a low-energy corticotomy to best preserve periosteal blood flow and a circular external frame suspended above and below the corticotomy which is pulled apart gradually, allowing the bone edges to regenerate bone in the corticotomy gap [5, 6]. Once the frame rings are further distracted until the targeted bone length is achieved, the intervening immature bone filling in the corticotomy gap ossifies. Once ossified, the circular frame is removed. The corticotomy and subsequent distraction osteogenesis is a technique that provides favorable biology to the injured limb by increased blood flow and eliciting the cascade of reparative processes like after fracture healing [52]. Gradual

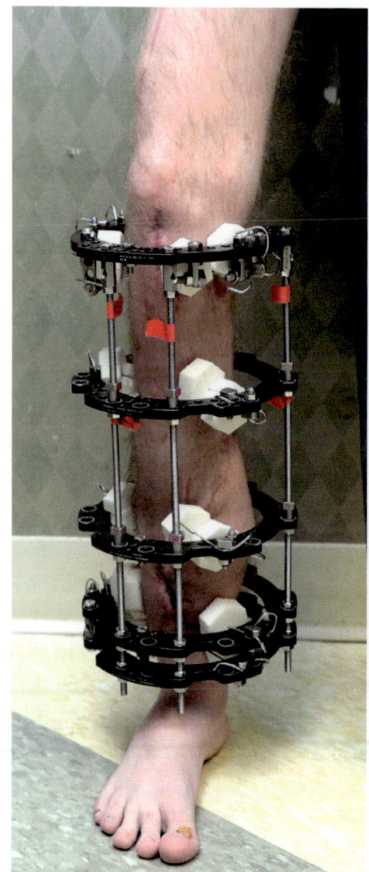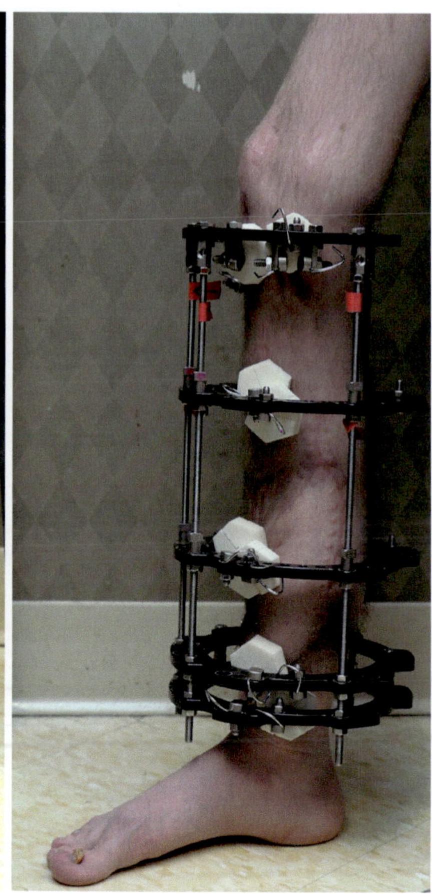

Fig. 9.1 Clinical photographs of a patient with a classic Ilizarov bone transport circular frame for an infected nonunion. The frame is suspended entirely with tensioned wires. Two levels of bone transport are achievable between the three spaced-out frame segments. Distally, the two closely spaced rings are useful to stabilize the distal frame to a small segment of distal tibial bone. Note the free flap coverage to the medial leg. (Used with permission from Rubin Institute for Advanced Orthopaedics, Sinai Hospital of Baltimore)

distraction also allows for soft tissue compliance of skin, muscle, and neurovascular structures [53]. While classically described by use of a circular, tensioned wire frame (Fig. 9.1), bone distraction can also be achieved by monolateral external fixation, hexapod circular frames, and now intramedullary lengthening/transport nails.

Bone Transport

Distraction osteogenesis methods can be used to distract bone at one site in order to move intervening bone toward a second site. By transporting a bone segment through a distracted corticotomy, a segmental defect can be filled. Once the transported bone meets the targeted host bone, this "docking" site then heals as would a fracture. Docking sites very commonly require a bone graft to promote healing, and this grafting procedure should be planned into the treatment schedule. Bone transport requires stabilization at the proximal and distal host segments and the intervening transported segment. A classic Ilizarov circular frame achieves bone transport by connecting suspended frame rings with threaded rods (Fig. 9.2). Nuts on the threaded rods are adjusted to slowly push the ring attached to the transported segment toward the docking site. The typical rate of distraction is 1 mm per day which is broken up into four frame adjustments, each 0.25 mm per adjustment. More rapid transport can result in poor bone regeneration and damage to soft tissue (nerve, vessels). Modifications to the classic Ilizarov frame include suspending the ring with half pins in addition to wires and using "clickers" along the rods to perform the gradual adjustment (Fig. 9.3).

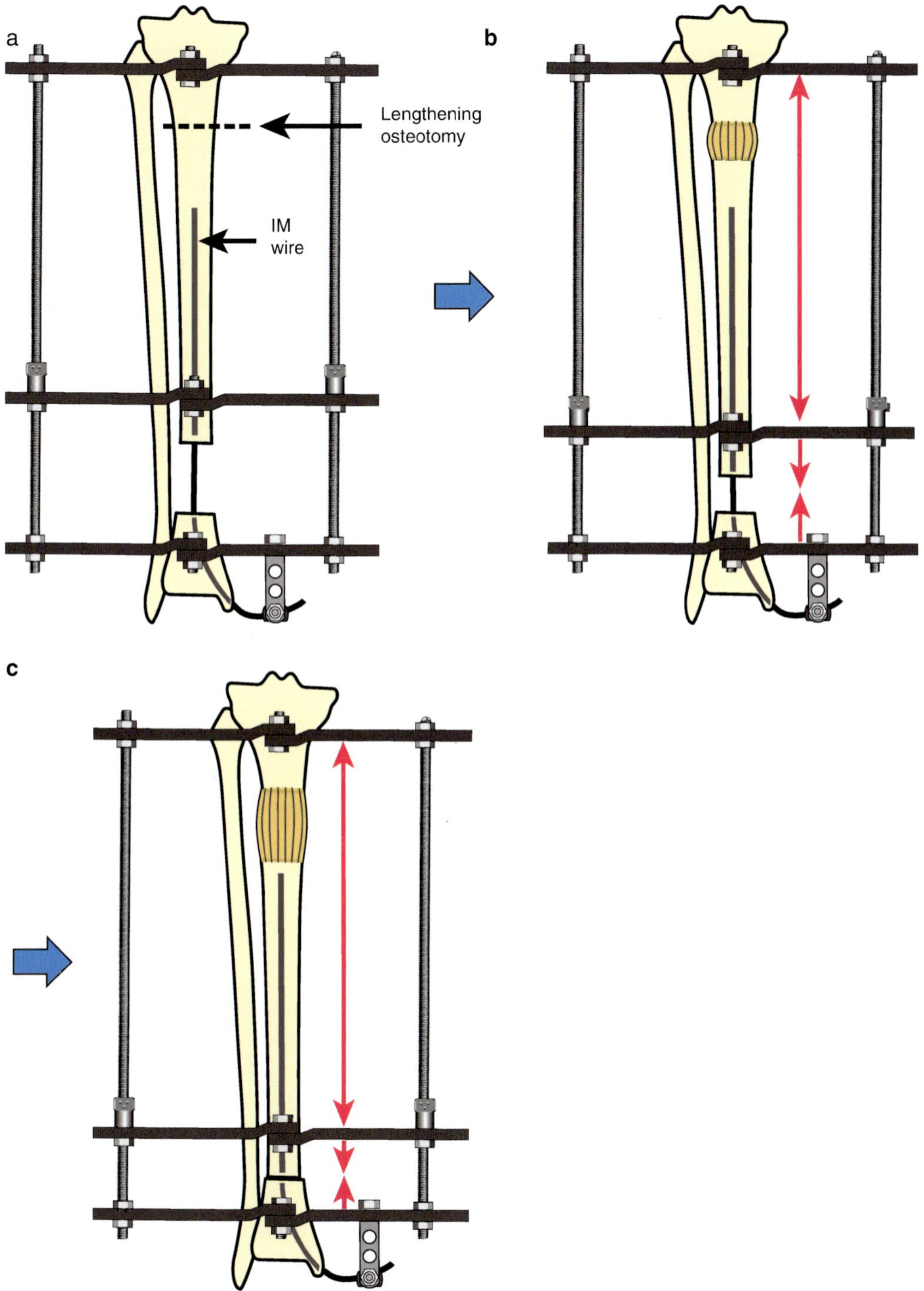

Fig. 9.2 Schematic of tibial bone transport for a tibial defect and intact fibula. (**a**) A proximal osteotomy is performed. (**b**) Long threaded rods between the proximal and middle rings are adjusted to lengthen the space between these top rings, while the threaded rods between the middle and distal rings are adjusted to shorten the distance between these bottom rings. (**c**) This results in the osteotomy being distracted while the bone loss distally is occupied by transported bone. A thin wire as depicted in (**a**) depicts one method to guide the transport while an alternative method is to use cables. (Used with permission from Rubin Institute for Advanced Orthopaedics, Sinai Hospital of Baltimore)

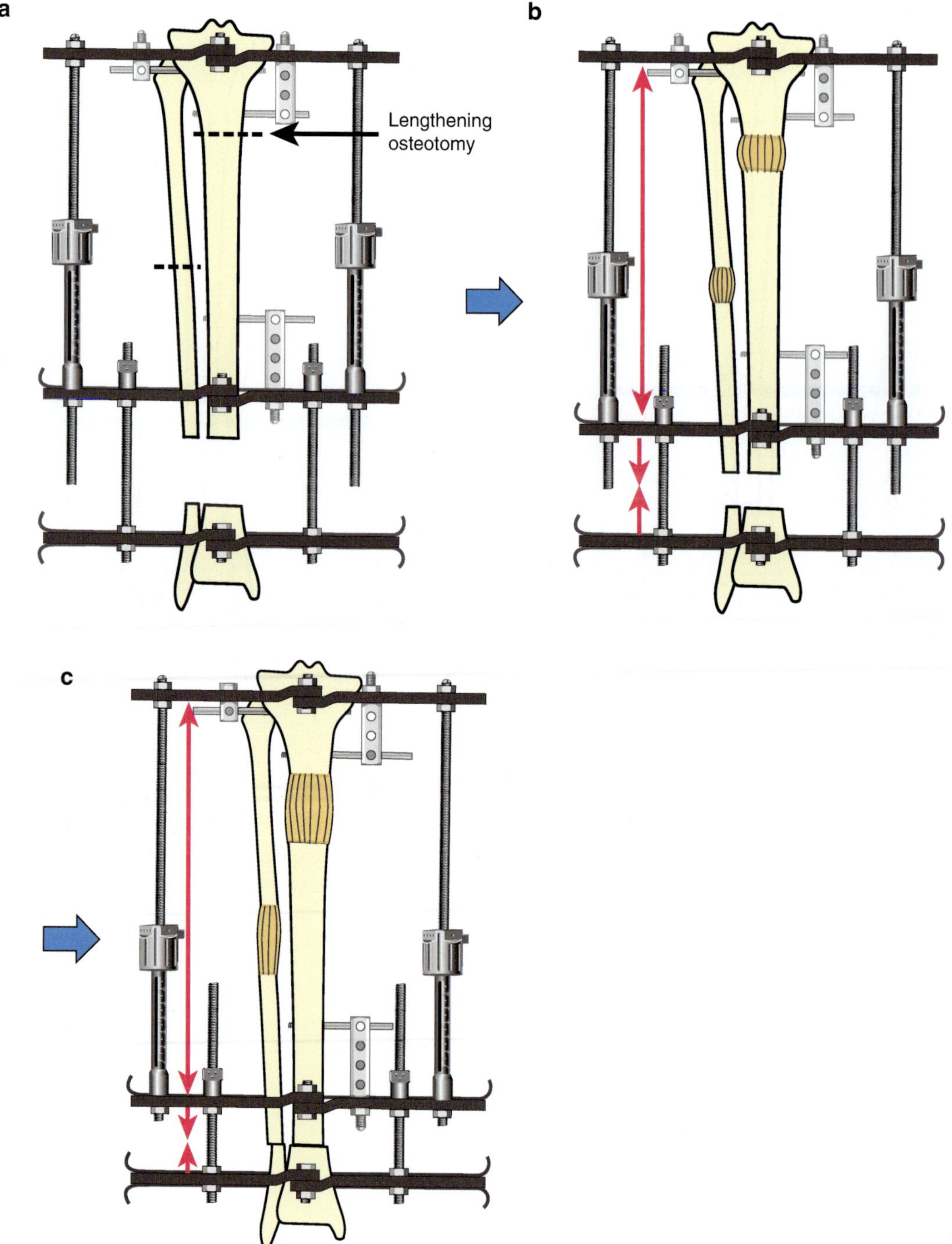

Fig. 9.3 Schematic of tibial bone transport for a tibial and fibular defect treated by simultaneous compression and distraction. (**a**) In this schematic, the fibula is also transported necessitating an osteotomy in the tibia and fibula. The rings are also fixed to the bone using a combination of thin wires and half pins. (**b**) Threaded rods are adjusted to lengthen the distance between the proximal and middle rings and shorten the distance between the middle and distal rings. The compression rate between the distal rings and the distraction rate between the proximal rings may be different: compression can easily be performed at 3–4 mm/day, while distraction should not exceed 1 mm/day. (**c**) This results in docked transport of both tibia and fibula. (Used with permission from Rubin Institute for Advanced Orthopaedics, Sinai Hospital of Baltimore)

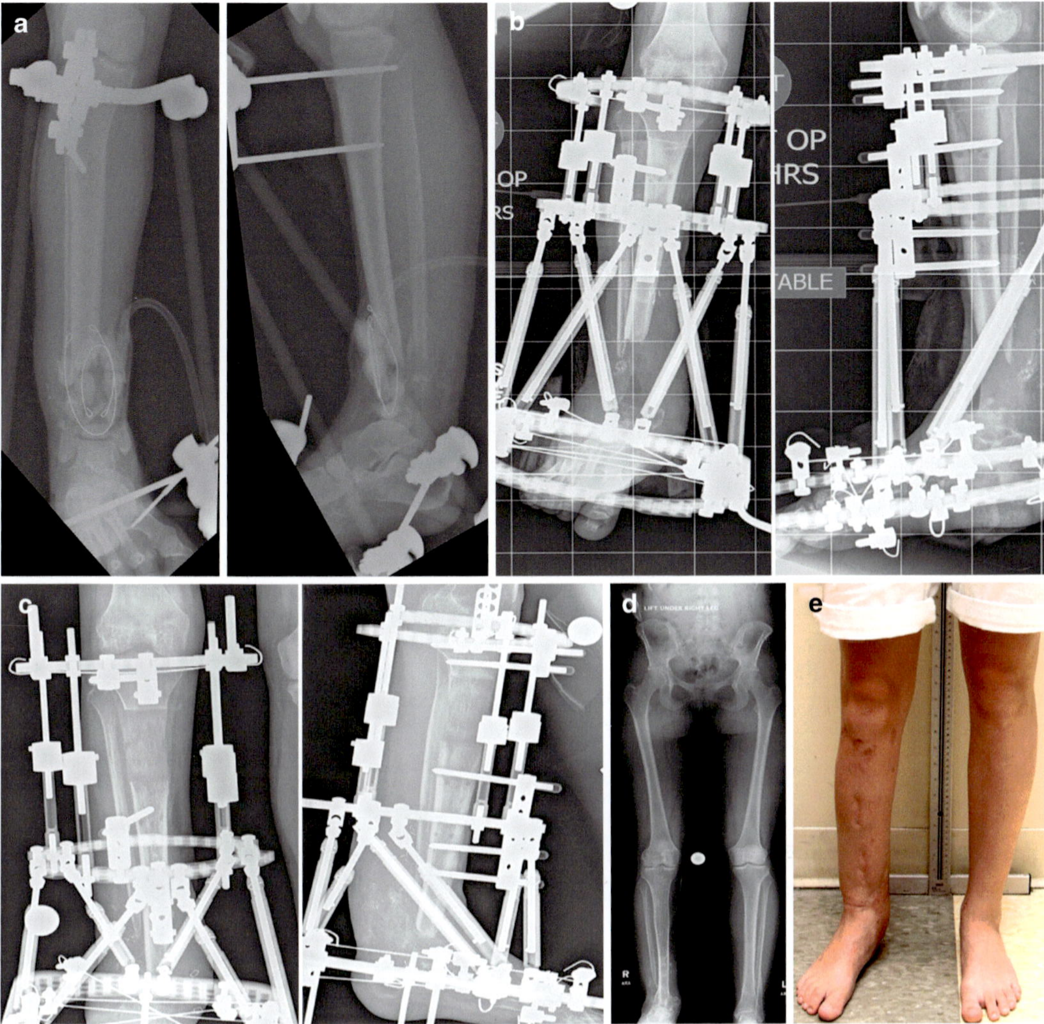

Fig. 9.4 Clinical example of hybrid frame used for bone transport. (**a**) Anteroposterior and lateral radiographs of a patient with distal tibia segmental bone loss after an ATV accident. Initial stabilization was achieved with a delta frame and antibiotic beads. (**b**) Anteroposterior and lateral radiographs of the patient following hybrid circular frame placement. Distraction will be performed from an osteotomy between the proximal and middle rings. The hexapod struts between the middle and distal rings will align the tibial-talar fusion. (**c**) Anteroposterior and lateral radiographs of the patient after the transport is completed proximally and fusion docked distally. (**d**) Erect leg anteroposterior radiograph and (**e**) clinical photograph of the patient following healing. Note the long column of healed regenerate bone. (Used with permission from Rubin Institute for Advanced Orthopaedics, Sinai Hospital of Baltimore)

Cable transport systems have also been used to lessen the drag on soft tissues that are seen with transverse wires and half pins [54].

Other frame configurations including monolateral and hexapod frames can also be used for bone transport. Hexapod frame offers the advantage of being able to correct angular or translational deformities that occur as the transported bone approaches the docking site (Fig. 9.4). One hybrid method is to perform the bulk of the bone transport with Ilizarov threaded rods and then convert the frame to a hexapod frame toward the completion of transport to fine-tune angular or translational corrections at the docking site [54].

Modifications to the classic Ilizarov bone transport methods have attempted to decrease

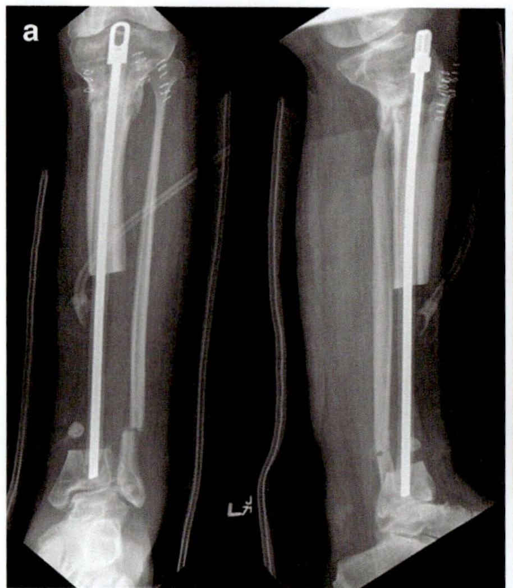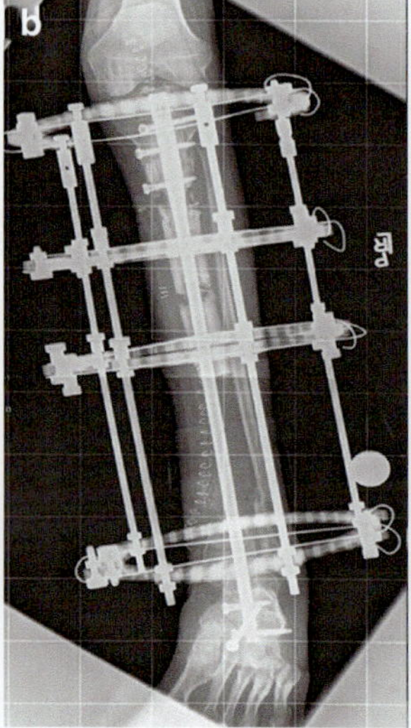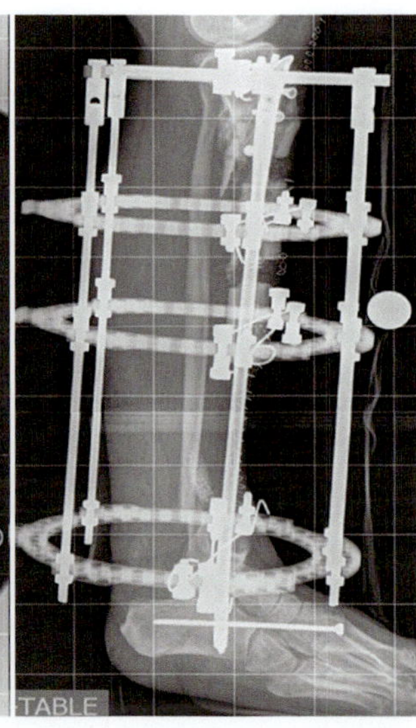

Fig. 9.5 Clinical example of a multilevel bone transport for a 14 cm post-infection segmental defect of the tibia. (**a**) Anteroposterior and lateral radiographs of defect stabilized with an antibiotic-coated rod constructed with an Ilizarov threaded rod. (**b**) Anteroposterior and lateral radiographs of the patient undergoing double-level bone transport over a conventional locked intramedullary nail. Note the distraction gap between the proximal and second rings and the second distraction gap between the second and third rings. The intramedullary nail stabilizes and guides the transported fragment. (Used with permission from Rubin Institute for Advanced Orthopaedics, Sinai Hospital of Baltimore)

transport time and healing time. One modification that does decrease transport time is to use multiple transport sites through more than one corticotomy [55, 56]. With both sites distracting, desired bone segment lengthening can be achieved faster; and the resultant two small distraction regenerates theoretically can heal more rapidly compared to one long regenerate (Fig. 9.5). While multifocal distraction may theoretically reduce "frame time," soft tissues may not tolerate a 1 mm per day distraction at both sites necessitating a slower distraction rate per site [54]. Additionally, slow regenerate bone formation may necessitate slowing the distraction rate.

Other modifications or alternatives to classic circular frame bone transport include performing the bone transport with a plate or nail in place to confer stability and potentially allow for faster frame removal [57–59]. Bone transport over a nail is particularly useful to guide transport trajectory and decrease docking site alignment adjustment (Fig. 9.6). In a pooled study of tibial lengthenings, patients with hardware in place (nail or plate) while undergoing lengthening with a circular frame had significantly less time in frame compared to patients treated with the frame alone (7 months versus 11 months) [59]. The sequential combination of external and intramedullayry fixation is also a viable strategy, with the external frame lengthening/correction completed first, followed by nailing at the time of frame removal [60]. Similarly, lengthening with a stabilizing plate in place or plating after lengthening confers similar advantages to decrease frame time [61, 62].

Acute Shortening and Deformation

Another application of distraction osteogenesis in the setting of trauma is intentional shortening and/or deformation of the extremity followed by gradual distraction to restore the limb length and correct deformity (Fig. 9.7). This is particularly useful in the setting of bone and soft tissue loss where acute shortening/deformation then allows for primary wound closure and as an alternative to flap coverage [63–65]. Because soft tissue is

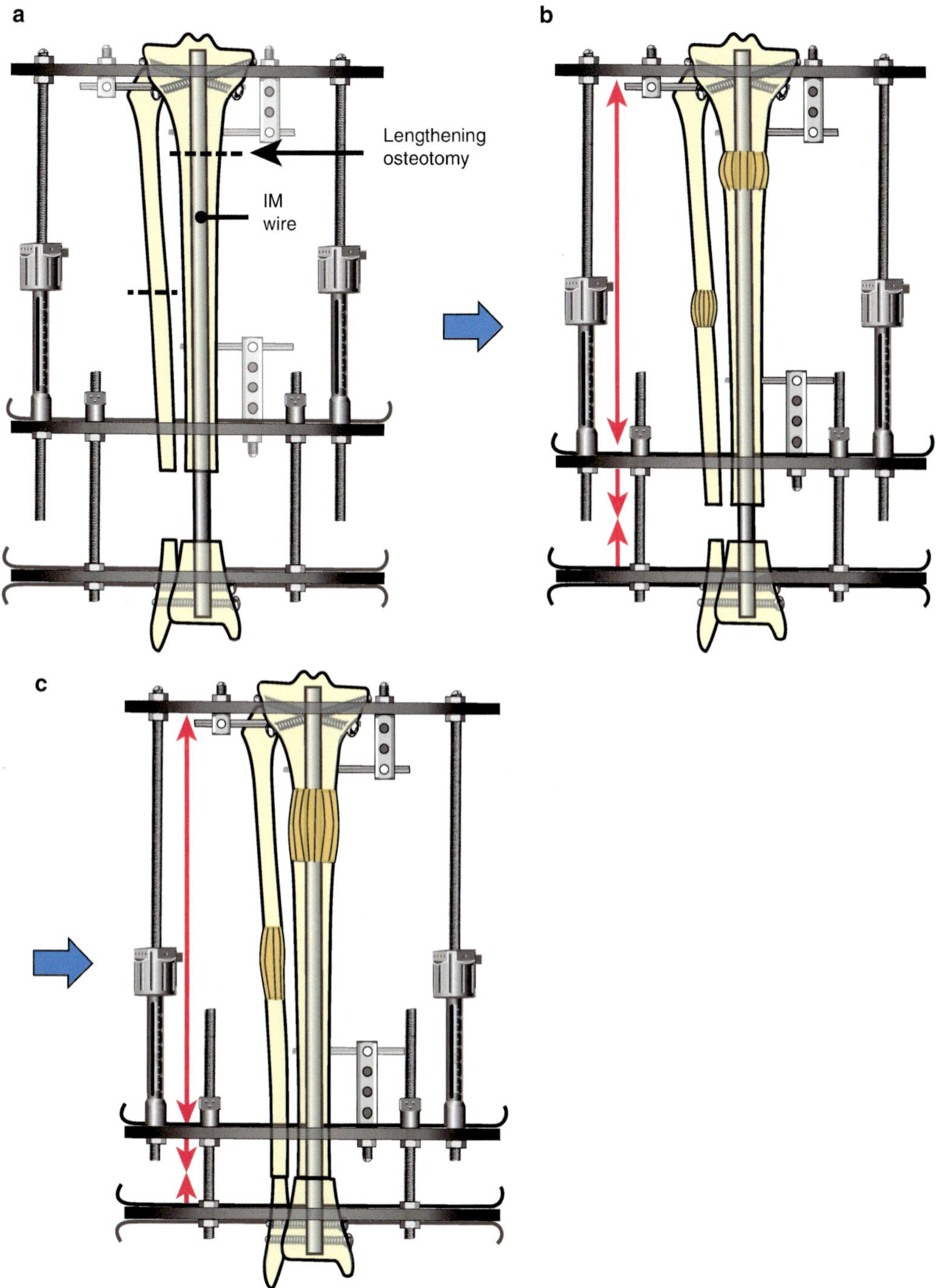

Fig. 9.6 Schematic of bone transport over a nail. (**a**) An intramedullary rod is locked with the bone out to length proximally and distally. (**b**) Ilizarov threaded rods with clickers are depicted transporting the bone distally from a proximal metadiaphyseal osteotomy. (**c**) With docking, the distal ring block is adjusted to apply compression at the docking site. The entire transport is stabilized and guided by the intramedullary rod. (Used with permission from Rubin Institute for Advanced Orthopaedics, Sinai Hospital of Baltimore)

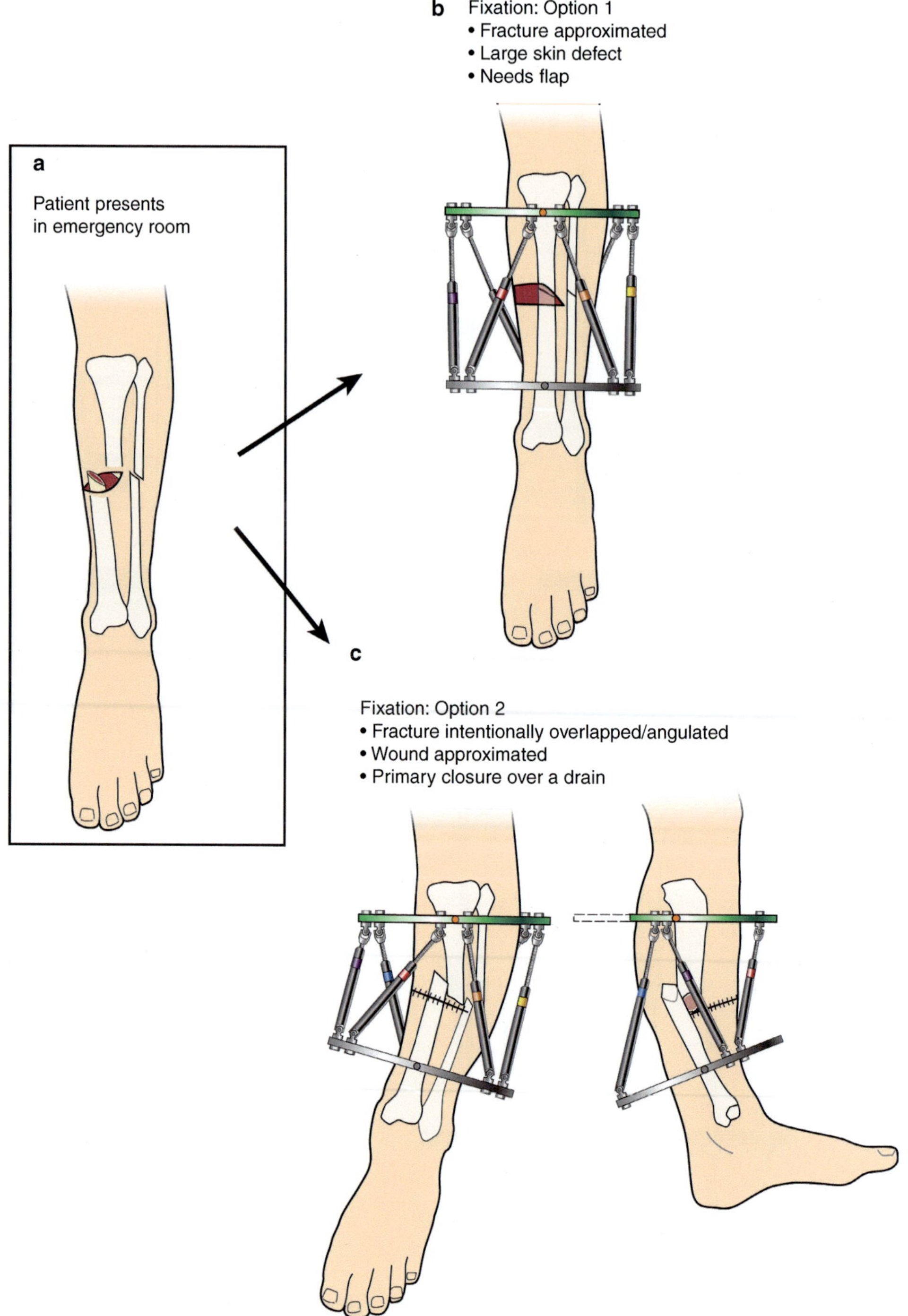

Fig. 9.7 Schematic of acute shortening for (**a**) composite bone and soft tissue injury. (**b**) The injury may be fixed with the bone out to length, rendering the soft tissue unclosable. (**c**) The injury may be fixed with the bone shortened and/or angulated to allow the soft tissue to be closed. After 3 weeks, the soft tissue envelope is suffi- ciently healed to begin distraction and realignment of the bone. (**d–f**) Anteroposterior and (**d–f**) lateral schematics of the circular hexapod frame gradually correcting the length and angulation after the soft tissue healing allows. (Used with permission from Rubin Institute for Advanced Orthopaedics, Sinai Hospital of Baltimore)

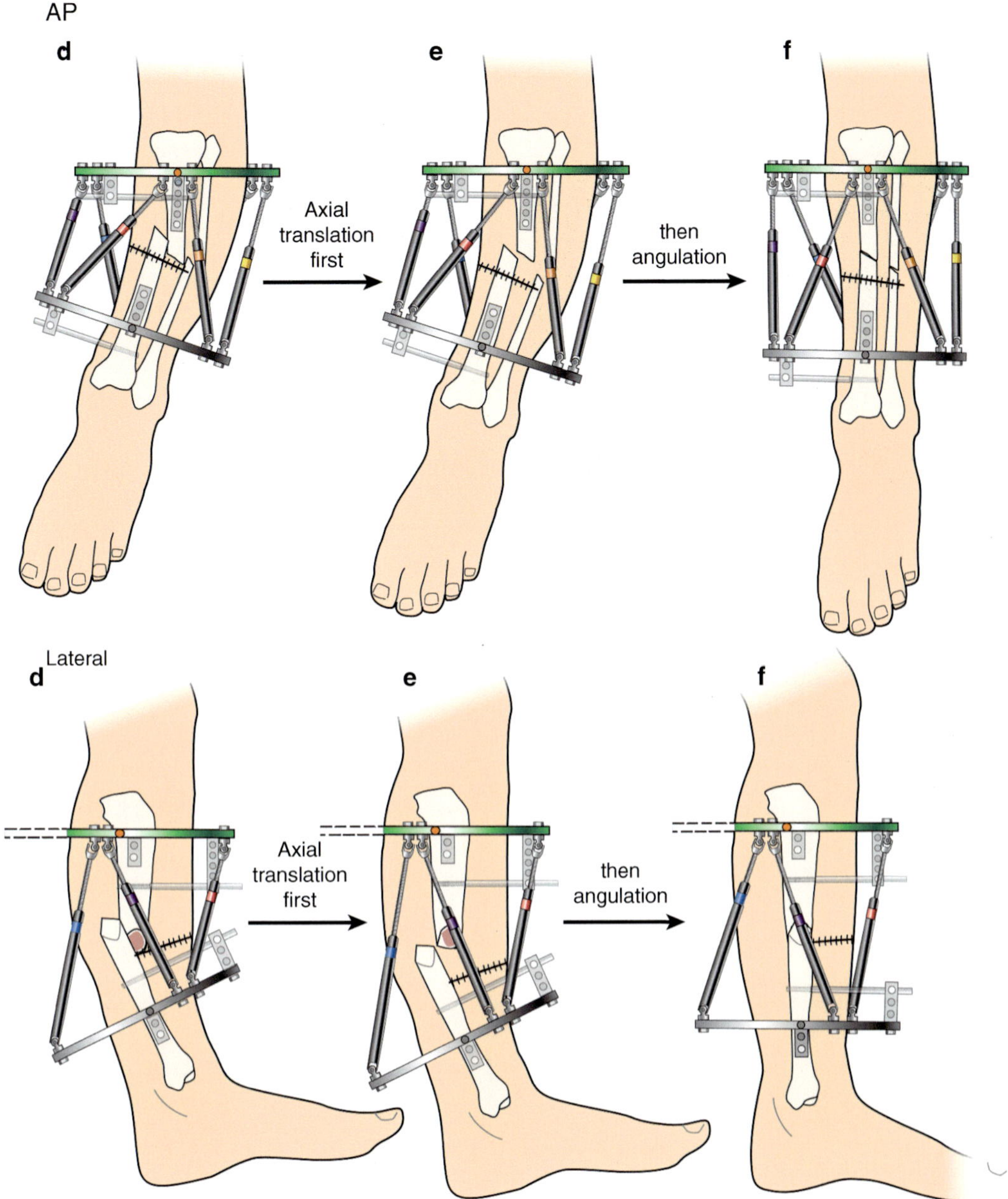

Fig. 9.7 (continued)

also amenable to gradual distraction, length and deformity correction following soft tissue healing is possible. Some authors suggest a limit to how much a limb can be acutely shortened with a suggested cut of 8 cm secondary to kinking or bending of intact vasculature [66]. Intraoperative vascular monitoring should be used during shortening/deformation procedures as changes in Doppler signal may define the limb's neurovascular structure toleration, particularly for imposed angulations [67]. Compared to bone transport for treatment of segmental tibial defects, acute shortening followed by distraction yields similar success rates with slightly fewer complications, particularly related to the soft tissue and potentially less subsequent bone grafting [68].

Internal Lengthening Techniques

Circular frame bone transport and lengthening is an exceptionally powerful tool; however, many surgeons and patients prefer not to use external devices if possible. Since the 1980s a number of telescoping internal lengthening nail iterations have been developed, initially driven by ratcheting mechanisms and more recently by an externally controlled magnetic drive mechanism [69–71]. Internal lengthening nails achieve bone transport as currently designed when used in combination with a plate to stabilize the transport. This technique is known as plate-assisted bone segment transport, or PABST. As currently designed these magnetic telescoping nails can be used to push bone by lengthening into a segmental gap (Fig. 9.8) or "pull" bone by shortening a pre-lengthened nail (Fig. 9.9). Newer designs permit transport without accessory plates, though experience as this time is limited.

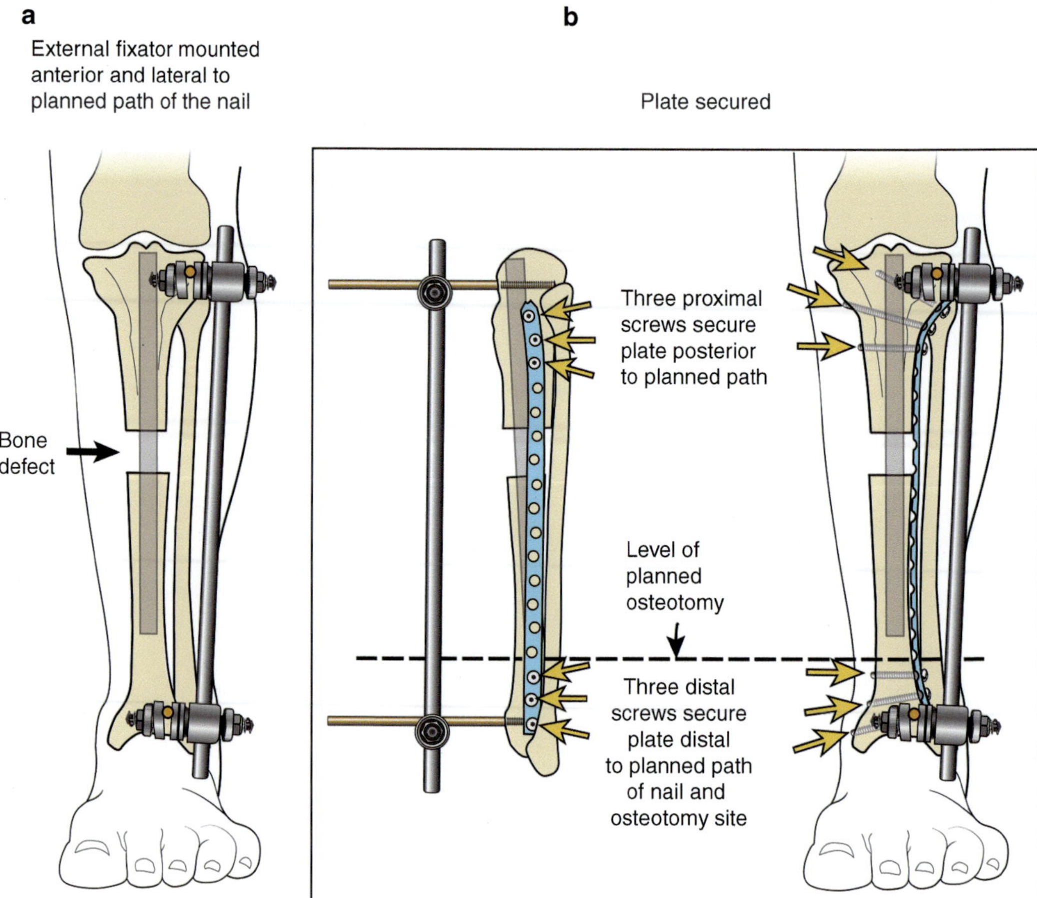

Fig. 9.8 Schematic of an internal lengthening nail/plate hybrid construct as a method to transport bone in the femur, so called plate-assisted bone segment transport (PABST). (**a**) The defect may be provisionally stabilized with an external fixator. (**b**) The definitive method to stabilize the bone while the transport is underway is with a long locking plate. (**c**) An osteotomy is made at least 4–6 cm from the telescoping end of the nail. (**d**) The nail is inserted and locked proximally and distally. Once the (**e**) external fixator is removed lengthening can begin. Note the thin portion of the nail telescoping out of the thicker portion of the nail. (**f**) Once the bone transport is completed, the docking site is allowed to heal with or without supplemental bone grafting. (Used with permission from Rubin Institute for Advanced Orthopaedics, Sinai Hospital of Baltimore)

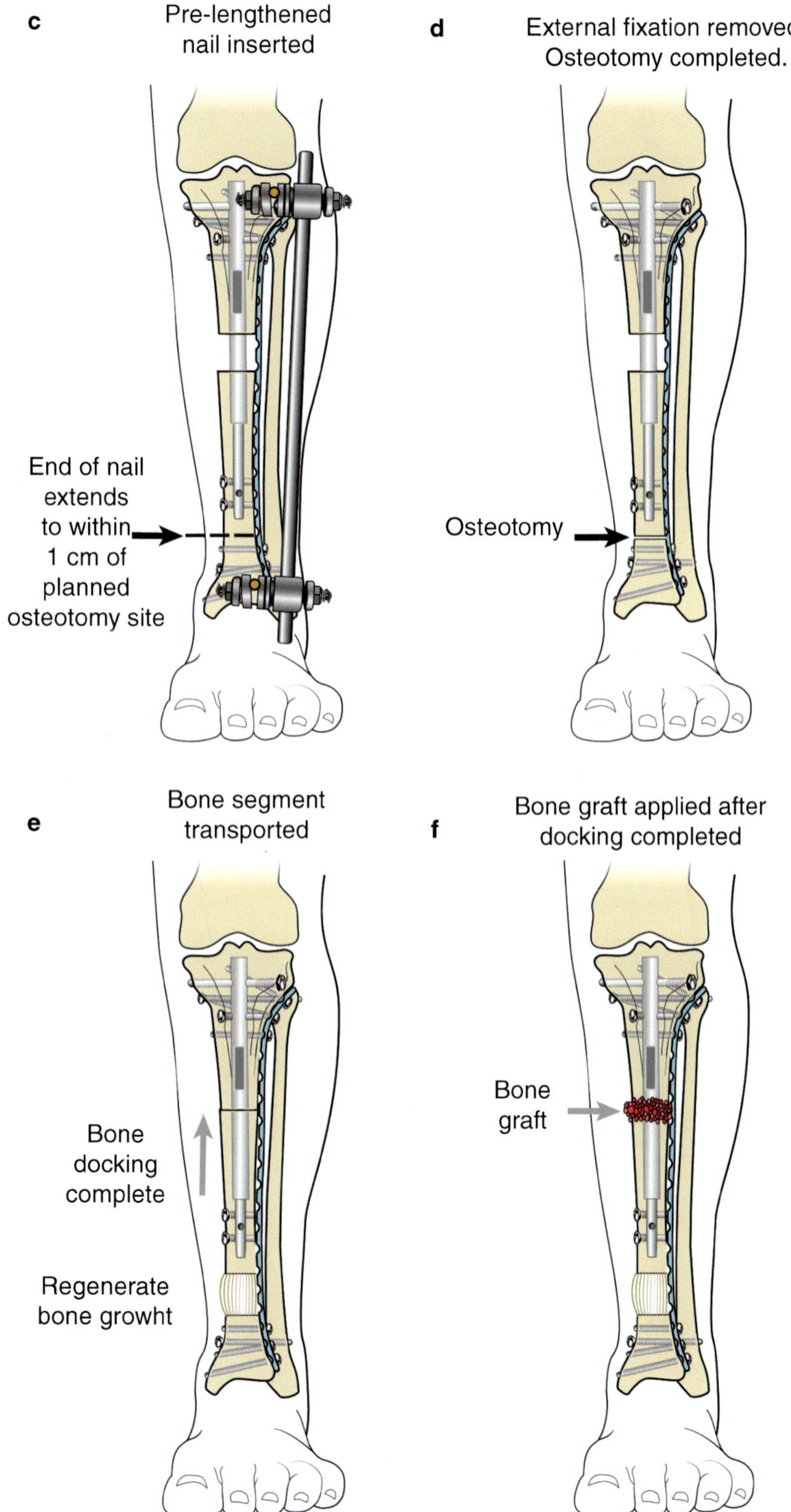

Fig. 9.8 (continued)

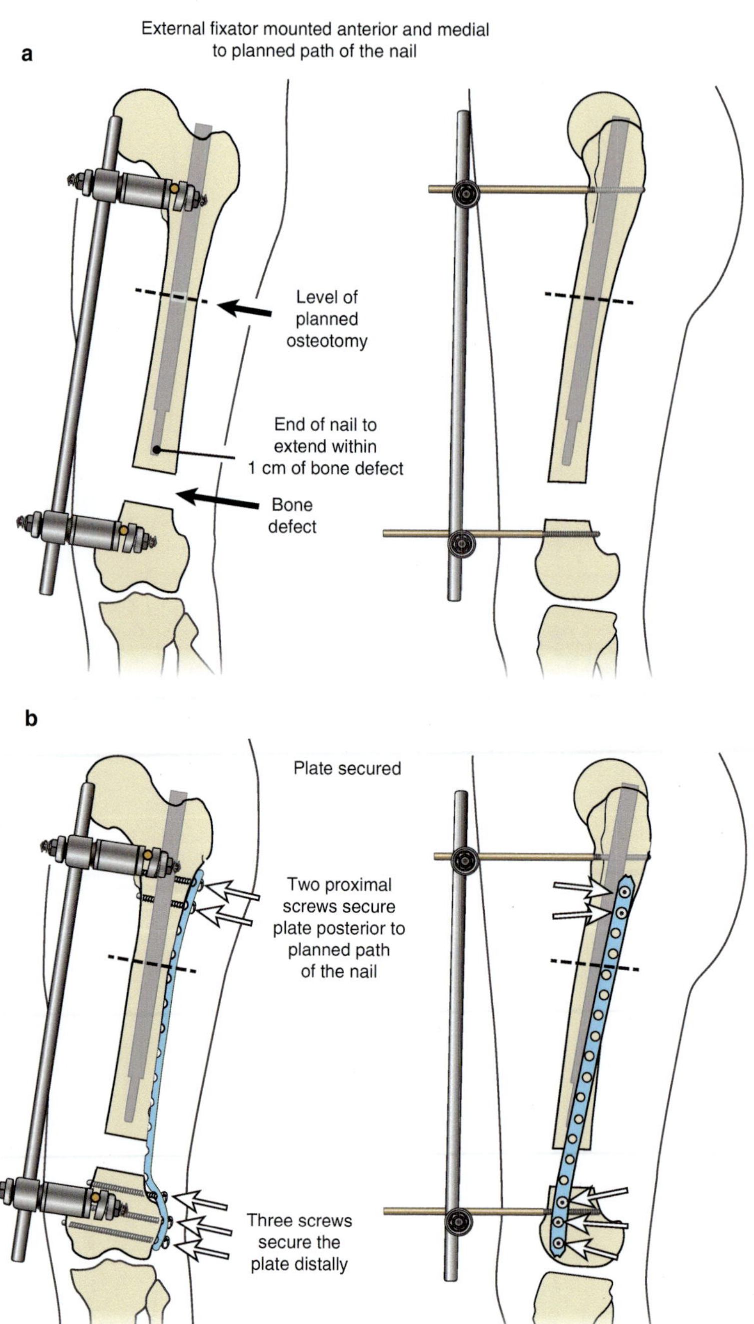

Fig. 9.9 Schematic of an internal lengthening nail as a method to transport bone in the tibia, so-called plate-assisted bone segment transport (PABST). (**a**) This example will depict how an osteotomy distal to the planned nail will be filled by "pulling" the transported bone proximally. (**b**) The defect may be provisionally stabilized with an external fixator. (**c**) The definitive method to stabilize the bone while the transport is underway is with a locking plate. (**d**) The telescoping internal lengthening nail is pre-lengthened on the back table the same distance that will be required to transport the bone. (**e**) An osteotomy is made distally at a favorable metadiaphyseal location and lengthening can begin. (**f**) The nail is then gradually shortened while "pulling" the transported bone segment into the diaphyseal defect. (**g**) Once the bone transport is completed, the docking site is allowed to heal with or without supplemental bone grafting. (Used with permission from Rubin Institute for Advanced Orthopaedics, Sinai Hospital of Baltimore)

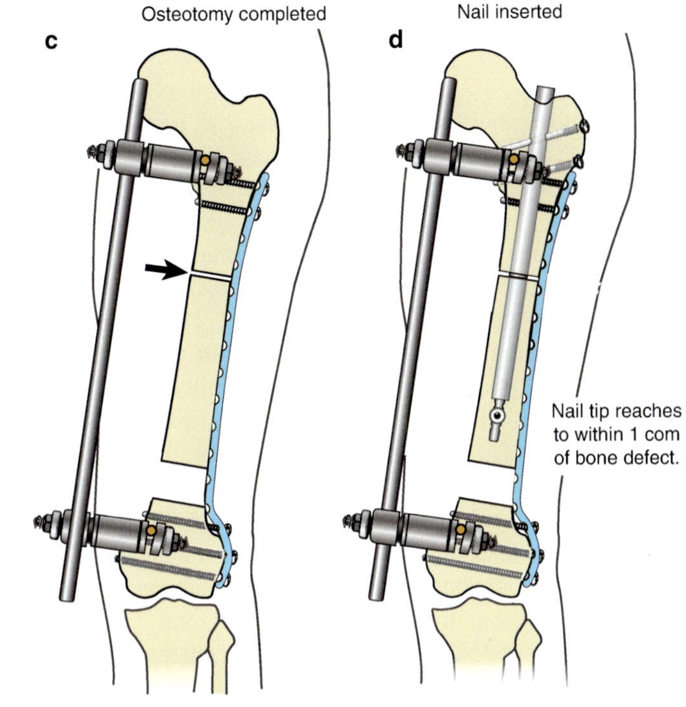

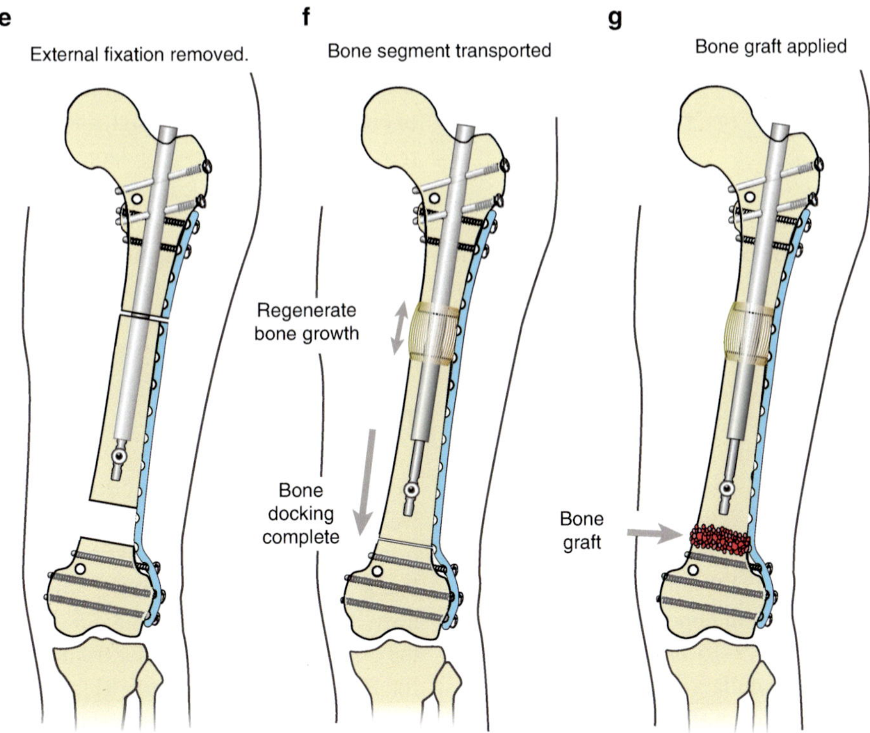

Fig. 9.9 (continued)

Evidence-Based Approach to Segmental Defects per Skeletal Site

Well-controlled studies on any of the abovementioned techniques are lacking with the bulk of the current peer-reviewed literature being case series and expert opinion (level IV and V evidence). Additionally, many case series describe combinations of techniques (e.g., induced membrane plus vascularized fibula graft, bone transport plus bone marrow aspirate concentrate, etc.), further confounding conclusions on individual approaches. It may be concluded that in the face of complex extremity reconstruction challenges, surgeons should use the tools that work best in their hands. Here below the authors have attempted to summarize the available data on useful techniques per skeletal site and continue to emphasize regard for the patient's physiology, meticulous soft tissue management, and proper understanding of the surgeon's skill set, institutional support, and patient's psychosocial support as critical to successful treatment and should influence the selected treatment plan.

Femur

For femoral defects <5 cm or for partial defects which do not involve the entire cortical width, induced membrane or other local grafting techniques work reliably. There are no large series of patients treated with induced membrane techniques in the femur; however, several small series describe high success rates for union. Wu et al. reported 19 cases with femoral bone loss averaging 5.5 cm (range 2–10.9 cm) [72]. All patients underwent internal fixation and autograft or auto- and allograft mixture placement following the induced membrane. All femora united. Yu et al. reported 13 cases with femoral bone loss averaging 9.8 cm (range 5–16 cm) [73]. All patients underwent intramedullary rod fixation for stabilization at the time of grafting following induced membrane. All femora united. Eight patients with femoral defects ranging from 1 cm to 25 cm underwent induced membrane technique fol-

lowed by autogenous bone grafting harvested by RIA. All but one femur healed by 1 year. In a small series of cases comparing induced membrane techniques versus bone transport in the femur, Tong et al. found that periarticular femoral defects were more amenable to induced membrane [75]. While a small series, this paper in particular highlights the application of induced membrane technique in periarticular areas which may not be treatable with external fixation and bone transport. The induced membrane at these sites allows for controlled grafting even up against subchondral bone.

Large defects are best treated with distraction osteogenesis. Circular external fixation, however, is challenging and poorly tolerated on the thigh. Therefore, hybrid frames or monolateral frames are an option. A systematic review by Kadhim et al. reported combined data on 96 cases indicating that monolateral frames used to bone transport femoral segmental bone defects yields 99% rate of union and good functional results in 94% [76]. Use of circular frames in this comparison resulted in a lower union rate (89%) and substantially worse function (57% good functional results). This review demonstrates the challenges of circular frames on the thigh and highlights that pins and wires traversing large muscle groups can result in more soft tissue problems including functional limitation. Monolateral bone transport in the femur is further supported by multiple studies including good to excellent results and high union rates [77–80].

Tibia

In contrast to the femur, circular fixation is a well-supported method for segmental reconstruction in the tibia. Monolateral fixators can be used but are associated with more iatrogenic deformity, residual shortening, and pin site infection in the tibia compared to circular frames, particularly for larger defects (>6 cm) [81]. Bone transport with circular fixation is also supported in systematic reviews including segmental bone defect cases [76, 82]. Kadhim et al. included 334 tibiae in their review, reporting a 99% union rate and good functional outcomes when segmental bone loss was treated with a combined circular frame bone transport plus internal stabilization with a nail or plate [76]. Other substantial series demonstrate positive results. For example, Yin et al. reported 91% union primary rate in 66 patients with tibial segmental defects averaging 6 cm (range 3–13 cm) [83]. The ununited tibiae were all successfully salvaged by bone grafting at the transport docking site. Peng et al. also report a 91% success rate in 58 patients with tibial infected nonunions resulting in an average 9 cm segmental defect (range 6–15 cm) [84]. Napora et al. reported the use of hexapod frames for tibial bone transport in 75 patients with average segmental bone loss of 5.4 cm [85]. All but five patients (93%) achieved successful union. In another study, 55 tibial nonunions were treated by either Ilizarov circular fixator or Taylor Spatial Frame hexapod fixator following nonunion resection. Union was achieved without additional surgery in 49/55 (89%) of patients [86]. Arslan et al. reported on eight pediatric patients with segmental bone loss associated with open tibia fractures with an average defect of 5.4 cm (range 4.5–8.5 cm) [87]. Additional, smaller studies support bone transport for tibial segmental bone loss [88–91].

Compared to induced membrane treatment, bone transport for tibial segmental defects was found to achieve similar union results as the abovementioned Tong et al. study [75]. Defect size averaged 6.7 cm (range 2.7–15.7 cm). One patient treated with induced membrane required one transport for eventual healing due to a recurrent infection. Functional outcomes did differ between the groups, favoring induced membrane technique for reasons cited related to prolonged frame time. Sadek et al. compared Masquelet to bone transport in patients with tibial nonunions with segmental bone loss less than 6 cm [93]. In this series of 30 patients, follow-up bone grafting was no different between treatments, and functional results related to foot/ankle range of motion were better in the induced membrane group [93]. Karger et al. reported union in 53 of 61 (87%) tibial defects treated with induced membrane [12]. Nineteen tibial nonunions

treated with induced membrane followed by RIA bone grafting resulted in 17/19 (89%) healed by 1 year [74]. Other reports suggest good outcomes with small or partial tibial defects treated with induced membrane method; however, most studies have mixed populations which do not always have bone and defect size clearly specified and surgical techniques not always described [94–97]. This is particularly pertinent for studies reporting on segmental defects following infection, as eradication of infection is a critical step prior to embarking on an induced membrane treatment [92, 98, 99]. Also pertinent to the tibia is the option to utilize the fibula as graft and/or supplement the bone healing by creating a synostosis between the tibia and fibula.

Humerus

The humerus is amenable to shortening and bone loss up to 3 cm may be treated with acute shortening. For larger segments, vascularized autograft or strut allograft with plate fixation has been reported in small case series. Kamrani et al. published a series of nine patients with distal humeral nonunions treated with vascularized radial forearm bone flap [100]. Eight of the nine patients healed without additional surgery; and all achieved functional improvements. Adani et al. published in 13 cases of vascular fibula graft for humeral segmental defects averaging 12.3 cm (range 10–16 cm) [101]. While five cases in this series required revision surgery, the authors reported good to excellent functional results in all patients. Ilizarov bone transport may be used in the humerus, though is thought to be less well tolerated than in the lower extremity. One series of ten patients with an average segmental human defect of 6 cm (range 3–9 cm) was reported to achieve excellent functional and radiographic results. Liu et al. published on acute shortening followed by humeral lengthenings averaging 9.5 cm (range 5.5–13.4 cm) resulting in 10 of 11 patients with successful healing [102, 103]. The induced membrane technique is also theoretically possible for the humerus, though only described in scattered case reports. One important caveat to using cement spacers in the humerus is that caution must be exercised to protect the radial nerve from the exothermic reaction that occurs as PMMA is setting.

Forearm

The induced membrane technique is well tolerated in the forearm. Prasarn et al. published a series of 15 forearms treated with the induced membrane and subsequent iliac crest bone grafting for defects averaging 2.1 cm (range 1–7 cm). All bones healed without infection [104]. Lou et al. published a smaller series of seven patients with larger defects (average 5.8 cm; range 4–8 cm), all of whom healed without infection and with good functional results [105]. Walker et al. likewise published a series of nine patients with defects averaging 4.7 cm (range 1.7–5.4 cm) treated with induced membrane and second stage bone grafting with RIA autogenous graft in eight patients and iliac crest autograft in one [106]. All patients healed with only patient requiring hardware revision. Vascularized fibula grafts and bone transport have also been reported in small series. Cano-Luis et al. published on 14 patients who underwent vascularized fibula graft for segmental defects ranging from 6 to 11 cm and including four cases where both the radius and ulna were reconstructed [107]. Twelve of 14 cases healed and functional results found to be satisfactory. Eleven of 12 patients in a series by Adani et al. healed bone defects ranging between 6 and 13 cm with vascularized fibular graft [108]. Two studies by Zhang et al. and Lui et al. reported on 16 cases and 21 cases, respectively, of bone transport in the forearm [109, 110]. Both series involved cases with segmental loss averaging approximately 3 cm (ranges 2.2–7.5 cm and 1.8–4.6 cm, respectively). All forearms in both series healed with four patients in the Lui et al. series requiring docking site grafting.

In summary, both bone transport and the Masquelet techniques can theoretically be used at each long bone segment for bone loss. However, the literature tends to support the application of bone transport for defects in the humerus and larger defects in the lower extremities while Masquelet technique is reasonably supported in the forearm and smaller and partial defects in the lower extremities (Table 9.1). The soft tissue status must always be considered and optimized, particularly as second stage Masquelet grafting and transport docking site bone grafting is planned at the onset of treatment. Given the complex nature of the injuries and conditions that result in segmental bone loss, it is also important that the patient's expectations for staged surgeries, multiple procedures, and likelihood of complications be appropriately managed. Finally, we emphasize the importance of a cumulative assessment of the overall patient physiology and psychosocial support and the surgeon's skill set and supportive healthcare team/services when formulating a treatment strategy for complex extremity injuries.

Table 9.1 Summary points of treatment options per bone segment based on supportive literature

	Bone transport	Masquelet technique
Humerus	Large defects (>5 cm) Hybrid, monolateral frames better tolerated	
Radius/ulna		Any sized defect Soft tissue envelope must be stable over spacer
Femur	Large defects (>5 cm) Hybrid, monolateral frames better tolerated	Small defect (<5 cm) Partial defects
Tibia	Large defects (>5 cm) Circular frames result in less deformity	Small defect (<5 cm) Partial defects Soft tissue envelope must be stable over spacer

Case 9.1: Bone Graft After Cement Spacer (Masquelet Technique)

History: A 36-year-old male sustained a right femur fracture in a bicycle accident 8 months prior which was treated with intramedullary nailing and complicated by surgical site infection. At the initial treating hospital, cultures obtained during one of the three subsequent irrigation and debridements were positive for *Staphylococcus aureus*. He was treated with 12 weeks of IV antibiotics. On exam, he had a chronic draining sinus over the right mid thigh and a gross limb length discrepancy right < left. He had palpable dorsalis pedis and posterior tibial artery pulses. Radiographs (Case Fig. 9.10) showed atrophic nonunion of the midshaft femur.

Treatment: The patient was taken to surgery where 11 cm of nonunion was resected and thorough soft tissue debridement performed. An antibiotic cement-coated intramedullary rod was placed for length and rotational stability. A PMMA spacer was then fashioned to fill the segmental defect (Case Fig. 9.11a). Eight weeks later, the spacer was removed and a new intramedullary nail was exchanged. The RIA reamer was used to harvest autograft from the contralateral femur, yielding about 40cc of graft material which was then placed in the defect held by the PMMA spacer and the area bone grafted using autograft obtained from the contralateral femur by RIA (Case Fig. 9.11b).

Outcome: The patient went on to heal the segmental defect with minimal limb length difference (Case Fig. 9.12).

> **Clinical Pearls and Pitfalls**
> - Persistent infection is associated with induced membrane graft failure. Assure that infection is adequately surgically and medically treated.
> - Inadequate soft tissue stabilization can promote recurrence of infection. An intramedullary nail stabilizes both the bone and soft tissue and allows for weight bearing and therapy participation between staged procedures.

Case 9.2 Bone Transport

History: A 17-year-old male sustained a left 3B open tibia fracture after being struck by a car. Initial stabilization, antibiotic spacer placement, and free flap coverage were performed at an outside hospital. He presented with provisional delta frame in place and stable, closed soft tissue envelope. His exam indicated palpable dorsalis pedis and posterior tibial artery pulses. Radiographs demonstrated segmental defect of the mid to distal tibia temporized with delta frame and antibiotic spacer (Case Fig. 9.13).

Treatment: He underwent debridement to an 8 cm total defect. A circular frame was fashioned with a 155 mm proximal 2/3 ring, two 155 mm full rings, and a 140 mm full ring distally using a combination of tensioned thin wires and half pins. The proximal tibio-fibular joints were stabilized. A proximal and distal tibial osteotomy was performed to achieve double-level transport of bone from both proximal and distal tibial segments to fill the midshaft bone loss (Case Fig. 9.14a). After 3 months of transport, the docking site was stabilized with the addition of half pins to the frame and bone grafted using autogenous graft obtained using the RIA reamer (Case Fig. 9.14b).

Outcome: After an additional 3 months, the frame was removed (Case Fig. 9.15a). The patient went on to heal without additional procedure (Case Fig. 9.15b).

> **Clinical Pearls and Pitfalls**
> - Two levels of distraction facilitate faster transport to fill in defect and less frame time. The distal and proximal osteotomies were both at metaphyseal areas of the bone rather than two proximal osteotomies which would have included a tibial diaphyseal distraction.
> - Frames can be modified during the treatment course if needed such as in this case where additional stability was warranted at the docking site at the time of bone grafting.
> - Failure to stabilize the tibio-fibular joints can result in migration of the fibula.

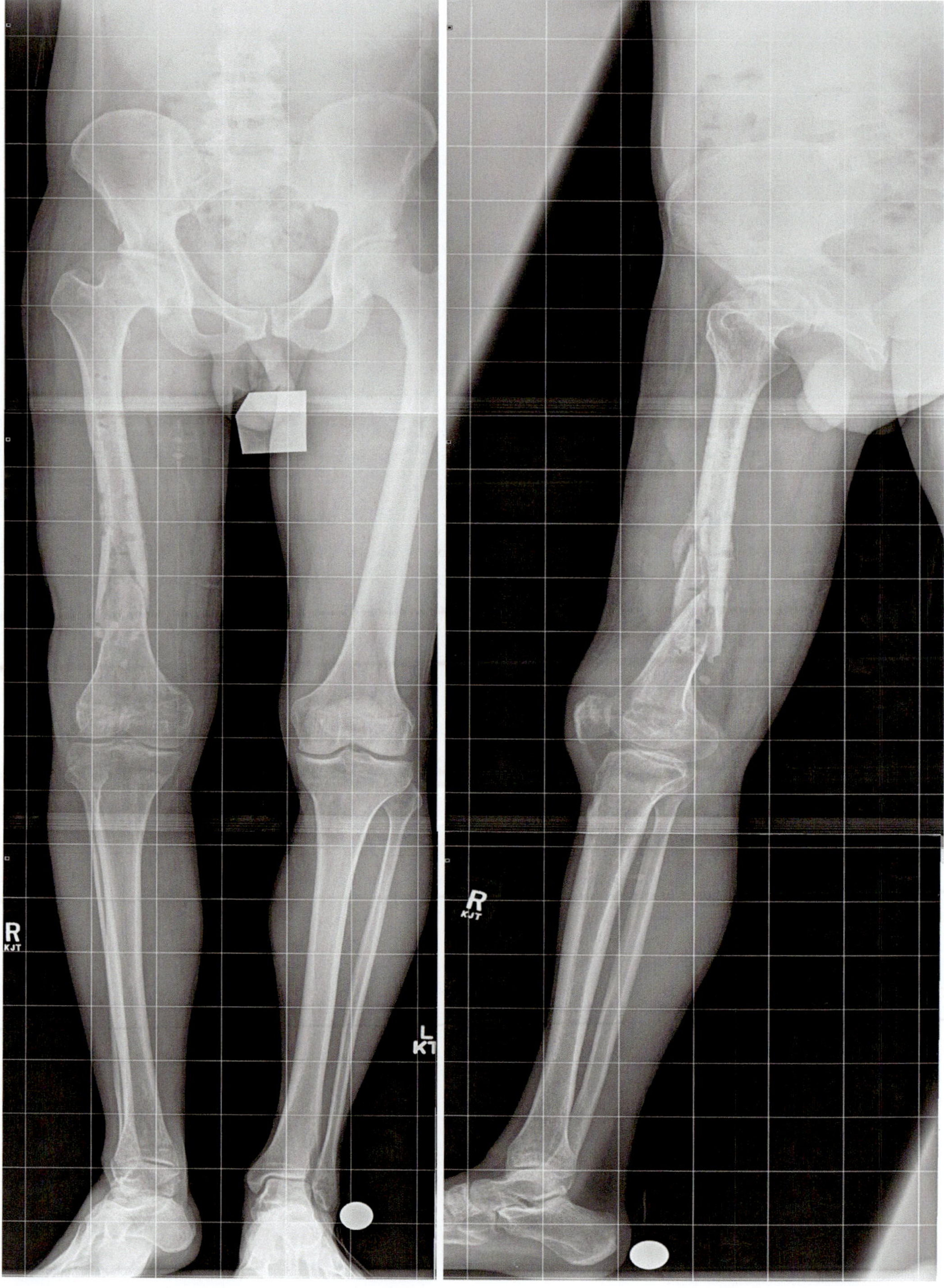

Fig. 9.10 Erect leg and long-leg lateral radiographs of a patient with infected nonunion of the midshaft, right femur, and resultant leg length discrepancy. (Used with permission from Rubin Institute for Advanced Orthopaedics, Sinai Hospital of Baltimore)

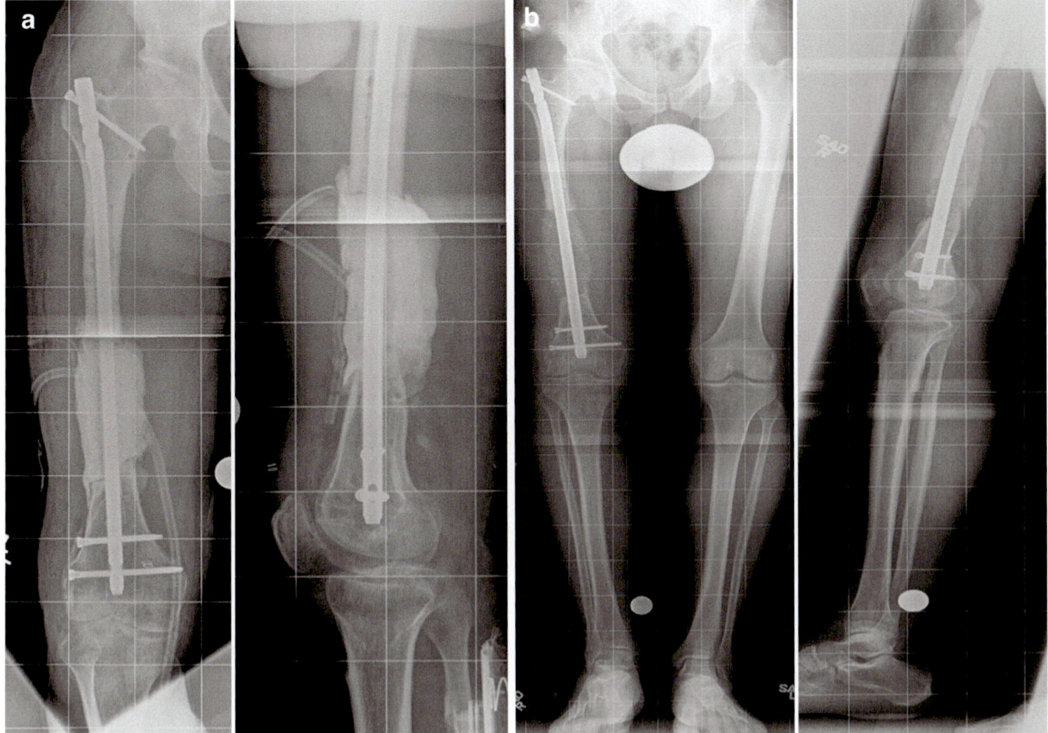

Fig. 9.11 Resection of the nonunion yielded an 11 cm defect. (a) The defect was first filled with a PMMA cement spacer using the Masquelet technique. (b) At the subsequent staged operation, the spacer was replaced with bone graft. (Used with permission from Rubin Institute for Advanced Orthopaedics, Sinai Hospital of Baltimore)

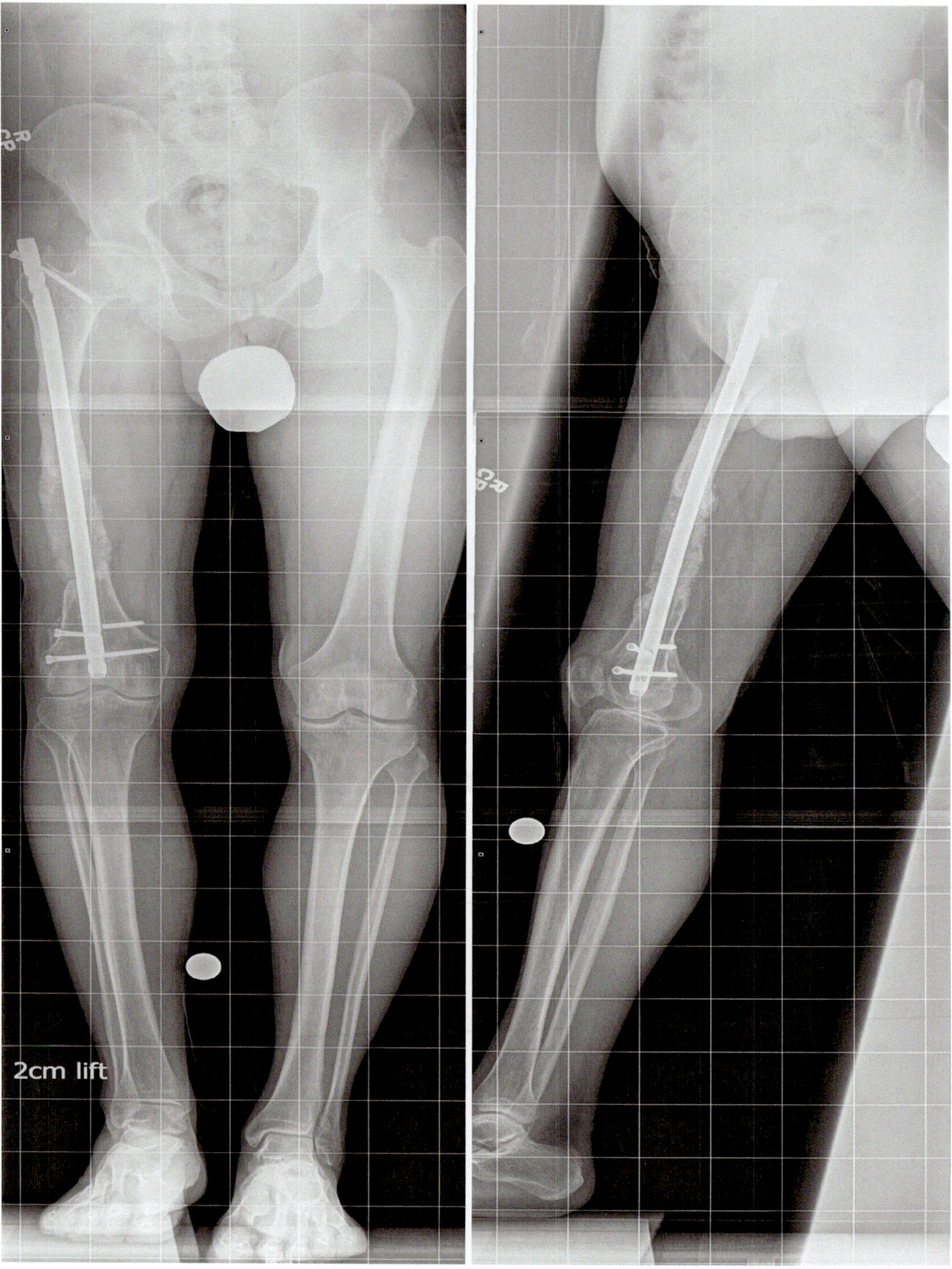

Fig. 9.12 Erect leg and long-leg lateral radiographs of the same patient with healed bone graft filling the segmental defect. (Used with permission from Rubin Institute for Advanced Orthopaedics, Sinai Hospital of Baltimore)

Fig. 9.13 Presenting radiographs with provisional external fixation and antibiotic spacer in place. (Used with permission from Rubin Institute for Advanced Orthopaedics, Sinai Hospital of Baltimore)

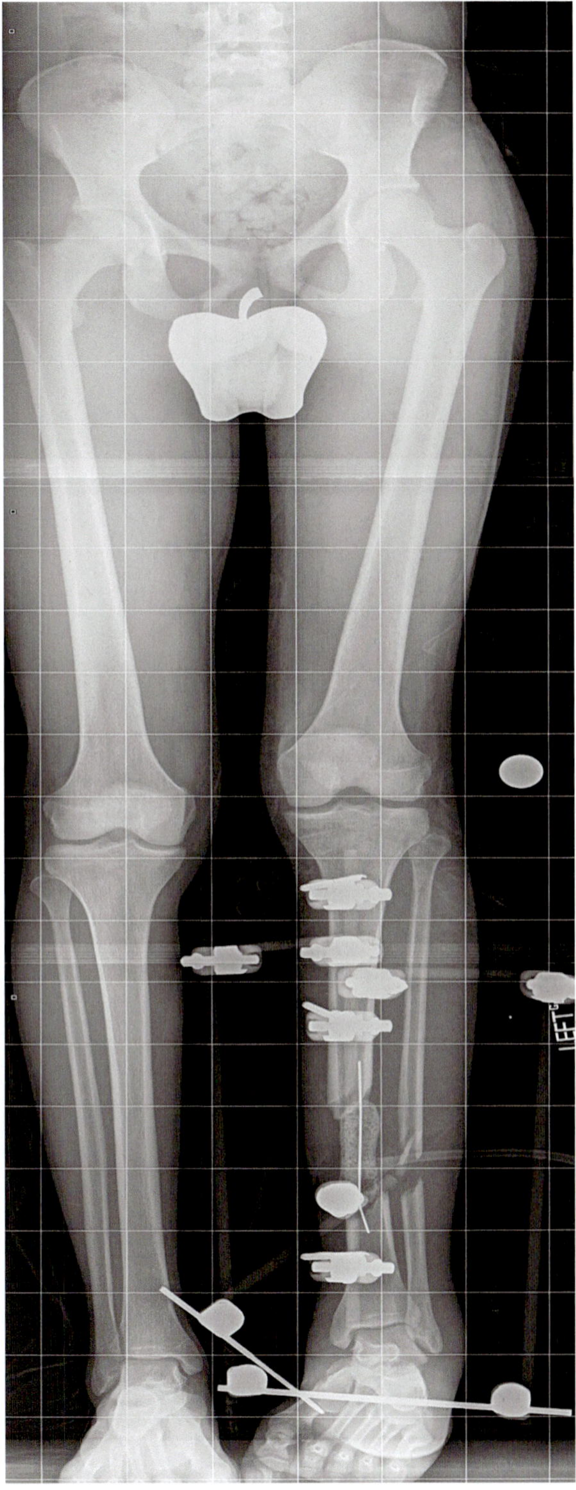

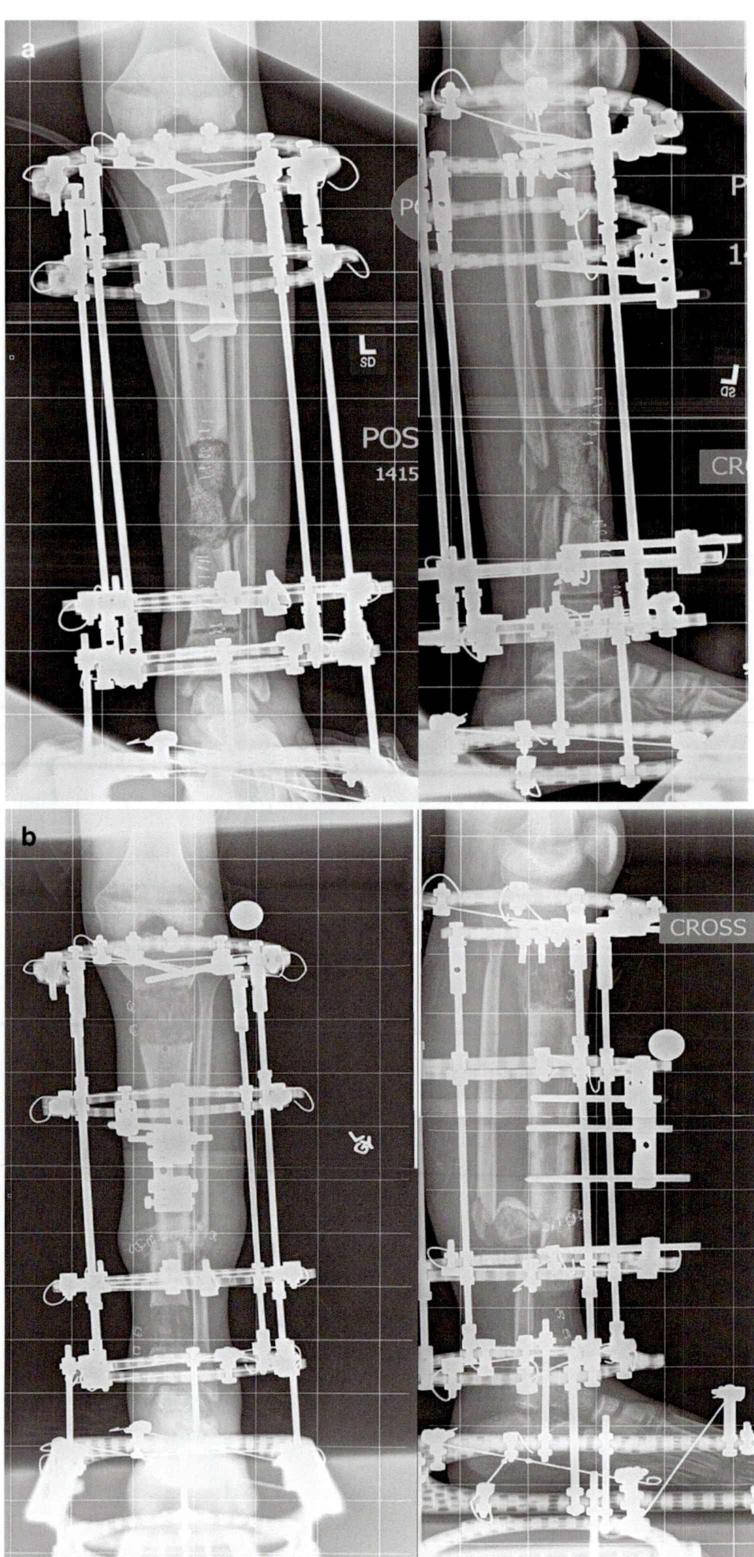

Fig. 9.14 (**a**) Anteroposterior and lateral radiographs of the double-level transport frame showing transport sites from osteotomies proximal and distal to the segmental defect. (**b**) Anteroposterior and lateral radiographs after the transport was completed and the mid-diaphyseal docking site was bone grafted. (Used with permission from Rubin Institute for Advanced Orthopaedics, Sinai Hospital of Baltimore)

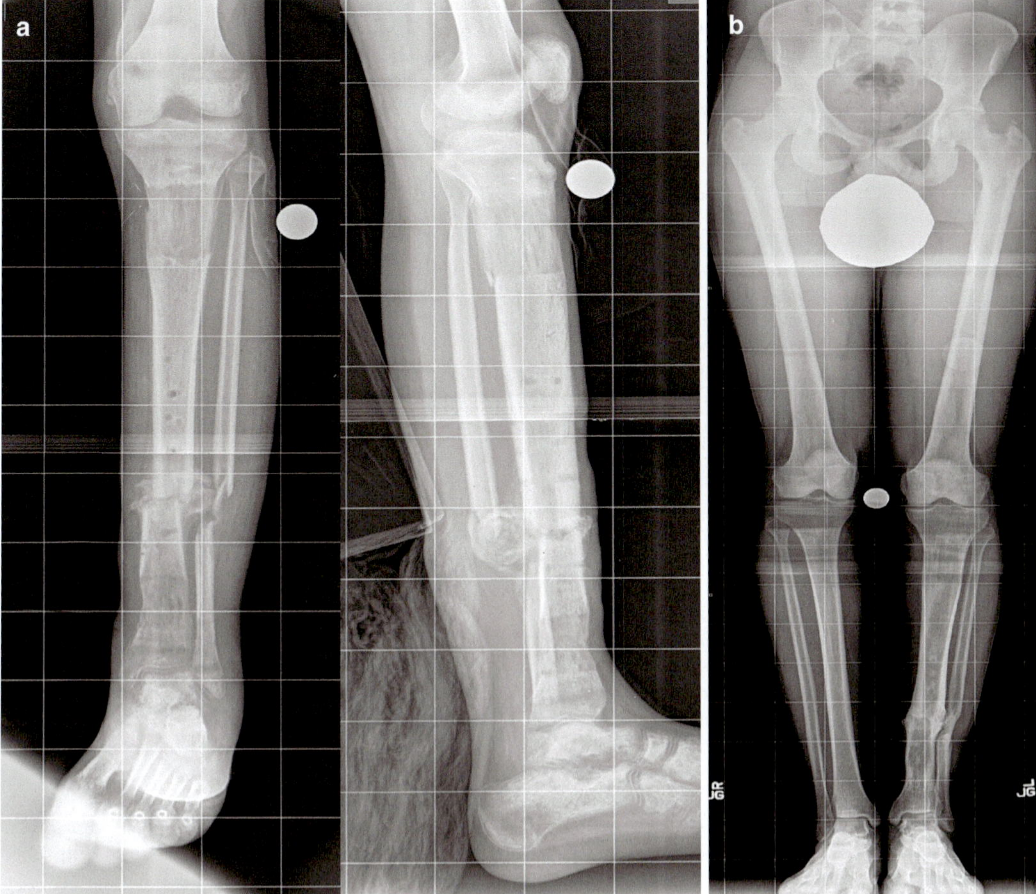

Fig. 9.15 (**a**) Anteroposterior and lateral radiographs of the bone after the circular frame was removed. Note the healing regenerate bone sites proximally and distally. (**b**) Final erect leg radiograph of the healed tibia. (Used with permission from Rubin Institute for Advanced Orthopaedics, Sinai Hospital of Baltimore)

References

1. Hernigou P. Bone transplantation and tissue engineering. Part II: bone graft and osteogenesis in the seventeenth, eighteenth, and nineteenth centuries (Duhamel, Haller, Ollier, and MacEwen). Int Orthop. 2015;39(1):193–204.
2. Meeder PJ, Eggers C. The history of autogenous bone grafting. Injury. 1994;25(Suppl 1):SA2–4.
3. Jordan CJ, Goldstein RY, McLaurin TM, Grant A. The evolution of the Ilizarov technique: part 1: the history of limb lengthening. Bull Hosp Jt Dis. 2013;71(1):89–95.
4. Green SA, Dahl MT. Historical background. In: Intramedullary limb lengthening. Principles and practice. Cham: Springer International Publishing; 2018. p. 1–14.
5. Ilizarov GA. The tension-stress effect on the genesis and growth of tissues. Part I. The influence of stability of fixation and soft-tissue preservation. Clin Orthop Relat Res. 1989;238:249–81.
6. Ilizarov GA. The tension-stress effect on the genesis and growth of tissues. Part II. The influence of the rate and frequency of distraction. Clin Orthop Relat Res. 1989;239:263–85.
7. Keating JF, Simpson AH, Robinson CM. The management of fractures with bone loss. J Bone Joint Surg Br. 2005;87:142–50.
8. Sanders DW, Bhandari M, Guyatt D, Heels-Ansdell D, Schemitsch EH, Swiontkowski M, Tornetta P 3rd, Walter S, Investigators SPRINT. Critical-sized defect in the tibia: is it critical? Results from the SPRINT trial. J Orthop Trauma. 2014;28(11):632–5.
9. Obremsky W, Molina C, Collinge C, Tornetta P 3rd, Sagi C, Schmidt A, Probe R, Ahn J, Nana A, Evidence-Based Quality Value and Safety Committee-Orthopaedic Trauma Association Writing Committee. Current practices in the management of open fractures among orthopaedic

trauma surgeons. Part B: management of segmental long bone defects. A surgery of Orthopaedic Trauma Association members. J Orthop Trauma. 2014;28:e203–7.

10. McClure PK, Alrabai HM, Conway JD. Preoperative evaluation and optimization for reconstruction of segmental bone defects of the tibia. J Ortho Trauma. 2017;31(Suppl 10):S16–9.

11. Davis KM, Griffin KS, Chu TG, Wenke JC, Corona BT, Mckinley TO, Kacena MA. Muscle-bone interactions during fracture healing. J Musculoskelet Neuronal Interact. 2015;15:1): 1–9.

12. Karger C, Kishi T, Schneider L, Fitoussi F, Masquelet SC, French Society of Orthopaedic Surgery and Traumatology (SoFCOT). Treatment of posttraumatic bone defects by the induced membrane technique. Orthop Traumatol Surg Res. 2012;98(1):97–102.

13. Rigal S, Merloz P, Le Nen D, Mathevon H, Masquelet AC, French Society of Orthopaedic Surgery and Traumatology (SoFCOT). Bone transport techniques in posttraumatic bone defects. Orthop Traumatol Surg Res. 2012;98(1):103–8.

14. Bosse MJ, MacKenzie EJ, Kellam JF, Burgess AR, Webb LX, Swiontkowski MF, Sanders RW, Jones AL, McAndrew MP, Patterson BM, McCarthy ML, Travison TG, Castillo RC. An analysis of outcomes of reconstruction or amputations after leg-threatening injuries. N Engl J Med. 2002;347(24):1924–31.

15. Lack WD, Karunaker MA, Anderame MR, Seymour RB, Sims S, Kellam JF, Bosse MJ. Type III open tibia fractures: immediate antibiotic prophylaxis minimizes infection. J Orthop Trauma. 2015;29:1): 1–6.

16. Chang Y, Bhandari M, Zhu KL, Mirza RD, Ren M, Kennedy SA, Negm A, Bhatnagar N, Naji FN, Milovanovic L, Fei Y, Agarwal A, Kamran R, Cho SM, Schandelmaiser S, Wang L, Jin L, Hu S, Zhao Y, Lopes LC, Wang M, Petrisor B, Ristevski B, Siemieniuk RAC, Guyatt GH. Antibiotic prophylaxis in the management of open fractures: a systematic survey of current practice and recommendations. JBJS Rev. 2019;7(2):e1.

17. Erdle NJ, Verwiebe EG, Wenke JC, Smith SC. Debridement and irrigation: evolution and current recommendations. J Ortho Trauma. 2016;30(Suppl 3):S7–S10.

18. Toogood P, Miclau T. Critical-sized bone defects: sequence and planning. J Orthop Trauma. 2017;31(Suppl5):S23–6.

19. Dedmond BT, Kortesis B, Punger K, Simpson J, Argenta J, Kulp B, Morykwas M, Webb LX. The use of negative pressure wound therapy (NPWT) in the temporary treatment of soft-tissue injuries associated with high-energy open tibial shaft fractures. J Orthop Trauma. 2007;21(1):11–7.

20. Liu DS, Sofiadellis F, Ashton M, MacGill K, Webb A. Early soft tissue coverage and negative pressure wound therapy optimizes patient outcomes in lower limb trauma. Injury. 2012;43(6):772–8.

21. Jenkinson RJ, Kiss A, Johnson S, Stephen DJ, Kreder HJ. Delayed wound closure increases deep-infection rate associated with lower-grade open fractures: a propensity-matched cohort study. J Bone Joint Surg Am. 2014;96(5):380–6.

22. Krug E, Berg L, Lee C, Hudson D, Birke-Sorensen H, Depoorter M, Dunn R, Jeffery S Duteille F, Bruhin A, Caravaggi C, Chariker M, Dowsett C, Ferreira F, Martinez JM, Grudzien G, Ichioka S, Ingemansson R, Malmsjo M, Rome P, Vig S, Runkel N, Martin R, Smith J, International Expert Panel on Negative Pressure Wound Therapy (NPWT-EP). Evidence-based recommendation for the use of negative pressure wound therapy in traumatic wounds and reconstructive surgery: steps towards an international consensus. Injury. 2011;42:S1–12.

23. Bhattacharyya T, Mehta P, Smith M, Pomahac B. Routine use of wound vacuum-assisted closure does not allow coverage delay for open tibia fractures. Plast Reconstr Surg. 2008;121(4):1263–6.

24. Baldwin P, Li DJ, Auston DA, Mir HS, Yoon RS, Koval KJ. Autograft, allograft, and bone graft substitutes: clinical evidence and indications for use in the setting of orthopacdic trauma surgery. J Orthop Trauma. 2019;33:203–13.

25. Shaw KA, Griffith MS, Shaw VM, Devine JG, Gloystein MD. Harvesting autogenous cancellous bone graft from the anterior iliac crest. JBJS Essent Surg Tech. 2018;8(3):e20.

26. Wenish S, Trinkaus K, Hild A, Hose D, Herde K, Heiss C, Kilian O, Alt V, Schnettler R. Human reaming debris: a source of multipotent stem cells. Bone. 2005;36:74–83.

27. Belthur MV, Conway JD, Jindal G, et al. Bone graft harvest using a new intramedullary system. Clin Orthop Relat Res. 2008;466:2973–80.

28. Yee MA, Hundal RS, Perdue AM, Hake ME. Autologous bone graft harvest using the reamer-irrigator-aspirator. J Orthop Trauma. 2018;32(Suppl 1):S20–1.

29. Dimitriou R, Mataliotakis GI, Angoules AG, Kanakaris NK, Giannoudis PV. Complications following autologous bone graft harvesting from the iliac crest and using the RIA: a systematic review. Injury. 2011;42(Suppl 2):S3–S15.

30. Dawson J, Kiner D, Gardner W, et al. The reamer-irrigator-aspirator as a device for harvesting bone graft compared with iliac crest bone graft: union rates and complications. J Orthop Trauma. 2014;28:584–90.

31. Calori GM, Colombo M, Mazza EL, Mazzola S, Malagoli E, Mineo GV. Incidence of donor site morbidity following harvest from iliac crest or RIA graft. Injury. 2014;45(Suppl 6):S116–20.

32. de Boer HH, Wood MB, Hermans J. Reconstruction of large skeletal defects by vascularized fibula transfer. Factors that influenced the outcome of union in 62 cases. Int Orthop. 1990;14(2):121–8.

33. Wang W, Yeung KWK. Bone grafts and biomaterials substitutes for bone defect repair: a review. Bioact Mater. 2017;2(4):224–47.

34. Rolvien T, Barbeck M, Wenisch S, Amling M, Krause M. Cellular mechanisms responsible for success and failure of bone substitute materials. Int J Mol Sci. 2018;19(10):e2893.

35. Allsopp BJ, Hunter-Smith DJ, Rozen WM. Vascularized versus nonvascularized bone grafts: what is the evidence? Clin Orthop Relat Res. 2016;474(5):1319–27.

36. Inzana JA, Schwarz EM, Kates SL, Awad HA. Biomaterials approaches to treating implant-associated osteomyelitis. Biomaterials. 2016;81:58–71.

37. McConoughey SJ, Howlin RP, Wiseman J, Stoodley P, Calhoun JH. Comparing PMMA and calcium sulfate as carriers for the local delivery of antibiotics to infected surgical sites. J Biomed Mater Res B. 2015; 103B;103:870–7.

38. Luo S, Jiang T, Yang Y, Yang X, Zhao J. Combination therapy with vancomycin-loaded calcium sulfate and vancomycin-loaded PMMA in the treatment of chronic osteomyelitis. BMC Musculo Skelet. 2016;7:502.

39. Govender S, Csimma S, Genant HK, Valentin-Opran A, Amit Y, Arbel R, BMP-2 Evaluation in Surgery for Tibial Trauma (BESTT) Study Group, et al. Recombinant human bone morphogenetic protein-2 for treatment of open tibial fractures: a prospective, controlled randomized study of four hundred and fifty patients. J Bone Joint Surg Am. 2002;84(12):2123–34.

40. Friedlaender GE, Perry CR, Cole JD, Cook SD, Cierny G, Muschler GF, Zych GA, Calhoun JH, LaForte AJ, Yin S. Osteogenic protein-1 (bone morphogenetic protein-7) in the treatment of tibial nonunions. J Bone Joint Surg Am. 2001;83(Suppl 1):S151–8.

41. Jones AL, Bucholz RW, Bosse MJ, Mirza SK, Lyon TR, Webb LX, Pollak AN, Golden JD, Valentin-Opran A, BMP-2 Evaluation in Surgery for Tibial Trauma-Allograft (BESTT-ALL) Study Group. Recombinant human BMP-2 and allograft compared with autogenous bone graft for reconstruction of diaphyseal tibia fractures with cortical defects. A randomized, controlled trial. J Bone Joint Surg Am. 2006;88(7):1431–41.

42. Garrison KR, Shemilt I, Donell S, Ryder JJ, Mugford M, Harvey I, Song F, Alt V. Bone morphogenetic protein (BMP) for fracture healing in adults. Cochrane Database Syst Rev. 2010;16(6):CD006950.

43. Hackl S, Hierholzer C, Friederichs J, Woltmann A, Buhren V, von Ruden C. Long-term outcome following additional rh BMP-7 application in revision surgery of aseptic humeral, femoral, and tibial shaft nonunions. BMC Musculoskeletal Disord. 2017;18(1):342.

44. Hernigou O, Poignard A, Beaujean F, et al. Percutaneous autologous bone-marrow grafting for nonunions: influence of the number and concentration of progenitor cells. J Bone Joint Surg Am. 2005;87:1430–7.

45. Schottle PC, Warner SJ. Role of bone marrow aspirate in orthopaedic trauma. Orthop Cli North Am. 2017;48(3):311–21.

46. Jager M, Herten M, Fochtmann U, Fischer J, Hernigou P, Zilkens C, Hendrich C, Krauspe R. Bridging the gap: bone marrow aspirate concentrate reduced autologous bone grafting in osseous defects. J Orthop Res. 2011;29(2):173–80.

47. Petri M, Namazian A, Wilke F, Ettinger M, Stubig T, Brand S, Bengel F, Krettek C, Berding G, Jagodzinski M. Repair of segmental long-bone defects by stem cell concentrate augmented scaffolds: a clinical and positron emission tomography-computed tomography analysis. Int Orthop. 2013;37(11):2231–7.

48. Gianakos A, Ni A, Zambrana L, Kennedy JG, Lane JM. Bone marrow aspirate concentrate in animal long bone healing: an analysis of basic science evidence. J Orthop Trauma. 2016;30(1):1–9.

49. Taylor BC, French BG, Fowler TT, Russell J, Poka A. Induced membrane technique for reconstruction to manage bone loss. J Am Acad Orthop Surg. 2012;20(3):142–50.

50. Masquelet AC. Induced membrane technique: pearls and pitfalls. J Ortho Trauma. 2017;31(Suppl 10):S36–8.

51. Yee MA, Mead MP, Alford AI, Hak DJ, Mauffrey C, Hake ME. Scientific understanding of the induced membrane technique: current status and future directions. J Orthop Trauma. 2017;31(Suppl 10):S3–8.

52. Eralp L, Kocaoglu M, Ozkan K, Turker M. A comparison of two osteotomy techniques for tibial lengthening. Arch Orthop Trauma Surg. 2004 Jun;124(5):298–300.

53. Beltran MJ, Blair JA, Rathbone CR, Hsu JR. The gradual expansion muscle flap. J Orthop Trauma. 2014;28(1):e15–20.

54. Quinnan SM. Segmental bone loss reconstruction using ring fixation. J Orthop Trauma. 2017;31(Suppl 10):S42–6.

55. Borzunov DY. Long bone reconstruction using multilevel lengthening of bone defect fragments. Int Orthop. 2012;36(8):1695–700.

56. El-Alfy B, El-Mowafi H, Kotb S. Bifocal and trifocal bone transport for failed limb reconstruction after tumour resection. Acta Orthop Belg. 2009;75(3):368–73.

57. Paley D, Herzenberg JE, Paremain G, Bhave A. Femoral lengthening over an intramedullary nail. A matched-case comparison with Ilizarov femoral lengthening. J Bone Joint Surg Am. 1997;79(10):1464–80.

58. Burghardt RD, Manzotti A, Bhave A, Paley D, Herzenberg JE. Tibial lengthening over intramedullary nail: a matched case comparison with Ilizarov tibial lengthening. Bone Joint Res. 2016;5(1):1–10.

59. Bernstein M, Fragomen AT, Sabharwal S, Barclay J, Rozbruch SR. Does integrated fixation pro-

Restoring Function: Tendon and Nerve Transfers

Keith T. Aziz, Jaimie T. Shores, and John V. Ingari

Introduction

Traumatic injury to the upper extremity can cause significant functional impairment, especially if there is neurologic injury causing loss of function due to muscle paralysis and sensory loss. Functional loss can also occur without neurologic injury if there is significant soft tissue loss – especially when there is sufficient damage to any part of the muscle, tendon, or myotendinous junction to render the muscle ineffectual. As always, treating any patient starts with a thorough physical exam and history. After a comprehensive understanding of all deficits is obtained, it is important to have a careful discussion with the patient to review goals in order to maximize satisfaction and outcomes when approaching reconstruction. This chapter will review principles and techniques available to the upper extremity

reconstructive surgeon, with a specific focus on restoring function through nerve and tendon transfers. While the focus of this chapter is on functional restoration, it is always important to recognize that osseous injury can further compound the complexity and considerations in managing the mangled extremity.

Nerve Transfers

History

The concept of nerve damage and repair has long been an area of focus – with one of the earliest descriptions of apposition of nerve ends to repair damaged nerves dating back to the seventh century, when Paul of Aegina described opposing nerve ends during wound closure [1]. A more comprehensive understanding of nerve injury began to emerge after Augustus Waller's experiment on transection of the hypoglossal nerve in an amphibian model – and it is for him that Wallerian degeneration is named [2]. Seddon was the first to publish a classification based on the scale of nerve injury – unfortunately likely being necessitated by World War II [3]. Seddon did acknowledge that his classification terms – neuropraxia, axonotmesis, and neurotmesis – were directly on the descriptions of Professor Henry Cohen of Liverpool [3]. As the understanding of

K. T. Aziz
Department of Orthopaedic Surgery, The Johns Hopkins University, Baltimore, MD, USA

J. T. Shores
Department of Plastic and Reconstructive Surgery, The Johns Hopkins University School of Medicine, Baltimore, MD, USA
e-mail: jshores3@jhmi.edu

J. V. Ingari (✉)
Hand Surgery Division, Department of Orthopaedic Surgery, Sinai Hospital of Baltimore, Baltimore, MD, USA

© Springer Nature Switzerland AG 2021
R. A. Pensy, J. V. Ingari (eds.), *The Mangled Extremity*, https://doi.org/10.1007/978-3-319-56648-1_10

nerve injury improved, there were corresponding improvements in nerve repair techniques that were developed [4, 5]. Sunderland expanded on the initial work of Seddon and further sub-divided neurotmesis and also provided significant insight into the importance of fascicular anatomy within peripheral nerves and made major contributions to mapping peripheral nerve fascicular anatomy [6–9]. Since the foundation established by Seddon and Sunderland's work, there has been a significant advancement in the understanding of the potential for nerve recovery after peripheral nerve injury – as well as a better understanding of when to consider nerve transfer to allow for gain of function.

Nerve transfer involves the coaptation of a healthy nerve to a recipient nerve with a goal of providing sensation or motor function to a distal target [10]. Flourens published some of the first nerve transfer outcomes using a rooster model in the early 1800s [11]. This work was followed by other animal model studies – specifically a canine model by Vulpian and Philipeaux [12]. Since much of the early literature on nerve transfers originated from France, it is perhaps not surprising that perhaps some of the earliest clinical reports of nerve transfer are found in the works of Létiévant in the late 1800s [13]. It was not long after that nerve transfers were attempted to treat brachial plexopathy, and Harris and Low reported on early functional outcomes using an intact nerve root for Erb's palsy [14]. Since these early reports, there have been several advancements in the field of nerve transfer, and other types of nerve transfer have been widely reported on [10, 15, 16]. When considering nerve transfers as a part of the reconstructive algorithm in managing upper extremity injury, the timing, zone of injury, availability of donor nerves, specific reconstructive goals, or other patient-specific factors must be carefully considered.

Principles of Nerve Transfer

When considering nerve transfer to restore function, it is important to recall an adage that is common when using any autograft – specifically that one is "stealing from Peter to pay Paul." If the functional gain from nerve transfer does not equal or exceed the functional deficit from the donor nerve, then it is necessary to consider alternative reconstructive options and discuss these at length with the patient. Ideally, the donor nerve or fascicles have redundant innervation – such that the donor deficit is minimal or negligible. The donor and recipient nerve type should be matched, such that motor nerve donors are used for motor nerve recipients and sensory nerve donors are used for sensory nerve recipients. When transferring motor nerves, it is important to have high donor to recipient axon ratios; Schreiber has recommended a ratio of donor to recipient axons of at least a 0.7:1 for optimal outcome [17]. When considering motor nerve transfers, it is optimal to use nerves or fascicles that are often "in phase" – as this will improve post-operative rehabilitation. Also, the same donor nerve should not be used to innervate two opposing muscles – as this would make functional rehabilitation almost impossible. The muscle strength of the donor nerve should be at least M4 based on the Medical Research Council (MRC) muscle grading system, as it is not uncommon to decrease in power after transfer [18, 19]. The donor nerve should reach its recipient in a tension-free manner and ideally is closely positioned to the recipient nerve. Additionally, it is important to ensure that there is not gross size mismatch between the donor and recipient nerves. When considering nerve transfer, it is imperative to ensure that the joints affected by the muscle target are supple and have accompanying osseous stability. Finally, one should always consider whether the intended nerve transfer would render alternative reconstructive options – such as tendon transfers – impossible.

There are some relative contraindications to nerve transfer when considering reconstruction in a mangled upper extremity. Notably, if there is extensive scar tissue in the region of intended transfer, it may render the dissection infeasible or impossible. Also related to scar tissue is the issue of a segmental nerve lesion or an extensive neuroma in continuity of the intended recipient nerve. There are some important considerations to be made with timing of nerve transfers, as poor outcomes have been observed if motor nerve transfers are attempted 12 months after injury [20, 21]. In the future though it may be possible to extend this window since Chao et al. have identified future targets to prevent motor endplate degradation [22]. Finally, it is important to consider neuroplasticity whenever attempting nerve transfers – as motor cortex plasticity is recognized as playing a role in functional outcomes [23, 24]. There is, however, no current widely accepted quantitative means of assessing neuroplasticity.

The Paralytic Shoulder

In the paralytic shoulder, there is often a loss of abduction, external rotation, or some combination of both abduction and external rotation. These two functions are required in order to provide stability to the shoulder to allow for the hand to be positioned in space. The axillary nerve (C5–C6) and the suprascapular nerve (C5–C6) both arise from upper cervical roots in the brachial plexus. Both nerves provide innervation to muscles that allow for abduction – the deltoid (axillary) and supraspinatus (suprascapular). Additionally, both nerves provide innervation to muscles that control external rotation with the teres minor (axillary) and infraspinatus (suprascapular). Because the roots are located at the most cephalad portion of the brachial plexus, it is not uncommon to see patients with a paralytic shoulder secondary to traction injuries.

Suprascapular Nerve Palsy

One of the most widely reported nerve transfer options available for suprascapular (SS) nerve injury involves transfer of the distal branch of the spinal accessory nerve (SAN) [25–27]. It is important to identify the distal branch of SAN in order to avoid denervation of the entire trapezius, as the distal branch only provides motor innervation to the inferior head of the trapezius [28, 29]. Transfer of the distal branch of the SAN to the SS nerve does not typically require an intercalated nerve graft. Surgical approach for SAN to SS

transfer can be done either through an anterior supraclavicular approach (Figs. 10.1 and 10.2) [25] or a posterior approach [30], allowing one to tailor the approach to avoid a field of contamination or injury. The SAN to SS transfer can often be accomplished by primarily coaptation of the SAN to the SS (Figs. 10.2, 10.3, 10.4, and 10.5). In a large series of SAN to SS transfers, a steep learning curve was observed – with a 25% failure

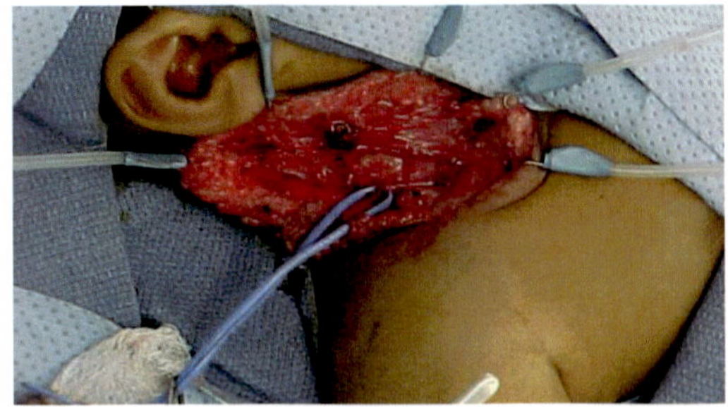

Fig. 10.1 Vessel loops around right suprascapular nerve. The patient (infant) is supine with the head turned to the contralateral side

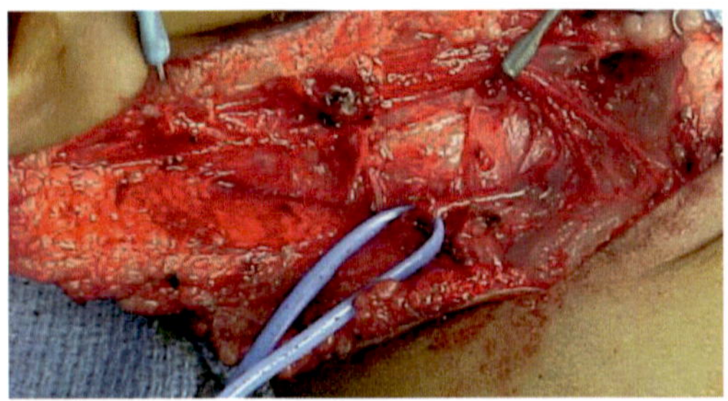

Fig. 10.2 Magnified view of suprascapular nerve, with vessel loops around nerve. Patient is supine with head turned to the contralateral side

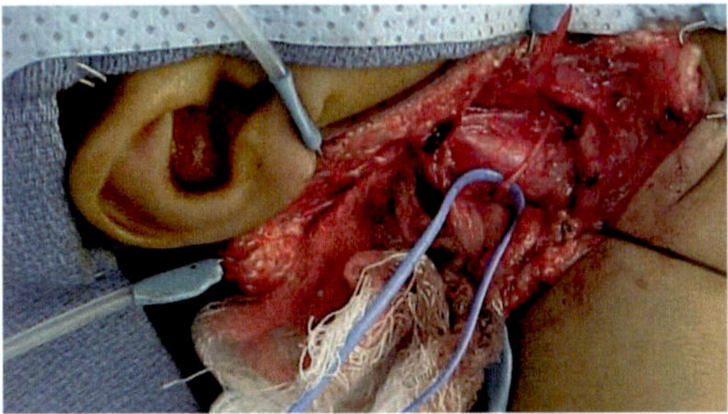

Fig. 10.3 Identification of the donor nerve, the spinal accessory nerve. Vessel loops around the spinal accessory nerve

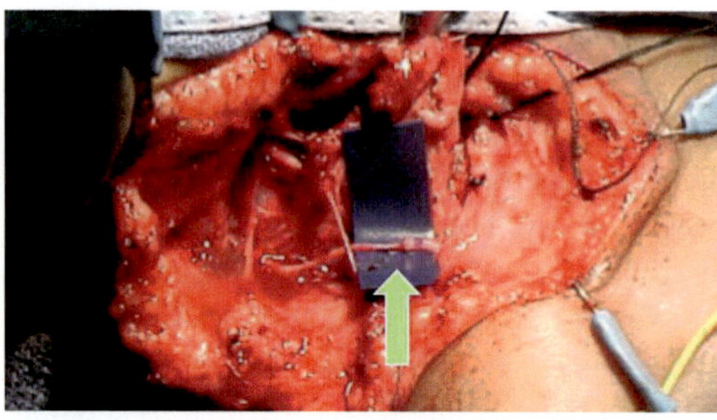

Fig. 10.4 Coaptation of the spinal accessory nerve to the suprascapular nerve. Arrow highlights coaptation

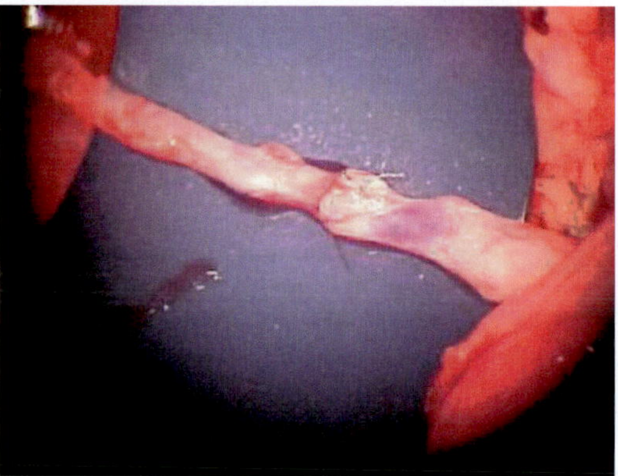

Fig. 10.5 Coaptation of the spinal accessory nerve to the suprascapular nerve under the microscope

rate observed in the first 2 years of a 10-year series, with a 5% failure rate observed in the remaining 8 years [25]. In this group, failure was defined as patients who gained less than 30° of active abduction.

The functional outcomes observed after SAN to SS nerve transfer have demonstrated a mean gain of abduction ranging from 30° to 80° [27, 31–33] and a mean gain in external rotation ranging from 13.3° to 71.2° [27, 31–33]. It is possible that some of the poor outcomes reported are a result of inadequate identification of SS nerve lesions [34]. There are three commonly identified locations for SS nerve injury, including the origin in the upper trunk, the scapular notch, the spinoglenoid notch, or any combination of the above injuries – and inadequate identification of any of these sites would significantly compromise outcomes [26].

In the event that SAN is not available, either secondary to prior trauma or prior harvest, there

are other donor nerves for SS nerve palsy that have been described. The phrenic nerve has also been utilized for SS nerve transfer, with the largest study describing a mean gain of abduction of 80° [35]. While additional nerve transfer options have been described, such as intercostal (IC) nerves and the ipsilateral hypoglossal nerve, both require the use of an intercalated nerve graft and demonstrate inferior outcomes [36, 37].

Axillary Nerve Palsy

In isolated axillary nerve palsy, the primary goal is to focus on reinnervation of the deltoid muscle. Several prior studies have demonstrated the importance of the deltoid in shoulder function, and even in rotator cuff-deficient patients, the deltoid has been shown to be able to adequately compensate and allow for some internal and external rotation [38]. The transfer of a motor branch of the radial nerve, specifically a branch to one of the heads of the triceps brachii, is an excellent option to assist in restoring deltoid function in the setting of an axillary nerve injury [39–41]. The radial nerve is often in close proximity to the axillary nerve because both arise from the posterior cord of the brachial plexus, and there is often good size match between the motor branches to the heads of the triceps brachii and the branches of the axillary nerve [34]. When determining the recipient site in the setting of axillary nerve palsy, it is recommended to select the anterior branch of the axillary nerve because Leechavengvongs et al. have demonstrated that even the posterior deltoid is innervated by the anterior branch in over 90% of cadaveric specimens [42]. The radial to axillary motor nerve transfer can be done from a posterior or anterior approach – though some have advocated for the anterior deltopectoral approach because of the extensile nature and ability to access alternative donor nerves (Figs. 10.6 and 10.7) [43, 44].

If the axillary nerve is injured as part of an upper brachial plexus injury (C5–C6), then it is recommended to perform a double transfer – such that a motor branch of the radial nerve is used to reinnervate the axillary nerve and the distal branch of SAN is used for the SS nerve. In double transfer patients, limited case series have

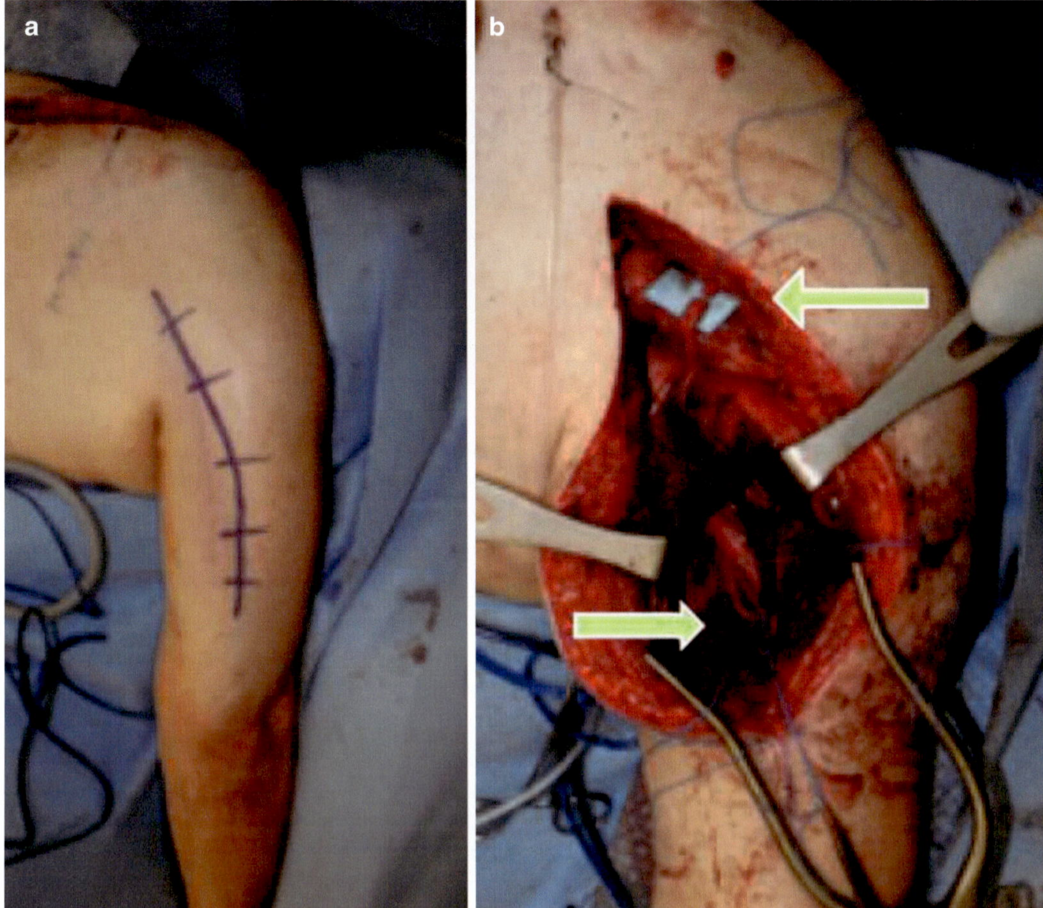

Fig. 10.6 (**a**) View of the incision for radial nerve to axillary nerve transfer, using the posterior approach; (**b**) appearance after approach and identification of the recipient axillary nerve (arrow from the right) and donor radial nerve (arrow from the left)

shown satisfactory outcomes in shoulder abduction and power [45].

If there is damage to the radial nerve or upper plexopathy that also involves C7 nerve root, the medial pectoral nerve can be transferred to the axillary nerve with reasonable function reported in a series of eight patients [46]. An anterior approach must be used if the median pectoral nerve is being transferred.

In the event that intraplexal motor branches cannot be transferred – especially in the setting of more extensive plexopathy – there are extraplexal transfers that have been described. Notably, it is possible to transfer the distal branch of the SAN to the axillary nerve [47]; however, this does require the use of an intercalated graft – and cannot be done in conjunction with SS nerve transfers [48]. The IC nerves have also been described as alternative extraplexal nerve transfer donors – though the outcomes of IC nerve transfers to the axillary nerve are somewhat varied [47, 48].

Restoring Elbow Function

Elbow Flexion

The restoration of elbow flexion is among the most important functional considerations when treating a patient with a mangled upper extremity [49, 50]. Restoring the ability to flex the elbow can enable patients to position the hand in space in a manner that significantly facilitates self-care

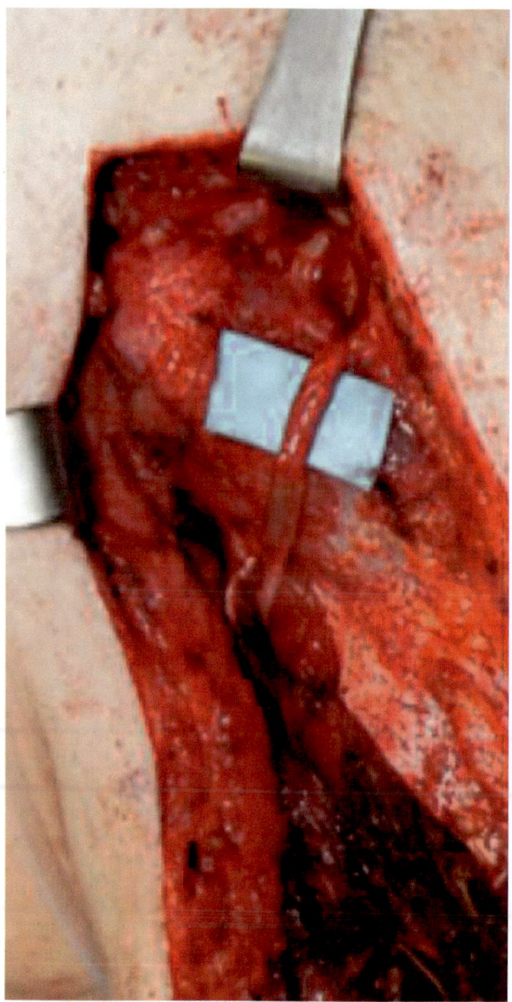

Fig. 10.7 Coaptation of the radial nerve motor branch to triceps to the axillary nerve

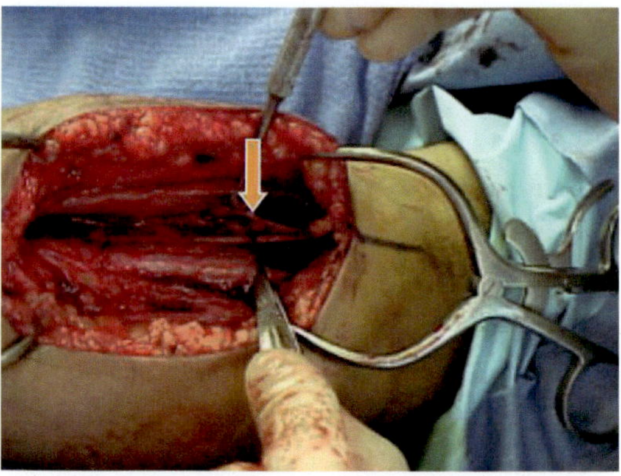

Fig. 10.8 Approach for Oberlin transfer – patient is supine with arm abducted. First step is identificaiton of musculocutaneous nerve (highlighted by arrow)

and increases patient independence. Elbow flexion is controlled by the musculocutaneous (MC) nerve and its terminal branches, which provide innervation to the biceps brachii and brachialis muscles.

One of the most widely reported nerve transfer options available for MC nerve injury was popularized by Oberlin et al. and involves transfer of fascicles of the ulnar nerve to the biceps brachii [51]. The eponym "Oberlin" is widely recognized, though it is important to make the distinction that the "Oberlin" involves only a sin-gle nerve transfer [52]. The donor fascicle is typically the motor fascicle to the FCU, and it is important to assess grip strength prior to sacrificing motor innervation to the FCU for transfer [52–54]. In order to identify the motor fascicle, a nerve stimulator should be used intraoperatively (Figs. 10.8, 10.9, and 10.10) prior to coaptation (Fig. 10.11). The "Oberlin" transfer has been extensively studied and has shown very good clinical outcomes [52–56] – with as many as 92% of patients achieving a grade M4 for elbow flexion in upper plexopathies in a select series [55]. When counseling patients on expected outcomes of the Oberlin transfer, it is important to recall that plexopathies involving C7 can decrease functional outcomes because of compromise to muscles that originate on the medial epicondyle.

Tung et al. described alternative nerve transfers to restore elbow flexion, where the brachialis is the recipient muscle [57]. If the brachialis is the sole distal target that is being innervated, it is important to recall that the brachialis functions solely as an elbow flexor, whereas the biceps acts as a flexor and supinator. The use of alternative donor nerves is useful in the event that an ulnar nerve fascicle cannot be utilized because of patient-specific factors, and Tung et al. outlined techniques using the branch of the median nerve, the medial pectoral nerve, IC nerves, and motor branches to the triceps brachii. The transfer of an

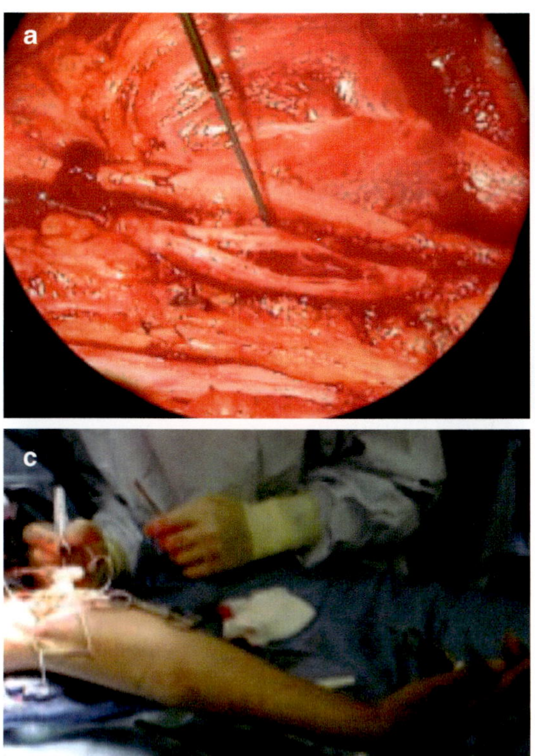

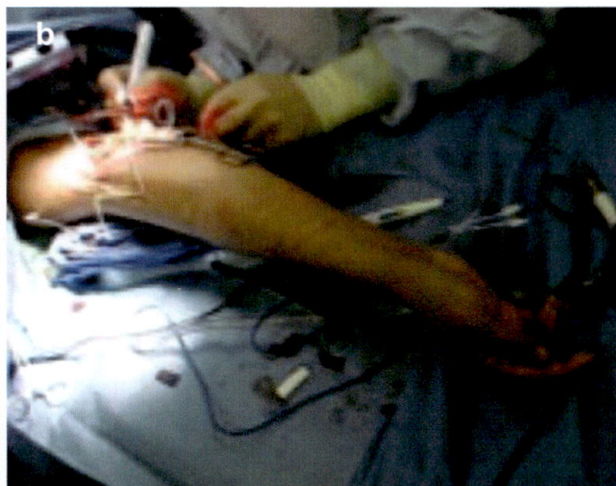

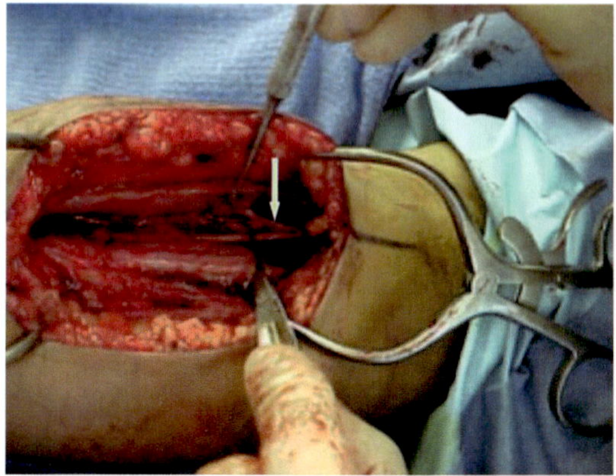

Fig. 10.9 (**a**) Identify ulnar nerve, grossly, and begin to dissect fascicles to identify motor nerve fascicles to the flexor carpi ulnaris (FCU); (**b**) stimulate FCU nerve fascicles to confirm; (**c**) visualize grossly firing of FCU (Arrow highlights flexion and ulnar deviation of wrist)

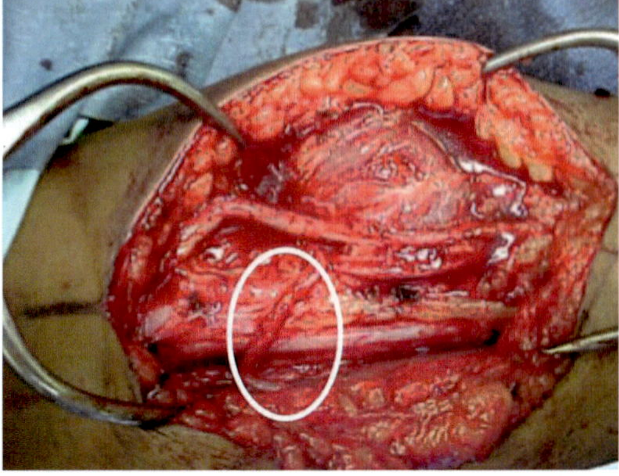

Fig. 10.10 Identify the motor branch of musculocutaneous nerve to the biceps brachii (highlighted by arrow)

Fig. 10.11 Coaptation of the ulnar nerve motor branch to the FCU to the motor branch to the biceps brachii of the musculocutaneous nerve

isolated median nerve motor fascicle, typically the branch to the FDS, has shown rates of grade M4 MRC power comparable to the "Oberlin" transfer [58]

Mackinnon et al. described the transfer of the median nerve motor fascicle to the FDS to the brachialis in conjunction with the "Oberlin" transfer [59]. Martins et al. compared the double transfer to a single transfer and found increased average flexion strength (5.6–4.14 kg) in double transfer groups [60, 61]. While a double transfer may improve flexion strength, it is important to cautiously interpret these results as patient plexopathies are not homogeneous. Further, the gain in flexion strength reported is unlikely to have any clinical significance, and does eliminate a donor fascicle for potential future reconstructive options.

In the event that there are no available intraplexal donors, there is literature that demonstrates reasonable outcomes using extraplexal donors. Intercostal nerve transfers have shown good outcomes in over 60% of patients as long as no intercalated nerve graft is used [62, 63]. Merrell demonstrated that the use of an intercalated nerve graft decreased the percentage of patients with at least antigravity elbow flexion from over 70% of cases without intercalary graft to 43% of cases with intercalary graft [63].

If not already being used to restore other functions, the distal branch of the SAN can also be transferred to restore elbow flexion. While the range of patients who achieved antigravity is quite varied in the available literature, ranging from 35% to almost 94%, most series suggest over 60% of patients will have good functional outcome of elbow flexion from distal SAN transfer to the MC nerve [33, 47, 64]. Finally, the phrenic nerve has also been used to restore elbow flexion – with over 80% of patient achieving antigravity function in two different series [65, 66]; however, the use of the phrenic nerve is not advised in patients with diaphragmatic or thoracic injuries (which can often be seen in patients with mangled extremities).

Maldonado et al. described another technique for restoring elbow flexion by use of innervated free gracilis transfer [67]. The use of free functional muscle transfer will be discussed in more detail in Chap. 12, but it should be recognized that the use of free innervated muscle transfer generates significantly less power in elbow flexion compared to extrinsic digital flexors (52% grade M3 or higher for elbow flexion compared to 85% grade M3 or higher for extrinsic digital flexion). Any reconstructive technique planning to employ free gracilis transfer should involve careful thought as to where the muscle will be deployed to gain maximal benefit.

Elbow Extension

Restoration of elbow extension is typically of low priority when seeking to restore function in a patient with brachial plexopathy. The exception is for patients who may require elbow extension for transfer (i.e., bed to chair). Otherwise, elbow extension can often be adequately achieved with gravity, and elbow extensors antagonize elbow flexion – which is among the most important functional considerations when treating a patient with a mangled upper extremity [49, 50]. In the absence of other injuries, some authors have argued that it is reasonable to consider nerve transfers for restoration of elbow extension to improve stability about the elbow, as well [68].

In patients with partial brachial plexus injuries, Bertelli et al. described the transfer of a fascicle of the ulnar nerve to the motor branch of the long head of the triceps brachii [69]. In their limited series, all five patients achieved grade M4 strength for elbow extension. The donor nerve described by Bertelli et al. is the same motor fascicle to the FCU in the ulnar nerve used in the "Oberlin" transfer. Oberlin et al. also reported on a similarly small series of patients using mostly a motor fascicle of the ulnar nerve with excellent results [70]. In their series, they also included one patient who underwent transfer of a median nerve fascicle to a branch of the triceps brachii with grade M5 power. The medial pectoral nerve has also been described as an intraplexal donor for nerve transfer to restore elbow extension [71]; however, in Flores et al.'s series, the recipient nerves included both the radial nerve and an isolated motor branch of triceps brachii – both with acceptable clinical outcomes [71].

A majority of literature focused on nerve transfers for elbow extension discusses the use of extraplexal donors – specifically IC nerves. Unfortunately, the literature on clinical outcomes of IC nerve transfer for elbow extension show extremely varied results. Studies show anywhere from 0% to 78% of patients achieve antigravity function with elbow extension [54, 68, 72, 73]. When using IC nerves for elbow extension, it may require more than a single IC nerve to achieve the desired outcome – though Gao et al. suggested that there is no difference between using two IC nerves versus three IC nerves [74]

Distal Reinnervation: The Hand and Wrist

Clinical outcomes following more distal nerve transfers contrast to the satisfactory results often seen with reinnervation of more proximal targets. Timing of nerve transfers aimed with restoring distal innervation also plays a larger role, since the longer distance needs to be traveled by transferred axons – which in turn necessitate a longer recovery time. When this longer time period is considered in the context of motor endplate degeneration, and the fact that any nerve transfer may compromise future tendon transfers, it becomes especially important to carefully decide the best course forward and council patients thoroughly.

Radial Nerve Palsy

When considering nerve transfers to restore functional deficits that occur secondary to radial nerve injury, it is important to identify the level of injury – as the approach to a nerve root injury differs from a posterior cord injury or high radial nerve injury. The focus of this section is distal reinnervation, which will address wrist and finger extensor deficits. Branches of the median nerve are well described to address motor deficits secondary to injury to the radial nerve, and several approaches are available.

Ray and Mackinnon described clinical outcomes following transfer of the motor fascicle of the FDS to the ECRB motor branch to restore

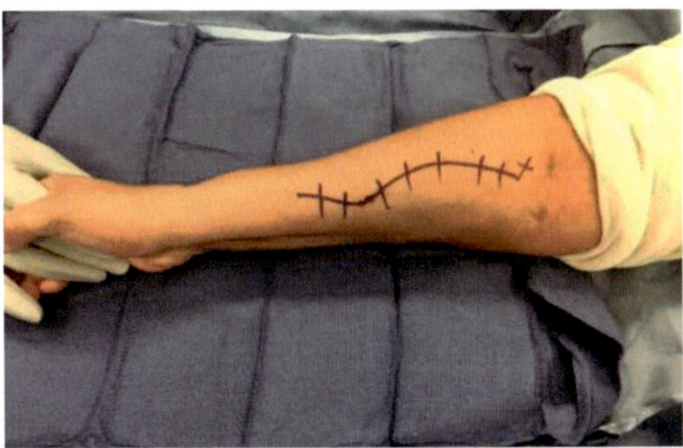

Fig. 10.12 View of the incision for transfer of the motor branch to the flexor carpi radialis (FCR) and the flexor digitorum superficialis (FDS) to the extensor carpi radialis brevis (ECRB) and posterior interosseous nerve (PIN) branches

wrist extension combined with a transfer of the motor fascicle of FCR to the PIN (Figs. 10.12, 10.13, and 10.14) [75]. In their series, only 1/19 patients did not recover at least antigravity wrist extension, while 14/19 had good or excellent recovery of finger and thumb extension [75].

Alternatively, Garcia-Lopez et al. described the use of the motor branch to the pronator teres to the ECRB motor branch to restore wrist extension [76]. Like Ray and Mackinnon, Garcia-Lopez et al. transferred the motor fascicle of FCR to the PIN for digital extension [75, 76]. In their series, Garcia-Lopez et al. found that all patients gained grade M4 wrist extension and thumb extension, with 4/6 patients also gaining grade M4 finger extension [76].

If the goal is to recover isolated wrist extension, or if the motor branch to the pronator teres and FDS are not available, Bertelli et al. have described the transfer of the pronator quadratus AIN motor branch to the ECRB [77]. In their series, 27/28 patients had successful reinnervation of the ECRB and could demonstrate antigravity wrist extension. Additionally, if the motor branch to FCR is not available, it is possible to transfer the motor branch of the supinator to the PIN to achieve digital and thumb extension. Li et al. described a series where the motor branch of the supinator was transferred to the PIN and with 3/3 patients who were available for follow-up showing grade M4 thumb and finger extension [78].

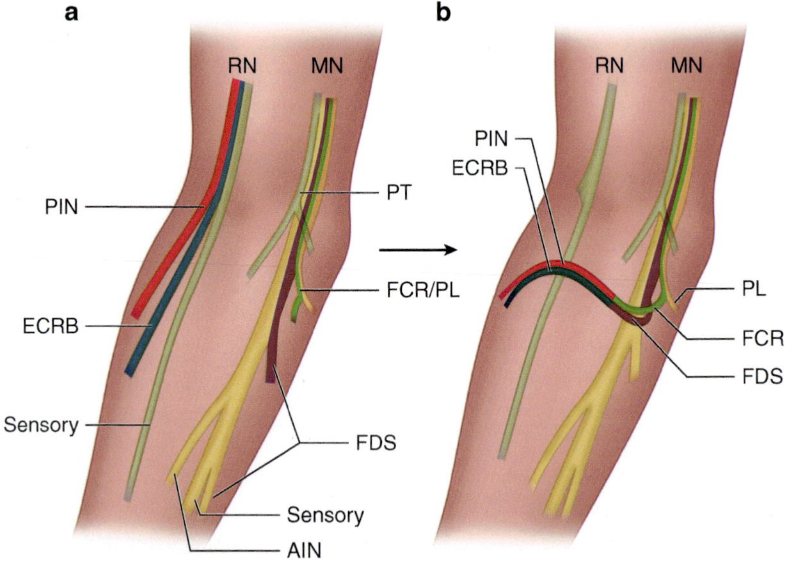

Fig. 10.13 Schematic figure demonstrating transfer of FDS and FCR motor branches to PIN and ECRB. (From Ray and Mackinnon [75])

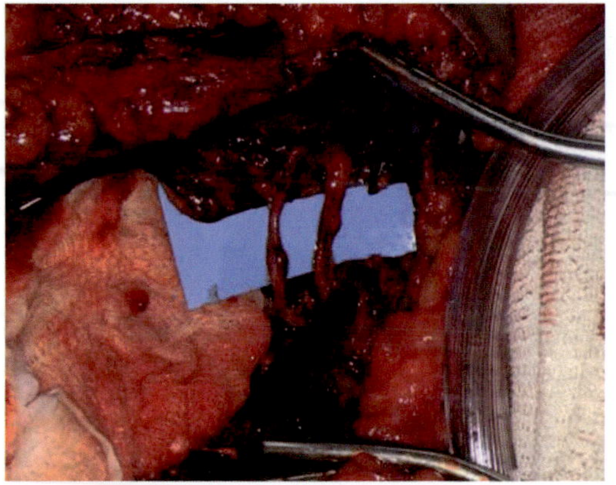

Fig. 10.14 Coaptation of the FDS and FCR motor branches to the ECRB and PIN branches

When deciding between different nerve transfer options, in addition to considering factors related to the field of injury and comfort of the surgeon, it is important to consider carefully the extent of plexopathy and roots involved. The nerve roots of the supinator involve C5–C6, while the nerve roots of the FCR involve C6–C7, and, for example, transferring the FCR motor branch would not yield the desired outcome in a patient with C6–C8 plexopathy.

Median Nerve Palsy

When restoring function in patients with median nerve palsy, the first priority should be directed at flexion of the thumb and index finger to restore pincer grasp function. Branches of the radial nerve have been used to reinnervate distal targets in median nerve deficits. In more proximal defects, the musculocutaneous nerve and contralateral cervical nerve root should be considered.

Bertelli described the transfer of the motor branch of ECRB to the AIN in a small series of four patients [79]. In his limited series, all four patients recovered at least grade M4 motor function and mean pinch strength of 2 kg [79]. In patients with more distal median nerve injuries, Li et al. described transfer of the motor branch of pronator teres to the AIN [78]. This is the same cohort as described above, but only two of three patients who followed up had satisfactory motor function recovery in the AIN distribution.

In the event that there are a complete median nerve palsy and absence of suitable distal motor donors, Ray et al. have described a series of cases where the motor branch to the brachialis is trans-

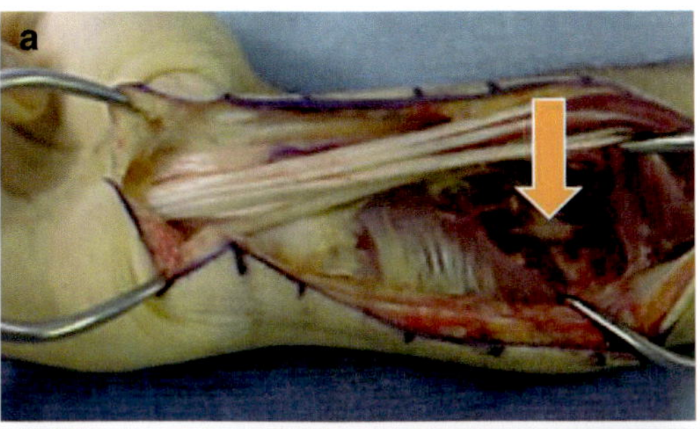

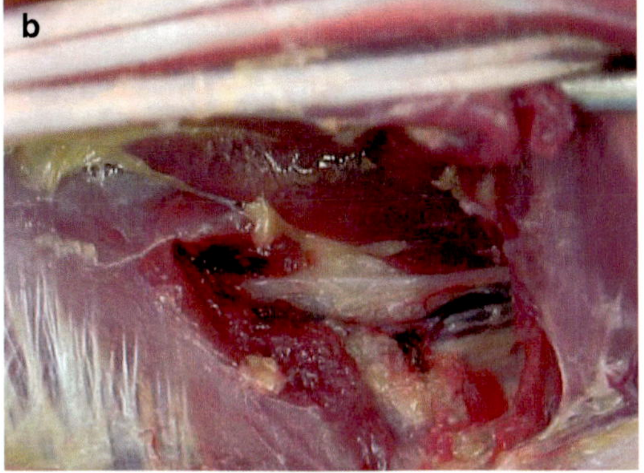

Fig. 10.15 (a) Identify the anterior interosseous nerve (AIN) motor branch to the pronator quadratus muscle (arrow highlights nerve entering pronator quadratus); (b) magnified view of AIN motor branch entering pronator quadratus

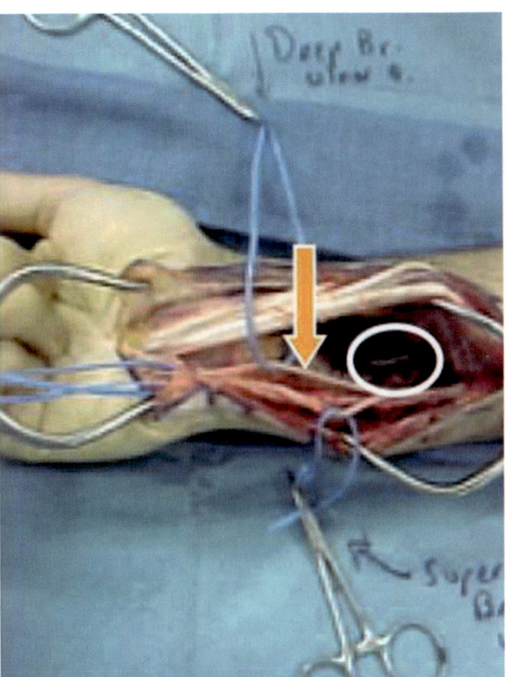

Fig. 10.16 Identify the deep branch of the ulnar nerve. Arrow highlights deep branch of ulnar nerve; circle highlights AIN branch to pronator quadratus. Vessel loops around superficial branch of ulnar nerve (located more ulnar than deep branch in photo)

ferred to the AIN [80]. In their limited series of four patients, all patients recovered grade M4 and mean pinch strength of 2.25 kg [80].

In the event of a complete brachial plexus avulsion, it is possible to transfer the contralateral C7 nerve root to the median nerve [81]; however, there is a great deal of variability in reported outcomes, with anywhere from 26% to 75% of patients achieving antigravity function with distal motor targets in the median nerve distribution [33, 82].

Ulnar Nerve Palsy

Nerve transfers available for the reinnervation of distal targets in the ulnar nerve distribution are fairly limited but do offer the advantage that the known nerve transfers do not compromise any potential future tendon transfers. Motor branches from both the radial and median nerves can be used as donors to reinnervate distal targets in the ulnar nerve distribution. The pronator quadratus motor branch from the AIN can be transferred to the deep branch of the ulnar nerve to recover intrinsic function (Figs. 10.15, 10.16, 10.17, and 10.18) [83]. Battiston et al. reported a series of patients, where 6/7 gained grade M4 power in distal targets [83].

If it is not possible to harvest the motor branch to the pronator quadratus, there are case reports detailing the transfer of the motor branch of the PIN to the ulnar nerve [84, 85]; however, at present no case series exist to guide surgeons and patients as to what might be expected beyond the successful case reports that have been described.

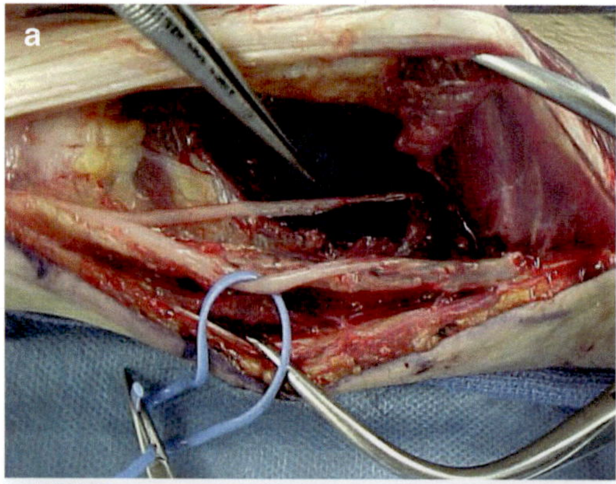

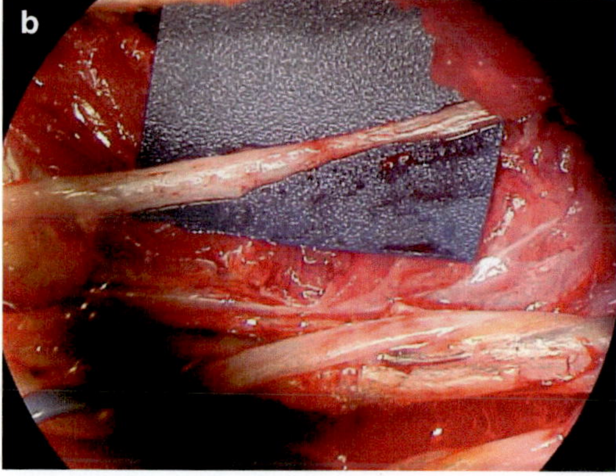

Fig. 10.17 (**a**) View of the coaptation between the AIN branch to the pronator quadratus; (**b**) view of coaptation between AIN branch and ulnar nerve under microscope

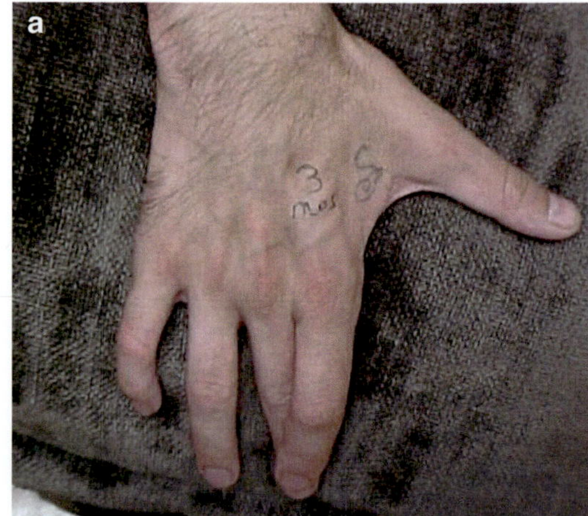

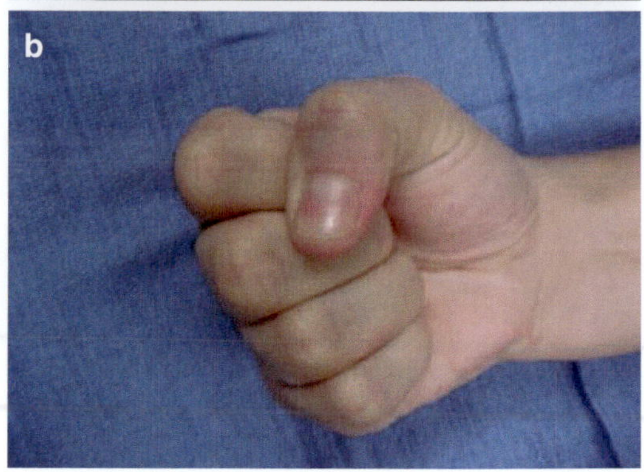

Fig. 10.18 (**a**) Clinical photo of outcome at 3 months – use of intrinsics to cross fingers; (**b**) demonstration of patient making a fist, showing no loss of thumb IP flexion as AIN transfer is done distal to innervation of flexor pollicis longus

Tendon Transfers

History

Nicoladoni described the earliest tendon transfers in the medical literature in 1881 [86]. The aim of early tendon transfers was to restore ambulatory function in a patient afflicted by poliomyelitis [86]. While early tendon transfers focused primarily on restoring ambulatory function to polio patients, World War I and World War II saw a significant increase in patients who sustained upper extremity injury with accompanying functional deficit [87–89]. Foundational principles of tendon transfers were first described by Mayer, and while there has been increased understanding in techniques and strategies to optimize outcomes, these principles are still important to consider [87]. Tendon transfers are meant restore function to non-functioning neuromuscular units, specifically by transferring the force generated by a functional neuromuscular unit to a non-functioning unit. When considering tendon transfers as a part of the reconstructive algorithm in managing upper extremity injury, the timing, zone of injury, availability of donor neuromuscular groups, specific reconstructive goals, strength, and other patient-specific factors must be carefully considered.

Principles of Tendon Transfer

As with nerve transfers, the adage stealing from Peter to pay Paul must be considered. The functional loss associated with harvesting a donor tendon must be less than the gain that is expected after transfer; ideally the donor tendon is expendable or redundant. Unlike in nerve transfers, it is important to consider the excursion of the donor unit when performing tendon transfers – as the myotendinous unit must be able to cause movement within an appropriately functional arc to the recipient site. Additionally, it is important to consider the force vector of the donor neuromuscular unit – and whether this force vector is appropriately in line with the intended recipient site. The joints affected by the intended recipient must also be supple and mobile and have a stable osseous environment. Strength of the donor tendon must be considered, as it is common to decrease the power of the tendon by one grade after transfer. It is also optimal to choose a donor neuromuscular unit that operates in phase, or synergistic, with the intended recipient, as this will facilitate rehabilitation. Finally, it is critical to consider the soft tissue environment. There must be a stable and pliable soft tissue bed, absent significant scaring, to allow for gliding of the donor tendon as it reaches its new recipient site. Unlike in nerve transfers, there is no "time limit" of an optimal window for tendon transfers, provided supple joints have been maintained in intended recipient region. Tendon transfers can be done many years after injury making this an attractive option for patients presenting late, who are no longer candidates for nerve transfer.

Median Nerve Palsy

High median nerve palsy describes injury or functional deficit beginning proximal to the elbow. In high median nerve palsy, there are several functional deficits that must be considered. There is loss of strength of both pronation and wrist flexion strength. There is also loss of thumb IP flexion, thumb opposition, and both DIP and PIP flexion at the index and long fingers. From the perspective of reconstruction with tendon transfers, the goals of reconstruction are primarily to restore thumb IP flexion, thumb opposition, and index and long finger DIP and PIP flexion. Since the FCU is intact, there is often adequate wrist flexion strength. Additionally, any loss in pronation can often be compensated for with the

brachioradialis or be overcome with shoulder motion.

Thumb opposition is perhaps the most important reconstructive goal to achieve, and several tendon transfers have been described to restore thumb opposition. Shin and Dao reviewed previously described opponensplasty techniques, with possible donor tendons including the FDS of the ulnar digits, the abductor digiti quinti, EDM, ECU, PL, ECRL, EIP, and EPL tendons [90]. When considering how to technically achieve thumb opposition, it is important to consider that opposition results from a combination of motions – notably pronation, MP joint flexion, and abduction. In order to replicate the aggregate vector that generates opposition, any muscle that originates in the forearm must be rerouted over a pulley to recreate the force vector of thumb opposition. Bunnell described the first pulley, using the pisiform as the fulcrum around which to reroute the force vector [91, 92]. Bunnell's pulley routes the FDS of the ring finger to the APB tendon by routing the FDS of the ring finger around the pisiform. Cooney et al. performed a biomechanical study of both FDS and ECRL opponensplasties and found that the Bunnell technique restored 40% of thenar strength while the ECRL restored 60% of thenar strength [93].

Burkhalter et al. were the first to describe the EIP to APB tendon transfer for restoration of thumb opposition. After harvesting the EIP, it is passed retrograde through the extensor retinaculum and then subcutaneously across the ulnar border of the hand and through the palm until it is attached to the APB stump (Figs. 10.19, 10.20, 10.21, and 10.22) [94]. Anderson et al. studied the clinical outcomes in a series of patients who underwent EIP opponensplasty, and 35/40 were able to at least oppose the tip of the index finger with the thumb [95].

When attempting to address index and long finger DIP and PIP flexion, it is important to assess all deficits. In the event that the ulnar nerve is intact, it is possible to perform a "sidecar" tenodesis to the FDP of the small and ring fingers to restore PIP and DIP flexion. When performing a "sidecar" tenodesis, it is important to position the digits in a normal resting cascade (Fig. 10.23).

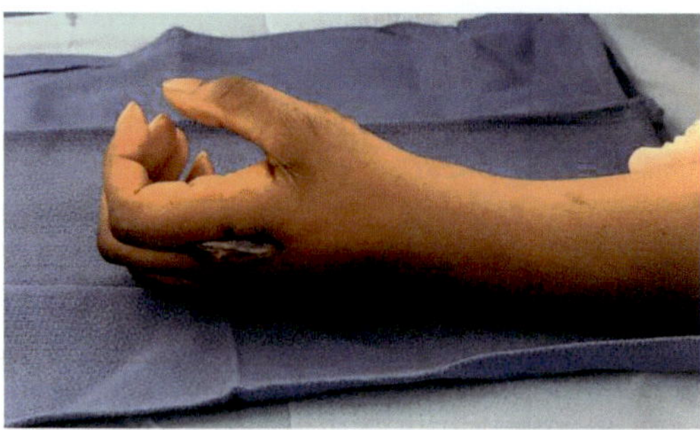

Fig. 10.19 Identification of extensor indicis proprius (EIP) tendon

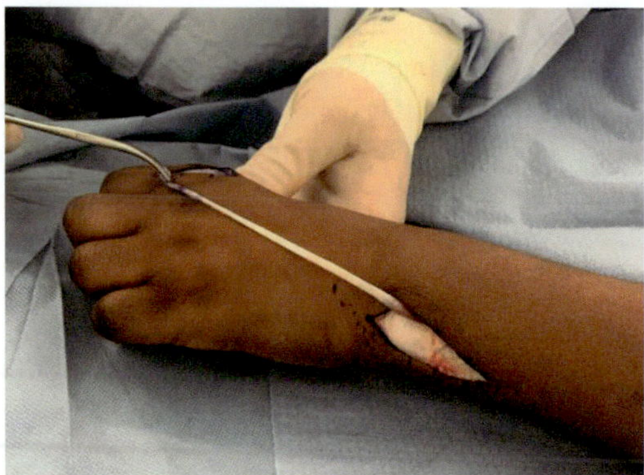

Fig. 10.20 Proximal dissection and harvest of EIP tendon to prepare reroute of tendon, with demonstration of tendon length and excursion

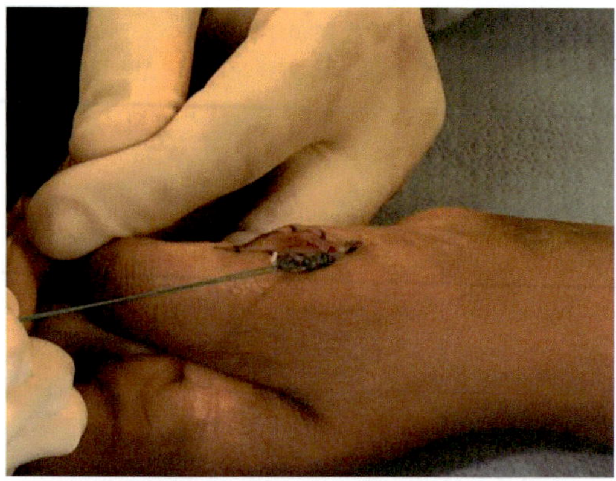

Fig. 10.21 Subcutaneously rerouted EIP to abductor pollicis brevis (APB tendon) insertion

If it is not possible to tenodese the index and long digits to the adjacent FDPs, then the ECRL has been described as a suitable donor for tendon transfer [96]. To restore thumb IP flexion, bra-

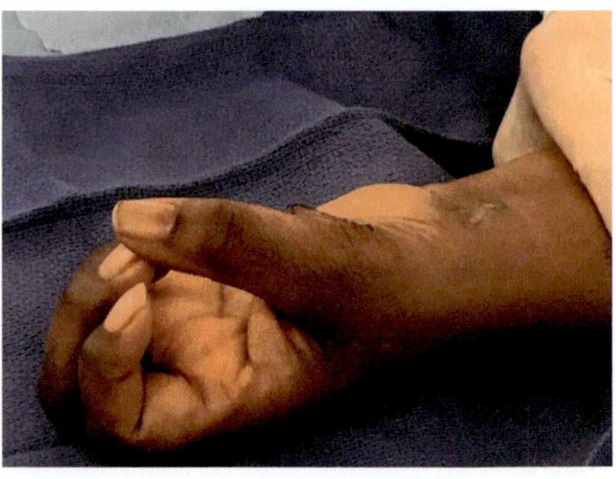

Fig. 10.22 Position of thumb after completion of transfer of EIP to APB, showing thumb in more pronated and palmarly abducted position at rest

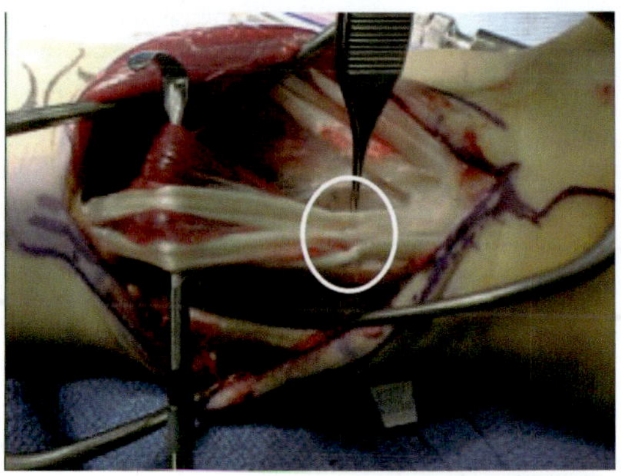

Fig. 10.23 Demonstration of "sidecar" or "hitch-hiking" tenodesis suturing all four slips of the flexor digitorum profundus side to side. It is important to restore the normal flexion "cascade" of the digits when this is performed

chioradialis can be harvested with the intended recipient the immediately adjacent FPL tendon [97]. If the brachioradialis is not available, it is possible to harvest either the ECRL or ECU tendons [97]. When suturing in the donor tendon to the FPL recipient site, tensioning is important – and the thumb MP and IP joints should be in 30° of flexion with the wrist in a neutral position.

Ulnar Nerve Palsy

Like median nerve palsies, ulnar nerve palsies can be classified as high or low – with high ulnar nerve palsies affecting muscle innervation proximal to the wrist joint. The deficits encountered in high ulnar nerve palsy include the weakness in wrist flexion, loss of PIP and DIP motion of the ring and small finger, loss of thumb adduction, and loss of hand intrinsic muscle function.

Loss of intrinsic function of the hand results in a muscle imbalance that causes a clawed appearance. In brief, the EDC function is unopposed because the intrinsic flexion forces at the MCP joint are absent – and the hand demonstrates hyperextension at the MCP joint with simultaneous IP flexion from extrinsic finger flexors. Typically clawing preferentially affects the ring and small fingers, because the lumbricals of the long and index finger receive some innervation from the median nerve. There are three techniques described for managing clawing of the digits – specifically the Zancolli lasso, the Stiles-Bunnell, and the Brand procedures [96, 98, 99].

The Zancolli lasso technique uses the FDS of the affected finger to restore MP flexion [100]. In brief, the FDS is transected proximal to its insertion, extricated from the flexor tendon sheath at the level of the MP joint, and sewn back onto itself over the A1 pulley. This creates MP flexion and slight IP joint extension when appropriately tensioned with the MCP joint in approximately 60° of flexion.

The Stiles-Bunnell transfer requires donation of the FDS of the long finger tendon only. The FDS of the long finger is transected just proximal to its insertion and extracted from the flexor tendon sheath. After removal, it is divided in half, and the halves are individually advanced through the lumbrical canal and sewn into the lateral band of the ring and small fingers (Fig. 10.24).

In both the Zancolli lasso and the Stiles-Bunnell transfer, there is risk of developing a post-operative swan neck deformity because the FDS no longer is contributing to PIP flexion.

If there is a desire to avoid a potential swan neck deformity, the Brand transfer can be performed. In the Brand transfer, either the FCR or ECRB is harvested. The donor tendon is then split into as many tails as are needed to address the clawing. Each tail is then attached to the radial lateral band of the affected finger – though often it is necessary to harvest free tendon graft to accommodate the added distance. Both the Brand

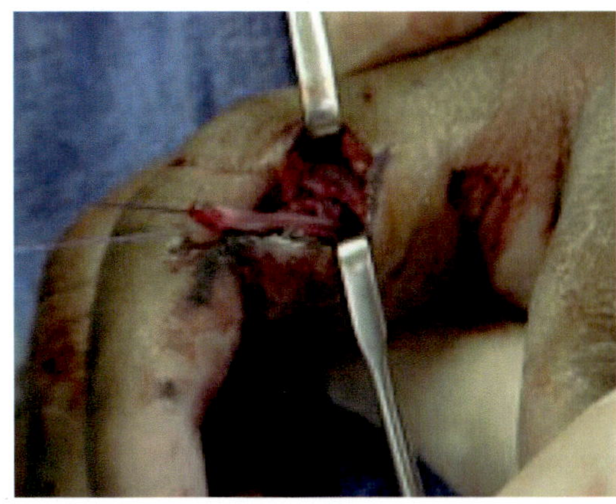

Fig. 10.24 Transfer of flexor digitorum superficialis (FDS) to radial aspect of lateral bands

transfer and the Zancolli lasso can be done if all four digits are affected by clawing, which is seen with a concomitant median nerve injury.

In executing pinch grip, there must be coordination of the adductor pollicis, the flexor pollicis brevis muscle, and the first dorsal interosseous muscle. In ulnar nerve palsy, the adductor pollicis is absent, and a tendon transfer must be performed to approximate normal function and restore pinch grip. It is possible to transfer the ECRB in an adductorplasty to restore thumb adduction. The ECRB is separated from its insertion, extracted from the extensor retinaculum, and then routed between the second and third metacarpals where it is attached to the adductor pollicis tendon palmarly.

Radial Nerve Palsy

Much like median and ulnar nerve palsies, the level of injury impacts the expected deficits seen in radial nerve palsy. If the injury is proximal to the elbow, the patient will have a high radial nerve palsy – with associated loss of innervation to the brachioradialis, ECRB, ECRL, EDC, ECU, EPL, and EIP. The functional consequence of a high radial nerve palsy includes inability to extend the wrist, inability to extend the fingers at the MP joints, and inability to radially abduct the thumb.

The most commonly performed tendon transfer for wrist extension involves transferring the pronator teres to the ECRB or ECRL [101, 102].

The PT is harvested from the radial aspect of the mid forearm, and mobilized, typically with a strip of periosteum to maximize length. It is then transferred radially and woven into the radial wrist extensors and can be routed into either the ECRL or ECRB or divided and routed into both wrist extensors (Figs. 10.26, 10.27, 10.28, 10.29, 10.30, and 10.31) [102]. It is important to tension the transferred myotendinous unit with the wrist in 45° of extension [102]. Thumb extension can be achieved either by transfer of the palmaris longus or the FDS of the ring finger to the EPL tendon. In some cases, the palmaris is absent or has already been harvested – which necessitates the use of the ring finger FDS. (Others have recommended using FDS of middle to maintain ring finger FDS, optimizing grip strength.) When performing the

tendon transfer to regain thumb extension, it may be easier to harvest the EPL from the dorsal wrist and then route the EPL tendon radially in the subcutaneous tissue (Figs. 10.25, 10.28, 10.29, 10.30, and 10.31) [102].

Jones et al. described transferring the FCR to restore finger extension at the MP joint [103].

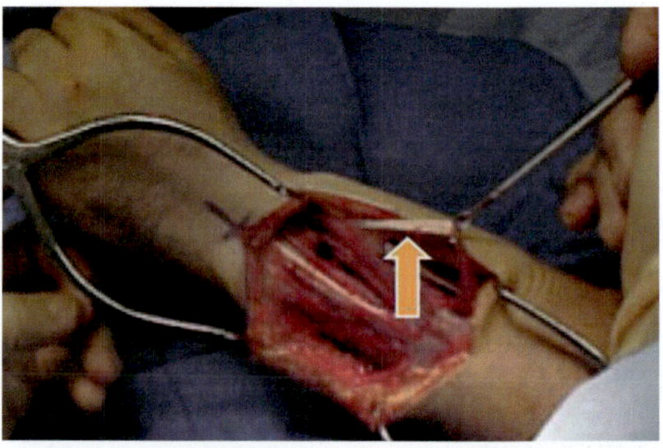

Fig. 10.27 Identification of extensor carpi radialis brevis (ECRB) tendon. Arrow indicates tendon; observe position of wrist in extension

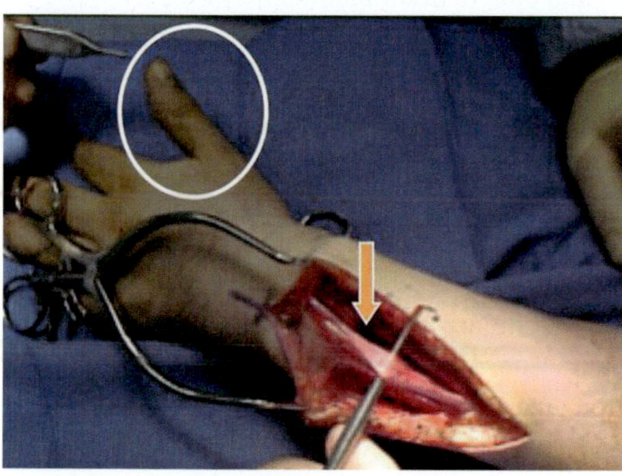

Fig. 10.25 Identification of extensor pollicis longus (EPL) tendon intraoperatively. Arrow highlights tendon, and circle highlights action after intraoperatively applying traction to tendon

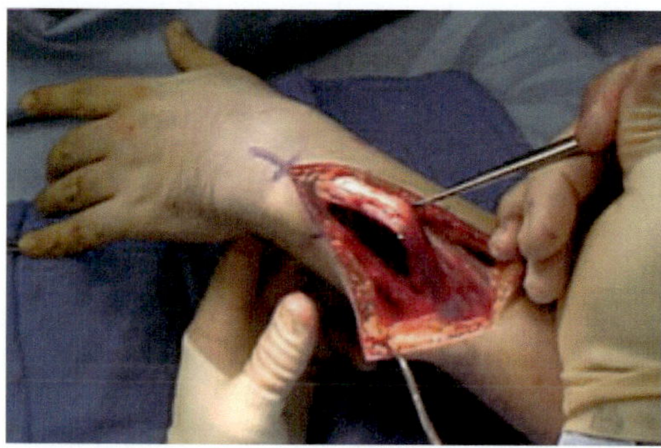

Fig. 10.26 Identification of extensor digitorum communis (EDC) tendons. Note extension of digits in photo

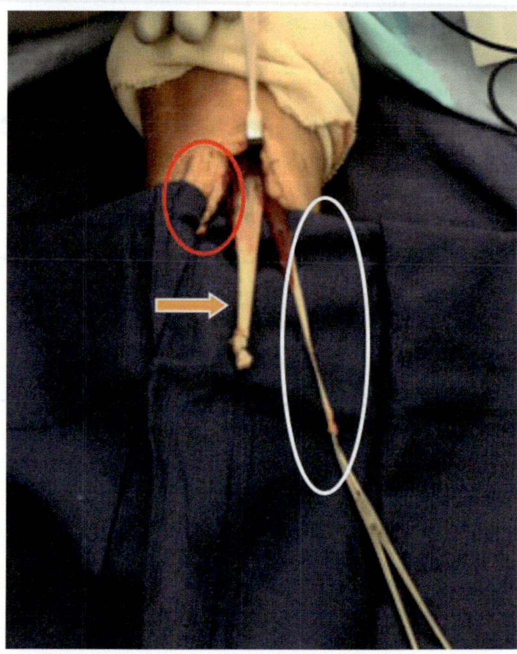

Fig. 10.28 Harvest of pronator teres (PT), flexor carpi radialis (FCR), and ring finger flexor digitorum superficialis (FDS). Arrow indicates FCR tendon, red circle indicates PT tendon, and white circle indicates ring finger FDS tendon

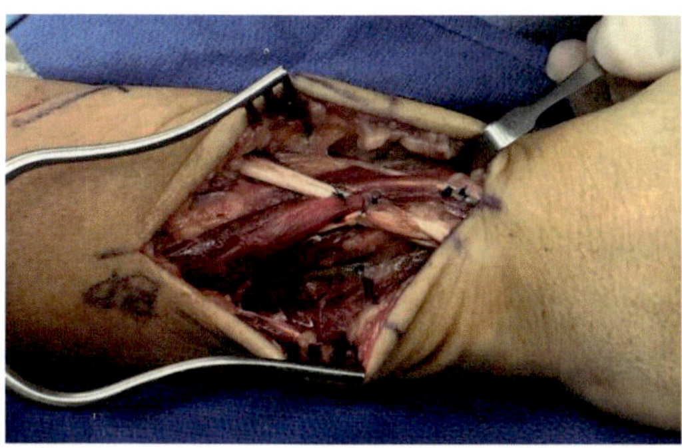

Fig. 10.29 Transfer of PT to ECRB, FCR to EDC, and FDS of ring finger to EPL using a Pulvertaft weave suture technique

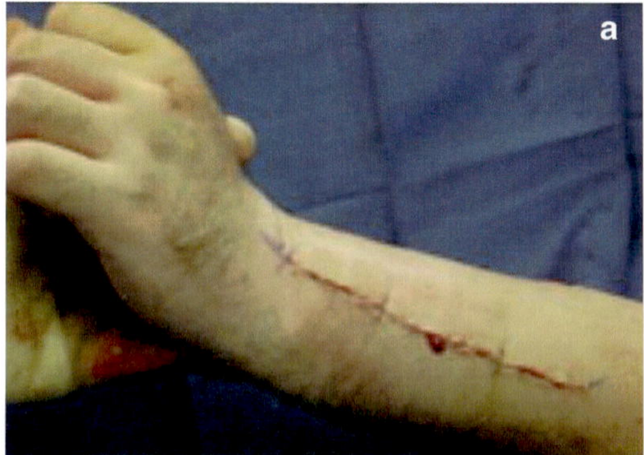

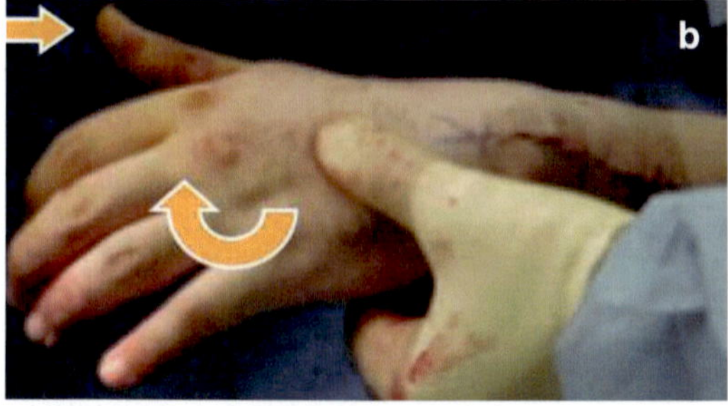

Fig. 10.30 (**a**) Intraoperative tenodesis test with wrist extended; (**b**) with wrist flexed

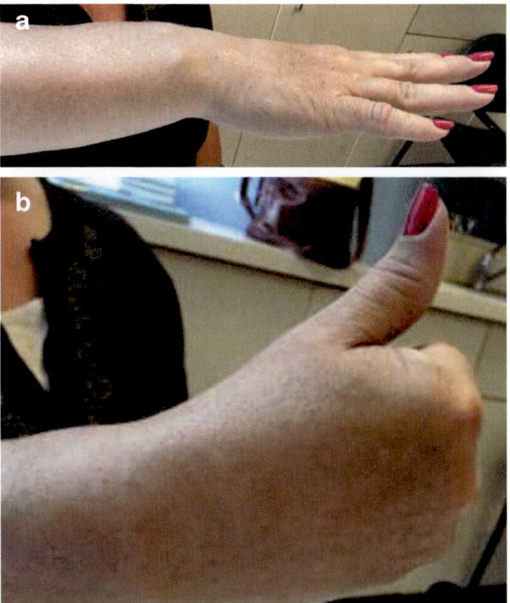

Fig. 10.31 Clinical outcome showing (**a**) digital extension and (**b**) thumb extension

EDC tendon. Tensioning is achieved with the wrist in neutral and the MP joints in full extension [105].

Elbow Flexion

As was discussed previously, the restoration of elbow flexion is among the most important functional considerations when treating a patient with a mangled upper extremity [49, 50]. The loss of elbow flexion is incredibly disabling – and several tendon transfers have been described to restore active elbow flexion. The donor muscles that have been described include the pectoralis major, latissimus dorsi, the Steindler flexorplasty (which involves transfer of the flexor-pronator mass onto the distal humerus), and the triceps brachii [106–111]. Transfer of the pectoralis major has been described in both a unipolar or bipolar fashion. In bipolar muscle transfer, both the origin and insertion of the pectoralis major are mobilized and relocated – and some prior literature suggests that a bipolar transfer is more mechanically advantaged because the axis of the transfer is more aligned with the axis of the elbow

Alternatively some studies have described harvesting the FCU and long finger FDS with the intent to deliver to the EDG, but there is risk of compromising the dart throwers motion if the FCU is harvested [104]. In FCR transfer, the tendon is divided distally at the wrist crease and then passed through the interosseous membrane – at which point it is affixed to the EDC tendon. Alternatively, the FCR can be routed radially in the subcutaneous tissue and then affixed to the flexors [107]. In a limited series of bipolar pectoralis tendon transfers, Botte et al. demonstrated that 4/4 patients achieved at least grade M3 power and a mean active range of motion from 25° to 125°.

Latissimus tendon transfers can also be monopolar or unipolar, but the transfer is considered to be more technically demanding than a pectoralis tendon transfer. There are some concerns that harvesting the latissimus dorsi could destabilize the shoulder, and it is important to recognize that the latissimus dorsi is often used as a tendon transfer in the paralytic shoulder. The literature on transfer of the latissimus dorsi tendon for restoration of elbow flexion suggests that a majority (roughly 74%) of patients achieve at least grade M4 elbow flexion, with a mean active flexion from 45° to 130° [112, 113]. Both the latissimus and pectoralis transfers may be utilized as a myocutaneous flap and offer the additional advantage of conferring soft tissue coverage in the setting of mangled extremity.

The Steindler flexorplasty and triceps to biceps transfers are additional options to restore elbow flexion. These transfers are less technically demanding than pectoralis major or latissimus dorsi transfer. The Steindler flexorplasty involves transferring the flexor-pronator mass more proximally onto the humerus – so that the flexor-pronator mass achieves both wrist and elbow flexion using a single muscle group. The Steindler flexorplasty is able to confer at least M4 power in a majority of patients (over 80% combined in two series), however, the active arc of motion smaller with mean active flexion and the mean arc ranging from 107° to 142° [114, 115]. Transferring the long head of the triceps to the biceps brachii is another means of restoring elbow flexion. In their series, Hoang et al. reported 5/7 patients achieved grade M4 motor function for elbow flexion – and the extension deficit as a result of the transfer was fairly minimal with a mean of 13° [116]. The mean active arc of motion achieved as a result of triceps to biceps transfer was 123°, with 3.3 kg flexion strength [116].

References

1. Paulus Aegeneta (Paul of Aegina). The seven books (Translated by F. Adams), vol. II. London: Sydenham Society; 1844–1847. p. 132–7.
2. Waller A. Experiments on the section of the glossopharyngeal and hypoglossal nerves of the frog, and observations of the alterations produced thereby in the structure of their primitive fibres. Edinb Med Surg J. 1851;76(189):369–76.
3. Seddon HJ. Peripheral nerve injuries. Glasgow Med J. 1943;139(3):61–75.
4. Seddon H. Advances in nerve repair. Triangle. 1968;8(7):252–9.
5. Campbell JB. Peripheral nerve repair. Clin Neurosurg. 1970;17:77–98.
6. Sunderland S. Nerves and Nerve Injury. Livingstone, LTD,. Edinburgh/London 1968.
7. Sunderland S. The anatomy and physiology of nerve injury. Muscle Nerve. 1990;13(9):771–84.
8. Sunderland S. Advances in diagnosis and treatment of root and peripheral nerve injury. Adv Neurol. 1979;22:271–305.
9. Sunderland S. The anatomic foundation of peripheral nerve repair techniques. Orthop Clin North Am. 1981;12(2):245–66.
10. Mackinnon SE, Novak CB. Nerve transfers. New options for reconstruction following nerve injury. Hand Clin. 1999;15(4):643–66. ix
11. Flourens P. Experiences sur la reunion ou cicatrisation des plaies de la moelle epiniere et des nerfs. Ann Sci Nat. 1828;13:113–22.
12. Dellon ES, Dellon AL. The first nerve graft, Vulpian, and the nineteenth century neural regeneration controversy. J Hand Surg Am. 1993;18(2):369–72.
13. Spicher C, Kohut G. Jean Joseph Emile Létiévant: a review of his contributions to surgery and rehabilitation. J Reconstr Microsurg. 2001;17(3):169–77.
14. Harris W, Low VW. On the importance of accurate muscular analysis in lesions of the brachial plexus and the treatment of Erb's palsy and infantile paralysis of the upper extremity by cross-union of nerve roots. Br Med J. 1903;2:1035.
15. Lee SK, Wolfe SW. Nerve transfers for the upper extremity: new horizons in nerve reconstruction. J Am Acad Orthop Surg. 2012;20(8):506–17.
16. Lien SC, Cederna PS, Kuzon WM. Optimizing skeletal muscle reinnervation with nerve transfer. Hand Clin. 2008;24(4):445–54. vii
17. Schreiber JJ, Byun DJ, Khair MM, Rosenblatt L, Lee SK, Wolfe SW. Optimal axon counts for brachial plexus nerve transfers to restore elbow flexion. Plast Reconstr Surg. 2015;135(1):135e–41e.
18. Paternostrosluga T, Grimstieger M, Posch M, et al. Reliability and validity of the Medical Research Council (MRC) scale and a modified scale for testing muscle strength in patients with radial palsy. J Rehabil Med. 2008;40(8):665–71.

19. Desai MJ, Daly CA, Seiler JG, Wray WH, Ruch DS, Leversedge FJ. Radial to axillary nerve transfers: a combined case series. J Hand Surg Am. 2016;41(12):1128–34.

20. Sakuma M, Gorski G, Sheu SH, et al. Lack of motor recovery after prolonged denervation of the neuromuscular junction is not due to regenerative failure. Eur J Neurosci. 2016;43(3):451–62.

21. Höke A. Mechanisms of disease: what factors limit the success of peripheral nerve regeneration in humans? Nat Clin Pract Neurol. 2006;2(8):448–54.

22. Chao T, Frump D, Lin M, et al. Matrix metalloproteinase 3 deletion preserves denervated motor endplates after traumatic nerve injury. Ann Neurol. 2013;73(2):210–23.

23. Dimou S, Biggs M, Tonkin M, Hickie IB, Lagopoulos J. Motor cortex neuroplasticity following brachial plexus transfer. Front Hum Neurosci. 2013;7:500.

24. Socolovsky M, Malessy M, Lopez D, Guedes F, Flores L. Current concepts in plasticity and nerve transfers: relationship between surgical techniques and outcomes. Neurosurg Focus. 2017;42(3):E13.

25. Bertelli JA, Ghizoni MF. Results of spinal accessory to suprascapular nerve transfer in 110 patients with complete palsy of the brachial plexus. J Neurosurg Spine. 2016;24(6):990–5.

26. Terzis JK, Kostas I. Suprascapular nerve reconstruction in 118 cases of adult posttraumatic brachial plexus. Plast Reconstr Surg. 2006;117(2):613–29.

27. Suzuki K, Doi K, Hattori Y, Pagsaligan JM. Long-term results of spinal accessory nerve transfer to the suprascapular nerve in upper-type paralysis of brachial plexus injury. J Reconstr Microsurg. 2007;23(6):295–9.

28. Kierner AC, Burian M, Bentzien S, Gstoettner W. Intraoperative electromyography for identification of the trapezius muscle innervation: clinical proof of a new anatomical concept. Laryngoscope. 2002;112(10):1853–6.

29. Kierner AC, Zelenka I, Burian M. How do the cervical plexus and the spinal accessory nerve contribute to the innervation of the trapezius muscle? As seen from within using Sihler's stain. Arch Otolaryngol Head Neck Surg. 2001;127(10):1230–2.

30. Colbert SH, Mackinnon SE. Nerve transfers for brachial plexus reconstruction. Hand Clin. 2008;24(4):341–61. v

31. Souza FH, Bernardino SN, Filho HC, et al. Comparison between the anterior and posterior approach for transfer of the spinal accessory nerve to the suprascapular nerve in late traumatic brachial plexus injuries. Acta Neurochir. 2014;156(12):2345–9.

32. Siqueira MG, Martins RS, Solla D, Faglioni W, Foroni L, Heise CO. Functional outcome of spinal accessory nerve transfer to the suprascapular nerve to restore shoulder function: results in upper and complete traumatic brachial plexus palsy in adults. Neurol India. 2019;67(Supplement):S77–81.

33. Bhatia A, Shyam AK, Doshi P, Shah V. Nerve reconstruction: a cohort study of 93 cases of global brachial plexus palsy. Indian J Orthop. 2011;45(2):153–60.

34. Leechavengvongs S, Malungpaishorpe K, Uerpairojkit C, Ng CY, Witoonchart K. Nerve transfers to restore shoulder function. Hand Clin. 2016;32(2):153–64.

35. Cardenas-mejia A, O'boyle CP, Chen KT, Chuang DC. Evaluation of single-, double-, and triple-nerve transfers for shoulder abduction in 90 patients with supraclavicular brachial plexus injury. Plast Reconstr Surg. 2008;122(5):1470–8.

36. Malessy MJ, Hoffmann CF, Thomeer RT. Initial report on the limited value of hypoglossal nerve transfer to treat brachial plexus root avulsions. J Neurosurg. 1999;91(4):601–4.

37. Hu S, Chu B, Song J, Chen L. Anatomic study of the intercostal nerve transfer to the suprascapular nerve and a case report. J Hand Surg Eur Vol. 2014;39(2):194–8.

38. Yian EH, Sodl JF, Dionysian E, Schneeberger AG. Anterior deltoid reeducation for irreparable rotator cuff tears revisited. J Shoulder Elb Surg. 2017;26(9):1562–5.

39. Jerome JT, Rajmohan B. Axillary nerve neurotization with the anterior deltopectoral approach in brachial plexus injuries. Microsurgery. 2012;32(6):445–51.

40. Lu J, Xu J, Xu W, et al. Combined nerve transfers for repair of the upper brachial plexus injuries through a posterior approach. Microsurgery. 2012;32(2):111–7.

41. Ren GH, Li RG, Xiang DY, Yu B. Reconstruction of shoulder abduction by multiple nerve fascicle transfer through posterior approach. Injury. 2013;44(4):492–7.

42. Leechavengvongs S, Teerawutthichaikit T, Witoonchart K, et al. Surgical anatomy of the axillary nerve branches to the deltoid muscle. Clin Anat. 2015;28(1):118–22.

43. Bauer AS, Rabinovich RV, Waters PM. The anterior approach for transfer of radial nerve triceps fascicles to the axillary nerve. J Hand Surg Am. 2019;44(4):345. e1–6.

44. Jerome JT. Long head of the triceps branch transfer to axillary nerve in C5, C6 brachial plexus injuries: anterior approach. Plast Reconstr Surg. 2011;128(3):740–1.

45. Estrella EP, Favila AS. Nerve transfers for shoulder function for traumatic brachial plexus injuries. J Reconstr Microsurg. 2014;30(1):59–64.

46. Ray WZ, Murphy RK, Santosa K, Johnson PJ, Mackinnon SE. Medial pectoral nerve to axillary nerve neurotization following traumatic brachial plexus injuries: indications and clinical outcomes. Hand (N Y). 2012;7(1):59–65.

47. Samardzić M, Rasulić L, Grujicić D, Milicić B. Results of nerve transfers to the musculocutaneous and axillary nerves. Neurosurgery. 2000;46(1):93–101.

48. Terzis JK, Barmpitsioti A. Axillary nerve reconstruction in 176 posttraumatic plexopathy patients. Plast Reconstr Surg. 2010;125(1):233–47.

49. Brophy RH, Wolfe SW. Planning brachial plexus surgery: treatment options and priorities. Hand Clin. 2005;21(1):47–54.

50. Shin AY, Spinner RJ, Steinmann SP, Bishop AT. Adult traumatic brachial plexus injuries. J Am Acad Orthop Surg. 2005;13(6):382–96.

51. Oberlin C, Béal D, Leechavengvongs S, Salon A, Dauge MC, Sarcy JJ. Nerve transfer to biceps muscle using a part of ulnar nerve for C5-C6 avulsion of the brachial plexus: anatomical study and report of four cases. J Hand Surg Am. 1994;19(2):232–7.

52. Oberlin C, Ameur NE, Teboul F, Beaulieu JY, Vacher C. Restoration of elbow flexion in brachial plexus injury by transfer of ulnar nerve fascicles to the nerve to the biceps muscle. Tech Hand Up Extrem Surg. 2002;6(2):86–90.

53. Bulstra LF, Shin AY. Nerve transfers to restore elbow function. Hand Clin. 2016;32(2):165–74.

54. Oberlin C, Durand S, Belheyar Z, Shafi M, David E, Asfazadourian H. Nerve transfers in brachial plexus palsies. Chir Main. 2009;28(1):1–9.

55. Sungpet A, Suphachatwong C, Kawinwonggowit V, Patradul A. Transfer of a single fascicle from the ulnar nerve to the biceps muscle after avulsions of upper roots of the brachial plexus. J Hand Surg Br. 2000;25(4):325–8.

56. Coulet B, Boretto JG, Lazerges C, Chammas M. A comparison of intercostal and partial ulnar nerve transfers in restoring elbow flexion following upper brachial plexus injury (C5-C6+/-C7). J Hand Surg Am. 2010;35(8):1297–303.

57. Tung TH, Novak CB, Mackinnon SE. Nerve transfers to the biceps and brachialis branches to improve elbow flexion strength after brachial plexus injuries. J Neurosurg. 2003;98(2):313–8.

58. Cho AB, Paulos RG, De Rresende MR, et al. Median nerve fascicle transfer versus ulnar nerve fascicle transfer to the biceps motor branch in C5-C6 and C5-C7 brachial plexus injuries: nonrandomized prospective study of 23 consecutive patients. Microsurgery. 2014;34(7):511–5.

59. Mackinnon SE, Novak CB, Myckatyn TM, Tung TH. Results of reinnervation of the biceps and brachialis muscles with a double fascicular transfer for elbow flexion. J Hand Surg Am. 2005;30(5):978–85.

60. Carlsen BT, Kircher MF, Spinner RJ, Bishop AT, Shin AY. Comparison of single versus double nerve transfers for elbow flexion after brachial plexus injury. Plast Reconstr Surg. 2011;127(1):269–76.

61. Martins RS, Siqueira MG, Heise CO, Foroni L, Teixeira MJ. A prospective study comparing single and double fascicular transfer to restore elbow flexion after brachial plexus injury. Neurosurgery. 2013;72(5):709–14.

62. Terzis JK, Kostopoulos VK. The surgical treatment of brachial plexus injuries in adults. Plast Reconstr Surg. 2007;119(4):73e–92e.

63. Merrell GA, Barrie KA, Katz DL, Wolfe SW. Results of nerve transfer techniques for restoration of shoulder and elbow function in the context of a meta-analysis of the English literature. J Hand Surg Am. 2001;26(2):303–14.

64. Songcharoen P, Wongtrakul S, Spinner RJ. Brachial plexus injuries in the adult. Nerve transfers: the Siriraj Hospital experience. Hand Clin. 2005;21(1):83–9.

65. Siqueira MG, Martins RS. Phrenic nerve transfer in the restoration of elbow flexion in brachial plexus avulsion injuries: how effective and safe is it? Neurosurgery. 2009;65(4 Suppl):A125–31.

66. Dong Z, Zhang CG, Gu YD. Surgical outcome of phrenic nerve transfer to the anterior division of the upper trunk in treating brachial plexus avulsion. J Neurosurg. 2010;112(2):383–5.

67. Maldonado AA, Kircher MF, Spinner RJ, Bishop AT, Shin AY. Free functioning gracilis muscle transfer with and without simultaneous intercostal nerve transfer to musculocutaneous nerve for restoration of elbow flexion after traumatic adult brachial panplexus injury. J Hand Surg Am. 2017;42(4):293.e1–7.

68. Terzis JK, Barmpitsioti A. Our experience with triceps nerve reconstruction in patients with brachial plexus injury. J Plast Reconstr Aesthet Surg. 2012;65(5):590–600.

69. Bertelli J, Soldado F, Ghizoni MF, Rodríguez-baeza A. Transfer of a terminal motor branch nerve to the flexor carpi ulnaris for triceps reinnervation: anatomical study and clinical cases. J Hand Surg Am. 2015;40(11):2229–2235.e2.

70. Oberlin C, Chino J, Belkheyar Z. Surgical treatment of brachial plexus posterior cord lesion: a combination of nerve and tendon transfers, about nine patients. Chir Main. 2013;32(3):141–6.

71. Flores LP. Reanimation of elbow extension with medial pectoral nerve transfer in partial injuries to the brachial plexus. J Neurosurg. 2013;118(3):588–93.

72. Zheng MX, Xu WD, Qiu YQ, Xu JG, Gu YD. Phrenic nerve transfer for elbow flexion and intercostal nerve transfer for elbow extension. J Hand Surg Am. 2010;35(8):1304–9.

73. Goubier JN, Teboul F. Transfer of the intercostal nerves to the nerve of the long head of the triceps to recover elbow extension in brachial plexus palsy. Tech Hand Up Extrem Surg. 2007;11(2):139–41.

74. Gao K, Lao J, Zhao X, Gu Y. Outcome after transfer of intercostal nerves to the nerve of triceps long head in 25 adult patients with total brachial plexus root avulsion injury. J Neurosurg. 2013;118(3):606–10.

75. Ray WZ, Mackinnon SE. Clinical outcomes following median to radial nerve transfers. J Hand Surg Am. 2011;36(2):201–8.

76. García-lópez A, Navarro R, Martinez F, Rojas A. Nerve transfers from branches to the flexor carpi radialis and pronator teres to reconstruct the radial nerve. J Hand Surg Am. 2014;39(1):50–6.

77. Bertelli JA, Ghizoni MF, Tacca CP. Results of wrist extension reconstruction in C5-8 brachial plexus palsy by transferring the pronator quadratus motor branch to the extensor carpi radialis brevis muscle. J Neurosurg. 2016;124(5):1442–9.

78. Li Z, Reynolds M, Satteson E, Nazir O, Petit J, Smith BP. Double distal intraneural fascicular nerve transfers for lower brachial plexus injuries. J Hand Surg Am. 2016;41(4):e15–9.

79. Bertelli JA. Transfer of the radial nerve branch to the extensor carpi radialis brevis to the anterior interosseous nerve to reconstruct thumb and finger flexion. J Hand Surg Am. 2015;40(2):323–328.e2.

80. Ray WZ, Yarbrough CK, Yee A, Mackinnon SE. Clinical outcomes following brachialis to anterior interosseous nerve transfers. J Neurosurg. 2012;117(3):604–9.

81. Terzis JK, Kokkalis ZT. Selective contralateral c7 transfer in posttraumatic brachial plexus injuries: a report of 56 cases. Plast Reconstr Surg. 2009;123(3):927–38.

82. Liu Y, Yang X, Gao K, et al. Outcome of contralateral C7 transfers to different recipient nerves after global brachial plexus avulsion. Brain Behav. 2018;8(12):e01174.

83. Battiston B, Lanzetta M. Reconstruction of high ulnar nerve lesions by distal double median to ulnar nerve transfer. J Hand Surg Am. 1999;24(6):1185–91.

84. Tung TH, Barbour JR, Gontre G, Daliwal G, Mackinnon SE. Transfer of the extensor digiti minimi and extensor carpi ulnaris branches of the posterior interosseous nerve to restore intrinsic hand function: case report and anatomic study. J Hand Surg Am. 2013;38(1):98–103.

85. Phillips BZ, Franco MJ, Yee A, Tung TH, Mackinnon SE, Fox IK. Direct radial to ulnar nerve transfer to restore intrinsic muscle function in combined proximal median and ulnar nerve injury: case report and surgical technique. J Hand Surg Am. 2014;39(7):1358–62.

86. Jeng C, Myerson M. The uses of tendon transfers to correct paralytic deformity of the foot and ankle. Foot Ankle Clin. 2004;9(2):319–37.

87. Mayer L. The physiological method of tendon transplants reviewed after forty years. Instr Course Lect. 1956;13:116–20.

88. Sammer DM, Chung KC. Tendon transfers: part I. Principles of transfer and transfers for radial nerve palsy. Plast Reconstr Surg. 2009;123(5):169e–77e.

89. Bunnell S. Surgery of the hand. Philadelphia: JB Lippincott; 1944. p. 295–300.

90. Shin AY, Dao KD. Tendon transfers for thumb opposition. Atlas Hand Clin. 2002;7(1):1–17.

91. Bunnell S. Opposition of the thumb. J Bone Joint Surg. 1938;22A:269.

92. Goldner JL, Irwin CE. An analysis of paralytic thumb deformities. J Bone Joint Surg Am. 1950;32-A(3):627–39.

93. Cooney WP, Linscheid RL, An KN. Opposition of the thumb: an anatomic and biomechanical study of tendon transfers. J Hand Surg Am. 1984;9(6):777–86.

94. Burkhalter W, Christensen RC, Brown P. Extensor indicis proprius opponensplasty. J Bone Joint Surg Am. 1973;55(4):725–32.

95. Anderson GA, Lee V, Sundararaj GD. Extensor indicis proprius opponensplasty. J Hand Surg Br. 1991;16(3):334–8.

96. Brand PW. Tendon transfers for median and ulnar nerve paralysis. Orthop Clin North Am. 1970;1(2):447–54.

97. Jones NF, Machado GR. Tendon transfers for radial, median, and ulnar nerve injuries: current surgical techniques. Clin Plast Surg. 2011;38(4):621–42.

98. Bunnell S. Tendon transfers in the hand and forearm. Instr Course Lect. 1949;6:106–10.

99. Brand P. Tendon grafting: illustrated by a new operation for intrinsic paralysis of the fingers. J Bone Joint Surg Br. 1961;43:444–53.

100. Zancolli E. Tendon transfers. In: Structural and dynamic bases of hand surgery. 2nd ed. Philadelphia: JB Lippincott Co; 1979. p. 159–206.

101. Brand PW. Clinical mechanics of the hand. St. Louis: CV Mosby; 1985. p. 127–65.

102. Chuinard RG, Boyes JH, Stark HH, Ashworth CR. Tendon transfers for radial nerve palsy: use of superficialis tendons for digital extension. J Hand Surg Am. 1978;3(6):560–70.

103. Jones A. Tendon fixation in unrecoverable musculospinal paralysis. J Orthop Surg. 1919;1:135–40.

104. Raskin KB, Wilgis EF. Flexor carpi ulnaris transfer for radial nerve palsy: functional testing of long-term results. J Hand Surg Am. 1995;20(5):737–42.

105. Boyes JH. Tendon transfers for radial palsy. Bull Hosp Jt Dis. 1960;21:97–105.

106. Clark JM. Reconstruction of biceps brachii by pectoral muscle transplantation. Br J Surg. 1946;34(134):180.

107. Carroll RE, Kleinman WB. Pectoralis major transplantation to restore elbow flexion to the paralytic limb. J Hand Surg Am. 1979;4(6):501–7.

108. Mayer L, Green W. Experiences with the Steindler flexorplasty at the elbow. J Bone Joint Surg Am. 1954;36-A(4):775–89.

109. Haninec P, Szeder V. Reconstruction of elbow flexion by transposition of pedicled long head of triceps brachii muscle. Acta Chir Plast. 1999;41(3):82–6.

110. Kawamura K, Yajima H, Tomita Y, Kobata Y, Shigematsu K, Takakura Y. Restoration of elbow function with pedicled latissimus dorsi myocutaneous flap transfer. J Shoulder Elb Surg. 2007;16(1):84–90.

111. Botte MJ, Wood MB. Flexorplasty of the elbow. Clin Orthop Relat Res. 1989;245:110–6.

112. Stern PJ, Carey JP. The latissimus dorsi flap for reconstruction of the brachium and shoulder. J Bone Joint Surg Am. 1988;70(4):526–35.

113. Vekris MD, Beris AE, Lykissas MG, Korompilias AV, Vekris AD, Soucacos PN. Restoration of elbow function in severe brachial plexus paralysis via muscle transfers. Injury. 2008;39(Suppl 3):S15–22.

114. Liu TK, Yang RS, Sun JS. Long-term results of the Steindler flexorplasty. Clin Orthop Relat Res. 1993;296:104–8.

115. Chen WS. Restoration of elbow flexion by modified Steindler flexorplasty. Int Orthop. 2000;24(1):43–6.

116. Hoang PH, Mills C, Burke FD. Triceps to biceps transfer for established brachial plexus palsy. J Bone Joint Surg Br. 1989;71(2):268–71.

elbow flexion. Elbow extension, arm abduction, and wrist and finger flexion and extension can also be targeted with FMT. Priorities should be determined and a staged approach followed in order to obtain maximal extremity function. Brachial plexus literature currently suggests the staged approach to achieve optimal function as well. The staged approach recommended by Doi is one of the well-accepted protocols [6].

Ultimately the staged reconstruction in a mangled extremity with minimal function may include up to six reconstructive steps that have been outlined by Doi [6]. First, a healthy tissue bed to accept the FMT is necessary to optimize outcomes. This may require serial debridements of the mangled extremity. Second, once the local soft tissue environment is stabilized, the shoulder girdle is stabilized. Third, elbow flexion can be restored with or without finger extension with a gracilis FFMT, depending on the distal attachment site. A potential fourth step would include using a second gracilis FFMT to power finger flexion [7]. Finally, adjunct procedures to re-innervate the triceps [8], fuse the wrist to improve finger range of motion, (Addosooki), or transfer intercostal nerves to the medial cord to provide sensibility of the hand [6] may be considered.

There are several diagnostic studies that may be considered after preparing the wound bed, which can aid in the success of a FMT. An MRI may be obtained, for example, to evaluate donor muscle viability. In addition, angiography may be considered to evaluate the vascularity of the FMT [9]. An angiogram is imperative for the recipient site to ensure that there is a viable inflow pedicle available in the mangled extremity. In traumatic injuries it is not uncommon to have had vascular injuries that may compromise available vascular pedicles for the free flap. An angiogram can help demonstrate patency of vessels and infer viability of surrounding tissues. For instance, a patent anterior interosseous artery by angiogram likely indicates a healthy anterior interosseous nerve, which can power a FFMT [9]. Finally, patient selection is key, as younger and more motivated patients are more likely to succeed due to improved neural regeneration. High levels of motivation are needed to sustain them through the difficult, therapy-intensive, post-operative period. One must be very cautious, then, in selecting an inflow pedicle in which a proximal vascular injury is, or was, suspected, such as in a scapulothoracic dissociation.

Free Functional Muscle Transfer Considerations

Nerve

In a mangled extremity, finding the ideal nerve to re-innervate the FFMT can be difficult. A thorough neurological exam to ensure the FFMT will be adequately powered is mandatory. In addition, pre-operative electrodiagnostic studies can add valuable information in determining the status of a proposed donor nerve. The donor should be a pure motor nerve, ideally with synergistic function to the proposed FFMT function. If possible, it is best to perform the coaptation as close as possible to the FFMT and without nerve graft [3]. Intraoperatively it is important to stimulate and assess the donor nerve with a nerve stimulator. If the appropriate muscle does not contract, the FFMT should not be raised. This is of particular importance with the obturator nerve in the gracilis FFMT after pelvic trauma [3]. If the patient has sustained a significant degree of trauma to the extremity and a complete neurological exam cannot be obtained, the spinal accessory and intercostal nerves 3–5 may be the most reliable motors to the FFMT [3]. Contralateral C7 transfers have been used in other countries, but are not commonly performed in the United States [10, 11]. Medial pectoral nerve with a nerve graft may be a last resort option [12].

Vascular

The FFMT vascular pedicle must be of reasonable length such that the anastomosis is free of tension. Finding a healthy vessel in a traumatic setting can be especially difficult. Subclavian or axillary artery injuries are common (10–25%) in traumatic brachial plexus injuries [13, 14].

However, even in these cases, the thoracoacromial and thoracodorsal arteries have been found to be reliable options for arterial anastomosis [15]. As mentioned previously, pre-operative imaging studies are readily available in the form of magnetic resonance angiogram (MRA), computed tomography angiogram (CTA), or even conventional angiography and should be obtained routinely. If needed, vein grafting may help provide enough length to ensure a tension-free repair away from the zone of injury. Arterial repair can be performed end to end if there is no size mismatch and adequate perfusion remains distally without the donor vessel. However, an end-to-side anastomosis may be advantageous as there is less concern regarding the caliber of vessels at the anastomosis, and distal perfusion would not be sacrificed. End-to-side repair may be the only available option in a mangled extremity with compromised vascularity. In addition, venous anastomoses are also critical as venous congestion is as likely to complicate the FFMT as arterial thrombosis [16].

Muscle

The free muscle transfer should be of sufficient strength, length, and excursion to power the desired function. The cross-sectional area of the muscle is proportional to the amount of force it is able to generate, while the excursion of the muscle is related to the length of its fibers [2]. Adequate tendon length or fascia must be present to anchor the FFMT in nearby tissue. The FFMT must be expendable and should ideally improve cosmesis in the recipient area, and should not lead to a demonstrable functional loss in the donor limb [3]. The donor muscle must have a healthy neurovascular pedicle for transfer. Lastly, there must be a well-functioning antagonistic force to balance the FFMT.

As a prime example, the gracilis is the most commonly utilized donor for FFMT [3]. The gracilis has been used to power elbow flexion but also can be utilized for finger flexion/extension [3, 12, 17]. The gracilis can be combined with the adductor longus [18] and even with the contralateral gracilis to increase function in a mangled extremity [6, 7]. Other common muscles used as FFMT in the traumatic setting include the latissimus dorsi and the gastrocnemius. Several FFMTs have been described for similar functions. For example, while the gracilis is the most commonly used FFMT for elbow flexion [18], the latissimus dorsi [19] and rectus femoris [20] have also been successfully utilized. In one retrospective comparison of 37 free latissimus and 28 gracilis FFMTs for restoration of elbow flexion, the authors found no difference in outcomes between the two FFMTs [21].

Free Functional Muscle Transfer in the Mangled Extremity: The Gracilis

The gracilis FFMT is versatile and has the potential to serve many functions in the mangled extremity (Table 11.1). The gracilis is an ideal FFMT as it may be harvested often far outside of the zone of injury; has sufficient power, excursion; and has a reasonable length and caliber of pedicle (Stevanovic). The gracilis is found in the medial thigh, posterior to the adductor muscles and anterior to the hamstrings. The muscle originates on the ischiopubic ramus and has a broad insertion on the superficial aspect of the pes anserinus on the medial aspect of the proximal tibia. The muscle is innervated by the anterior branch of the obturator nerve and supplied by a branch of the medial femoral circumflex artery. It functions to adduct and flex the hip, both functions which are primarily driven by other muscle groups, making it an ideal donor. In the past a reliable skin flap was difficult to obtain; however, with increasing the amount of fascia taken, one can sustain a very reliable skin flap in addition to the muscle.

To harvest the gracilis, the patient is placed in the supine position. The mangled upper extremity is placed on a hand table, and the contralateral lower extremity can be placed in the frog-leg position. This will allow two surgical teams to work concurrently. A skin marker is used to draw a line from the ischiopubic ramus to the medial

Table 11.1 Common function of gracilis transfers with attachment origin and insertion (O/I), artery, vein, and nerve donor

FFMT function	O/I	Artery	Vein	Nerve
Elbow flexion	Clavicle to Ulna	1. Thoracoacromial 2. Brachial	1. Brachial VC 2. Thoracoacromial VC	1. Musculocutaneous 2. Axillary 3. Spinal accessory 4. 3.4 + 5 intercostal
Elbow extension	Lateral scapula to Olecranon	1. Profunda brachii 2. Thoracodorsal	1. Profunda VC 2. Thoracodorsal VC	1. Radial 2. Intercostal 3. Spinal accessory with graft
Shoulder Abduction	Acromion and clavicle to Proximal humerus	1. Thoracoacromial 2. Thoracodorsal	1. Thoracoacromial VC 2. Cephalic 3. Thoracodorsal VC	1. Musculocutaneous 2. Axillary
Finger flexion/ extension	Medial/Lateral epicondyle to Pulvertaft weave into tendon	1. Radial 2. AIA	Radial VC	1. AIN (flexion) 2. PIN (extension)

VC vena comitantes, *AIA* anterior interosseous artery, *AIN* anterior interosseous nerve, *PIN* posterior interosseous nerve

aspect of the proximal tibia. Along this line, primary branch of the medial femoral circumflex artery perfuses the gracilis 8 cm distal to the ischiopubic ramus. The gracilis can be differentiated from the adductors as the gracilis is more posterior and the tension of the muscle changes with flexion and extension of the knee. There is secondary perforator to the gracilis found more distally in the muscle, which can be clipped once the dominant vessel is identified. Once identified, the primary proximal pedicle can be traced to the medial femoral circumflex artery to obtain a donor of 4–6 cm in length [22]. The axis of the skin paddle should be 2 cm posterior to the ischiopubic-pes anserine line [3]. While raising a skin paddle is not required, the recipient site may require skin coverage in the mangled extremity as well. Increasing the size of the fascia obtained around the muscle will increase the success of a viable skin paddle as well as minimize post-operative scarring and adhesions, leading to optimal functional success. It is important, prior to harvesting the gracilis, to mark the muscle at 5 cm intervals with normal resting tension on the muscle so that one can retension the muscle when insetting at the transferred location.

Venous outflow may be augmented by raising an anterior branch of the saphenous vein with the skin paddle. Typically, the gracilis is divided distally first and then proximally, and the pedicle is harvested last [3]. Once harvested the microscope

is introduced to the surgical field. The artery is typically anastomosed first, followed by the vein, and finally the nerve is coapted as close to the FFMT as possible. Once perfusion is established, the tension of the muscle can be set. For restoring elbow flexion, typically the distal third of the clavicle is used proximally, and the proximal ulna is used distally. Once the muscle is tensioned to its original resting length via the 5 cm markers with the elbow in extension, the elbow is then flexed to reduce muscle tension while securing the FFMT. The muscle may be secured with bone anchors, heavy suture, or bone tunnels to provide the desired function.

Post-operatively the patient is monitored as a standard free tissue transfer per the preference of the surgeon. Signs of impending failure include loss of Doppler signal, poor color, temperature drop, loss of turgor, and presence of petechial hemorrhage on the skin paddle [4]. It should be noted that monitoring the skin flap alone is insufficient as muscle has a lower tolerance for ischemia than the skin [2]. Dodakundi and colleagues reported three cases of gracilis FFMTs in which the skin paddle was perfused but the transferred muscle was not viable. Each of these cases was re-explored acutely and all three had arterial thromboses. Even after revision microsurgical re-anastomosis, two of the three showed delayed innervation of a small area of muscle, and one muscle demonstrated no innervation [16]. The authors maintain that the most accurate method to evaluate the muscle flap is to use an implantable electrode to monitor compound muscle action potentials [16] while others use implantable Doppler probes [2]. Critical ischemia time for muscle has been reported as short as 6 hours, and the time from ischemia to re-exploration is highly predictive of flap salvage [23]. After 2 hours of muscle ischemia, even if re-prefused, the FFMT may not function well [4]. In addition, up to 15% of FFMT fail – either from vascular congestion, arterial thrombosis, or non-functional muscle [24]. For these reasons, we recommend bedside Doppler checks by a reliable member of the surgical team every hour for 48 hours.

After 48 hours, the flap may be monitored every 4 hours until discharge after 5 days. Upon discharge, the elbow should be immobilized at 90° of flexion for 8 weeks. While immobilized the patient is encouraged to work on finger and wrist exercises. The patient is observed for spontaneous muscle function, at which point they are permitted to attempt to flex the elbow. Additionally, electromyography is useful in determining the status of muscle re-innervation.

Functional Muscle Transfer in the Mangled Extremity: The Latissimus dorsi

The latissimus dorsi rotational muscle transfer is a robust option for patients with massive soft tissue defect and associated loss of elbow flexion. A latissimus dorsi rotational muscle transfer may adequately cover the wound and provide function in a single rapid reconstructive stage. The latissimus dorsi is an ideal pedicled rotation flap as the muscle is large and easily mobilized, muscle function is expendable in most patients and contains a long neurovascular pedicle (thoracodorsal), and the donor defect can often be covered with limited morbidity [25]. Consideration of other options in the wheelchair-bound patient who will rely on the upper body strength for transfers is warranted. The latissimus can be rotated to cover abdominal, upper extremity, and thoracic wounds [26] and can be used to power

the shoulder elevation [27], adduction [28], and external rotation [29] and elbow flexion [30]. In a review of four patients having undergone a latissimus rotation procedure with an average soft tissue defect of 161cm², Stevanovic et al. reported that all four achieved M4 elbow flexion strength and an average elbow arc of motion of 126° [30]. In the setting of mangled upper extremities with soft tissue loss, other case series have reported achieving M4 elbow flexion in 60–75% of patients [31, 32] and an average flexion-extension arc of 100° [33–37].

Outcomes

It is somewhat difficult to pinpoint outcomes following FMT as the literature is comprised of multiple series with very heterogeneous populations and cases, with many described techniques [38]. Several different outcome measures have also been described [2, 3]. Furthermore, there is a disconnect between clinician's physical exam and histology of the FFMT. One histologic analysis of neurovascular muscle flaps found that only 46% of muscle graded M4 were completely innervated.

In one of the first FFMT reports, after 2 years of gracilis FFMT for restoration of elbow flexion using three intercostal nerves, 78% of patients achieved M4 strength [39]. Later, Barrie and colleagues (35) used the gracilis FFMT for single function alone in 18 patients (17 elbow flexion and 1 finger flexion) and for dual function in 9 cases. Seventy-nine percent of the single function cohort and 63% of the dual function cohort achieved M4 or greater strength. On average, patients in this study had EMG-discernable re-innervation at an average of 5 months and final elbow arch of motion of 105°. In the dual function cohort, the authors additionally secured the gracilis to the wrist extensors to indirectly activate finger flexion through the tenodesis effect. The authors concluded that more reliable results can be obtained when a single muscle is used to restore a single function. The authors also correlated poor compliance with physical therapy with adhesions and lower rates of success.

Similarly, in a review of 18 staged wrist fusions in the setting of a staged double gracilis FFMT, DASH scores improved, and finger range of motion improved once the wrist arthrodesis was completed [7]. Although in the mangled extremity a surgeon may attempt to have one FFMT power multiple functions, best results may be achieved with the simplest pre-operative goals.

In a report of 33 patients undergoing gracilis FFMT for restoration of elbow flexion, Kay and colleagues also reported that 21/33 achieved M4 strength. However, while 92% of those with an obstetric brachial plexus palsy achieved M4, only 31% adults with a traumatic injury achieved these results (Kay). Surgeons would do well to council their patients in the setting of a mangled extremity that while FFMT offers a potential avenue when few options remain, success is certainly not guaranteed.

Complications

The most significant acute complications include FFMT arterial thrombosis or venous congestion (15%) [24]. Outside of the acute phase, most common complications may be related to adhesions and post-operative stiffness [2, 3]. Up to a third of gracilis FFMT will need secondary tenolysis [6]. In addition, donor site morbidity can present even with non-critical donor structures. In a review of 459 intercostal nerve harvests in 153 patients, 15% of patients experienced a complication. These included pleural tear (9.1%), wound infection, pleural effusion, acute respiratory distress syndrome, and seroma. Ipsilateral rib fractures and harvesting three instead of two intercostal nerves were associated with a higher likelihood of complication [40].

Conclusion

In the setting of a mangled extremity, there may be few reconstructive options available to salvage function. For these cases, a FMT may both provide wound coverage and extremity func-

tion. The patient ideally should be young and motivated and understand the guarded results, potential complications, and long road to rehabilitation.

References

1. Gangurde BA, Doi K, Hattori Y, Sakamoto S. Free functioning muscle transfer in radiation-induced brachial plexopathy: case report. J Hand Surg W.B. Saunders. 2014;39(10):1967–70.
2. Fischer JP, Elliott RM, Kozin SH, Levin LS. Free function muscle transfers for upper extremity reconstruction: a review of indications, techniques, and outcomes. J Hand Surg W.B. Saunders. 2013;38(12):2485–90.
3. Seal A, Stevanovic M. Free functional muscle transfer for the upper extremity. Clin Plast Surg Elsevier. 2011;38(4):561–75.
4. Stevanovic M, Sharpe F. Functional free muscle transfer for upper extremity reconstruction. Plast Reconstr Surg. 2014;134(2):257e–74e.
5. Bishop AT. Functioning free-muscle transfer for brachial plexus injury. Hand Clin Elsevier. 2005;21(1):91–102.
6. Doi K, Hattori Y, Yamazaki H, Wahegaonkar AL, Addosooki A, Watanabe M. Importance of early passive mobilization following double free gracilis muscle transfer. Plast Reconstr Surg. 2008;121(6):2037–45.
7. Addosooki A, Doi K, Hattori Y, Wahegaonkar A. Role of wrist arthrodesis in patients receiving double free muscle transfers for reconstruction following complete brachial plexus paralysis. J Hand Surg W.B. Saunders. 2012 Feb 1;37(2):277–81.
8. Bulstra LF, Rbia N, Kircher MF, Spinner RJ, Bishop AT, Shin AY. Spinal accessory nerve to triceps muscle transfer using long autologous nerve grafts for recovery of elbow extension in traumatic brachial plexus injuries. J Neurosurg Am Assoc Neurol Surg. 2017;75:1–7.
9. Zuker RM, Manktelow RT. Functioning free muscle transfers. Hand Clin Elsevier. 2007 Feb 1;23(1):57–72.
10. Chen L, Gu Y-D, Hu S-N, Xu J-G, Xu L, Fu Y. Contralateral C7 transfer for the treatment of brachial plexus root avulsions in children—a report of 12 cases. J Hand Surg W.B. Saunders. 2007 Jan 1;32(1):96–103.
11. Gu YD, Zhang GM, Chen DS, YAN J-G, CHENG X-M, CHEN L. Seventh cervical nerve root transfer from the contralateral healthy side for treatment of brachial plexus root avulsion. J Hand Surg. SAGE Publications Sage UK: London, England. 2016;17(5):518–21.
12. Kay S, Pinder R, Wiper J, Hart A, Jones F, Yates A. Microvascular free functioning gracilis transfer with nerve transfer to establish elbow flexion. British J Plast Surg Churchill Livingstone. 2010;63(7):1142–9.

13. Gupta A, Jamshidi M, Rubin J. Traumatic first rib fracture: is angiography indicated? Review of 750 cases. Cardiovasc Surg. 1995 Sep;3:9–9.

14. Sturm JT, Perry JF. Brachial plexus injuries from blunt trauma–a harbinger of vascular and thoracic injury. Ann Emerg Med. 1987 Apr;16(4):404–6.

15. Hattori Y, Doi K, Sakamoto S, Satbhai NG. Complete avulsion of brachial plexus with associated vascular trauma. Plast Reconstr Surg. 2013 Dec;132(6):1504–12.

16. Dodakundi C, Doi K, Hattori Y, Sakamoto S, Yonemura H, Fujihara Y. Postoperative monitoring in free muscle transfers for reconstruction in brachial plexus injuries. Tech Hand Up Extrem Surg. 2012 Mar 1;16(1):48–51.

17. Terzis JK, Kostopoulos VK. Free muscle transfer in posttraumatic plexopathies part II: the elbow. Hand (N Y). Springer-Verlag. 2009;5(2):160–70.

18. Chuang DCC, Strauch RJ, Wei F-C. Technical considerations in two-stage functioning free muscle transplantation reconstruction of both flexor and extensor functions of the forearm. Microsurg Wiley-Blackwell. 1994;15(5):338–43.

19. Vekris MD, Beris AE, Lykissas MG, Korompilias AV, Vekris AD, Soucacos PN. Restoration of elbow function in severe brachial plexus paralysis via muscle transfers. Injury Elsevier. 2008 Sep 1;39(3):15–22.

20. Wechselberger G, Hussl H, Strickner N, Pülzl P, Schoeller T. Restoration of elbow flexion after brachial plexus injury by free functional rectus femoris muscle transfer. Br J Plast Surg Churchill Livingstone. 2009;62(2):e1–5.

21. Terzis JK, Barmpitsioti A. Secondary shoulder reconstruction in patients with brachial plexus injuries. Br J Plast Surg Churchill Livingstone. 2011;64(7):843–53.

22. Barrie KA, Steinmann SP, Shin AY, Spinner RJ, Bishop AT. Gracilis free muscle transfer for restoration of function after complete brachial plexus avulsion. Am Assoc Neurol Surg. 2007;16(5):1–9. https://doi.org/10.3171/foc.2004.16.5.9.

23. Mirzabeigi MN, Wang T, Kovach SJ, Taylor JA, Serletti JM, Wu LC. Free flap take-back following postoperative microvascular compromise: predicting salvage versus failure. Plast Reconstr Surg. 2012;130(3):579–89.

24. Adams JE, Kircher MF, Spinner RJ, Orthop MTA. Complications and outcomes of functional free gracilis transfer in brachial plexus palsy. Acta Orthop Belg. 2009;75(1):8–13.

25. Ma C-H, Tu Y-K, Wu C-H, Yen C-Y, Yu S-W, Kao F-C. Reconstruction of upper extremity large soft-tissue defects using pedicled latissimus dorsi muscle flaps – technique illustration and clinical outcomes. Injury Elsevier. 2008 Oct 1;39:67–74.

26. Bostwick JI, Nahai F, Wallace JG, Vasconez LO. Sixty Latissimus Dorsi Flaps. Plast Reconstr Surg. 1979 Jan 1;63(1):31.

27. Oh JH, Tilan J, Chen Y-J, Chung KC, McGarry MH, Lee TQ. Biomechanical effect of latissimus dorsi tendon transfer for irreparable massive cuff tear. J Shoulder Elbow Surg Mosby. 2013;22(2):150–7.

28. Gündeş H, Buluç L, Çırpıcı Y, Şarlak AY. Loss of pectoral muscles: treatment with latissimus dorsi muscle rotational flap. J Shoulder Elbow Surg Elsevier. 2006 Sep 1;15(5):e13–5.

29. Ghosh S, Singh VK, Jeyaseelan L, Sinisi M, Fox M. Isolated latissimus dorsi transfer to restore shoulder external rotation in adults with brachial plexus injury. Bone Joint J. 2013;95-B(5):660–3.

30. Stevanovic MV, Cuéllar VG, Ghiassi A, Sharpe F. Single-stage reconstruction of elbow flexion associated with massive soft-tissue defect using the latissimus dorsi muscle bipolar rotational transfer. Plast Reconstr Surg Glob Open. 2016;4(9):e1066.

31. Cambon-Binder A, Belkheyar Z, Durand S, Rantissi M, Oberlin C. Elbow flexion restoration using pedicled latissimus dorsi transfer in seven cases. Chir Main Elsevier Masson. 2012;31(6):324–30.

32. Schoeller T, Wechselberger G, Hussl H, Huemer GM. Functional transposition of the latissimus dorsi muscle for biceps reconstruction after upper arm replantation. Br J Plast Surg Churchill Livingstone. 2007;60(7):755–9.

33. Germann G, Steinau HU. Functional soft-tissue coverage in skeletonizing injuries of the upper extremity using the ipsilateral latissimus dorsi myocutaneous flap. Plast Reconstr Surg. 1995 Oct;96(5):1130–5.

34. Hochberg J, Fortes da Silva FB. Latissimus dorsi myocutaneous flap to restore elbow flexion and axillary burn contracture: a report on two pediatric patients. J Pediatr Orthop. 1982;2(5):565–8.

35. Mordick T, Britton EN, Brantigan C. Pedicled latissimus dorsi transfer for immediate soft-tissue coverage and elbow flexion. Plast Reconstr Surg. 1997;99(6):1742–4.

36. O'Ceallaigh S, Ali KSAM, O'Connor TPF. Functional latissimus dorsi muscle transfer to restore elbow flexion in extensive electrical burns. Burns Elsevier. 2005;31(1):113–5.

37. Stern PJ, Carey JP. The latissimus dorsi flap for reconstruction of the brachium and shoulder. J Bone Joint Surg Am. 1988;70(4):526–35.

38. Nicoson MC, Franco MJ, Tung TH. Donor nerve sources in free functional gracilis muscle transfer for elbow flexion in adult brachial plexus injury. Microsurg Wiley-Blackwell. 2017;37(5):377–82.

39. Chung DC, Carver N, Wei FC. Results of functioning free muscle transplantation for elbow flexion. J Hand Surg Am. 1996;21(6):1071–7.

40. Kovachevich R, Kircher MF, Wood CM, Spinner RJ, Bishop AT, Shin AY. Complications of intercostal nerve transfer for brachial plexus reconstruction. J Hand Surg WB Saunders. 2010;35(12):1995–2000.

The Psychological Impact of the Mangled Limb

12

Manas Nigam and Ryan Katz

Introduction

There should be no overlooking the emotional and social pain experienced by patients with upper extremity trauma. In addition to physical dysfunction, deformity, and disability, victims of extremity injuries often develop psychological maladies such as depression, anxiety, and post-traumatic stress disorder (PTSD).

Many patients endure a crisis of identity as they must either cope and adapt with their injury and "new self" or succumb to the patient role. It is the job of the clinician to recognize potential psychological barriers to a speedy recovery. Failure to do so can severely compromise the overall surgical result.

To date, there is a paucity of literature examining the psychologic consequences of upper extremity injury and how this affects the patient, the treatment, and the recovery. Moreover, the existing body of literature is varied and covers a breadth of topics rarely tailored to the surgeon or trauma providers. For victims of mangling upper extremity injuries, there exists no current standard of care for which psychiatric outcomes should be measured or reported, and for many providers, there exists only a tenuous understanding of the role psychiatric manifestations may play in treatment and recovery.

At least one third of patients with hand injuries experience symptomatic PTSD, depression, or signs of a mood disorder which can be detected clinically as early as 1 month after injury. Some patients experience a combination of disorders, particularly PTSD and depression [1]. Upper extremity injuries can lead to a decreased quality of life, an altered body image, communication difficulty, and withdrawal from society. A significant percentage of these patients – up to a third – endorse suicidal ideation [1–11].

To shine light on this corner of upper extremity trauma, often overlooked, we attempt to summarize the existing literature in the following domains: chronic pain; coping; self-efficacy; identity; depression; anxiety; PTSD; and social consequences.

Pain

Pain, an unavoidable consequence of trauma, can severely complicate rehabilitation and recovery. The severity of upper extremity pain is directly associated with the likelihood of disability in injured patients, and the presence and duration of pain has negative effects on both short- and long-term outcomes following extremity injury and treatment [12–15].

M. Nigam
Department of Plastic and Reconstructive Surgery,
MedStar Georgetown University Hospital,
Washington, DC, USA

R. Katz (✉)
The Curtis National Hand Center, MedStar Union
Memorial Hospital, Baltimore, MD, USA

© Springer Nature Switzerland AG 2021
R. A. Pensy, J. V. Ingari (eds.), *The Mangled Extremity*, https://doi.org/10.1007/978-3-319-56648-1_12

Chronic pain has been shown to be correlated with numerous psychiatric conditions including depression, anxiety, and post-traumatic stress disorder; all of which can further complicate attempts at post-injury rehabilitation [16, 17]. Ultimately, pain is a complex process with significant implications for an individual's recovery and long-term psychological well-being. Through empathy, the provider should, to the best of their ability, understand and anticipate the pain experience of their patients. This, itself, can be of therapeutic benefit.

Theory of Pain

The theoretical framework of the pain phenomenon has been the subject of much investigation [17]. Current theory differentiates between nociception, which is the automatic detection of and physiologic response to noxious stimuli, tissue injury, or impending tissue injury, and the experience of pain (i.e., the unpleasant emotional and sensory experience associated with injury) [18]. The amount of pain experienced between different patients with the same injury can vary greatly. Ultimately, pain is a *subjective* experience dependent on the nociceptive response to a physical insult which, in turn, is further modified by other variables such as psychological well-being, coping skills, and social factors. A number of theories have been advanced to help explain patients' variable responses to pain.

One of the first attempts to integrate nociception with subjective pain was the "gate control theory" proposed by Melzack and Wall, who argued that afferent pain signals from sensory nerves could be modulated by efferent signaling from the central nervous system [19]. These efferent signals, dependent on certain psychosocial variables, such as anxiety or depression, were described as capable of either amplifying or attenuating the afferent signals, thus linking nociception, pain, and the patient's psychosocial state. Melzack later proposed the "neuromatrix model of pain" which added individual stress and the function of the stress-regulatory systems as important modulators and amplifiers of subjective pain [20].

The most contemporary and accepted theory of pain however is the "biopsychosocial model," which challenges the traditional "biomedical model" of medicine (where disease and suffering were purely a function of specific pathophysiology) and instead argued that biological, psychological, social, and cultural factors all play a dynamic and integrated role in modulating the interpretation of pain signaling [21]. This chapter explores the interplay of these factors with regard to subjective pain, recovery, and outcomes following treatment in patients with upper extremity injuries.

Acute and Chronic Pain

While *acute pain* is sudden in onset and may be expected to last through the duration of illness, *chronic pain* is defined as ongoing or recurrent pain lasting for greater than 3 to 6 months or a duration beyond the typical and expected course of healing for an injury [17]. Given the pain of injury, the pain associated with the repair, and the expectation of pain while recovering, it is not surprising that about half of patients with extremity trauma will experience moderate to severe acute pain at the time of hospital discharge [22, 23].

Acute pain of high intensity has been shown to be a risk factor for the development of chronic pain, and strikingly, one recent review estimated that up to 86% of extremity trauma patients with acute pain eventually develop chronic pain at 6 months following injury and beyond [16, 24]. Furthermore, another study demonstrated that 77% of patients reported persistent pain up to 84 months following limb-threatening extremity trauma. These studies highlight both long duration of suffering and the high risk for developing chronic pain experienced by these patients [25].

Chronic pain following upper extremity trauma can alone severely limit physical function and social reintegration and has been reported to be a risk factor for disability and loss of productivity following injury [26, 27]. Besides physical limitations, chronic pain has been associated with a number of psychiatric conditions including depression, anxiety, and PTSD [28]. Several authors have examined the relationship between pain and affective conditions (e.g., depression, anxiety) in extremity trauma patients. One longitudinal study reported that pain predicted the development of anxiety and depression for up to one year following extremity trauma [29]. The same authors have shown a correlation between pain and negative affective mood symptoms on function; they propose a model where the presence of negative affective disorders, such as pain and anxiety, modulate the negative effect of pain on extremity function, with the latter having a greater influence on disability later in the course of recovery [30].

The association between pain, affect, and function further highlights the notion that pain and psychiatric conditions should be identified early and addressed in the treatment plan for the patient to have the best possible outcome. Chronic pain is costly not just to the individual, but to society at large. In the United States, it is estimated up to 100 million people suffer from chronic pain, including pain associated with musculoskeletal disease, and that the cost of chronic pain was $560 to $635 billion in 2010 (accounting for healthcare expenditures, days of work missed, hours of work lost, and lower wages) [31]. To put these numbers into context, the annual cost of chronic pain was greater than the individual costs of heart disease, cancer, and diabetes and of cancer and diabetes combined. In Canada, chronic pain is the leading cause of disability among adults of working age, and it is estimated that 60% of people with chronic pain, including those with extremity trauma, will eventually lose their jobs and income or experience a reduction in work responsibilities [32].

Chronic Pain: Pathogenesis and Susceptibility

Although acute pain is a reversible process, prolonged and unrelieved acute pain may ultimately lead to the development of irreversible chronic pain. This appears to occur through permanent changes in neuronal structure, connectivity, and function. One theory regarding the pathogenesis of chronic pain implicates inflammation and neuronal sensitization [16]. It is thought that pro-

longed inflammation secondary to tissue injury can sensitize peripheral nociceptive neurons to both a lower firing threshold and a higher intensity response to injury (primary hyperalgesia). In the absence of a continued pain stimulus or inflammatory process, peripheral sensitization is a likely normal response to injury and is reversible. Sensitization of the central nervous system appears to become permanent however after exposure to intense, noxious peripheral stimuli. During this process, inputs from areas without tissue damage can induce pain without nociception (secondary hyperalgesia) or can modify nonpainful peripheral signals to make the patient experience pain (allodynia).

Distinct anatomic changes to the central nervous system following extremity trauma have been noted in a mouse chronic pain model that utilizes tibial fractures to stimulate pain. Interestingly, mice with tibial fractures demonstrate nociceptive sensitization in their injured limbs and develop memory impairment and increased levels of anxiety. These changes correlate with structural alterations in mouse brain architecture which involve the dendritic architecture of the amygdala, hippocampus, and perirhinal cortex [33]. The findings of this study further underline the complex association between acute and chronic pain, affective symptoms, and brain function.

Recent evidence has suggested that certain individuals may be susceptible to the development of chronic pain. From a genetic standpoint, the catechol-o-methyltransferase (COMT) gene, the 5-hydroxytryptamine receptor 2A (HTR2A) gene, and solute carrier family 6 member 4 (SLC6A4) gene have been implicated in the development of chronic pain, lending credence to the idea that the condition may be heritable [16]. Perhaps not surprising, all three aforementioned genes are also implicated in psychiatric disorders. This includes an association between alcohol use disorder and opiate addiction with COMT; major depressive disorder and obsessive compulsive disorder with HTR2A; and anxiety and obsessive compulsive disorder and SLC6A4, among others [34]. Functional MRI (fMRI) studies have also contributed to the theory of chronic pain susceptibility with one recent study demonstrating a higher level of functional connectivity to emotion-related circuitry in chronic pain patients than in those who recovered without chronic pain. This suggests that some individuals may be at risk for developing chronic pain from persistent nociception [35]. Ultimately, protracted exposure to painful stimuli in conjunction with genetic susceptibility and unique brain connectivity is thought to enable transformation from acute to chronic pain. Though research is still nascent, future genetic and fMRI screening may be able to identify individuals who are at risk for developing chronic pain following extremity trauma so that appropriate interventions may be initiated before chronic pain develops [35].

Chronic Opioid Use

The number of deaths due to opioid abuse now surpasses the number of deaths due to motor vehicle accidents in most of the United States. The increase in deaths corresponds to an increase in the number of opioid users, opioid abusers, and the number of prescriptions filled [36, 37]. A study of Medicaid patients found that trauma patients prescribed opioids were 1.4 times more likely to persist in opioid usage compared with those not prescribed opioids. Up to 60% of patients with trauma continue to experience pain related to their surgery, and about 10–20% of trauma patients who used opioids persisted in their use [38–40] [41]. , Risk factors for continued opioid use after surgery include presence of significant pain earlier in the disease course, catastrophic thinking, anxiety, post-traumatic stress disorder, and depression [42, 43].

Long-term opioid abuse often begins with treatment of acute pain. [44–47] Of all medical specialties, surgeons are among the highest prescribers of opioids [44–50]. Factors associated with prolonged opioid use after elective hand surgery include arthritis, nerve compression, youth, female gender, a large number of comorbidities, lower income, mental health disorders, and tobacco dependence or abuse. Interestingly patients undergoing elective procedures actually had *higher* rates of opioid abuse than did those

undergoing trauma-related surgeries (though trauma patients had a higher average number of prescriptions per patient) [40].

Opiates work on "reward centers" that affect the motivational state of a patient [51]. Opiates provide an analgesic effect, a sense of well-being and an indifference to ongoing pain. It is thought that opiates (and other addictive drugs) usurp the neural systems that otherwise direct the patient to satisfy urges such as hunger, thirst, and sex. From a neurobiological standpoint, it remains unexplained why only some individuals exposed to opioids become chronic opioid users.

In a complex topic on which there is much ongoing research, opioids are thought to cause increased firing of the reward dopaminergic neurons of the ventral tegmental area of the brain. This area stimulates other structures (such as the nucleus accumbens, amygdala, and prefrontal cortex) that provide the user with emotional support. This then affects the perceived reward of different behaviors. Three theories are put forth to explain addiction: (1) failure to reestablish homeostasis after prolonged exposure to a substance; (2) change in the salience, or desire of a substance, regardless of the effects; and (3) aberrant learning and memory mechanisms establishing drug "habits."

Psychological Concepts

Coping

Coping describes an individual's response to a stressor, such as pain, and is a form of personal resiliency. Coping strategies can either be adaptive, where patients assume an active role in managing their pain and rehabilitation, or nonadaptive, where patients adopt a pessimistic mindset and passive approach to their therapy and relegate themselves to a sick role. Adaptive coping strategies are associated with personality traits such as optimism, extraversion, and agreeableness. Nonadaptive coping is associated with neuroticism. Both are dependent on the severity of stress experienced by the patient and are influenced by the psychosocial environment [52].

A patient's ability or inability to cope with trauma influences a number of specific measurable outcomes including pain severity and disability [17]. One study determined that nonadaptive thoughts and inadequate coping strategies influenced the patient's personal goals of rehabilitation as well as their perception of advice offered by hand therapists resulting in overall greater disability [53].

Administering a validated tool such as the Negative Pain Thoughts Questionnaire (NPTQ) after trauma and before beginning rehabilitation can help identify patients at risk for poor coping strategies. This can allow the treating team the opportunity to offer the patient counseling and a balanced treatment plan.

Self-Efficacy

Self-efficacy refers to an individual's belief that they are capable of successfully executing a behavior to achieve a certain outcome. Higher levels of individual self-efficacy have been demonstrated to be associated with improved tolerance of pain including lower pain intensity and less pain disability [17]. Self-efficacy also appears to be related to functional outcomes in patients with extremity trauma. One study, which examined predictive variables for physical function and pain intensity following orthopedic trauma, noted that self-efficacy significantly correlated with physical function [54]. Thus, the association between self-efficacy, pain tolerance, and functional outcomes further underscores the complex interplay between variables of the biopsychosocial model and the need to address patients holistically.

Identity

Identity can be defined as an individual's self-construal or how one perceives and understands themself. A traumatic upper extremity injury can affect not just a patient's function and appearance but their entire world view. The trauma can distort their physical identity and perception of self (body image); these psychological effects may be a greater source of suffering for patients than functional limitations and can have profound effects on their personal lives complicating their recovery in often overlooked ways [55].

While patients may express satisfaction with overall medical and surgical treatment following extremity trauma, they frequently have unmet psychiatric needs that exacerbate their suffering. One study, which examined individuals with reconstructed or amputated extremities several years after the inciting traumatic incident, noted that while patients described their overall lives as "normal," they experienced largely untreated psychological trauma that negatively impacted their perception of self and their ability to recuperate [56]. Some patients stated that their new handicaps made them unable to play with their children or grandchildren, making them feel older than their actual age and as if they were unable to express love and affection for their family [56]. Others noted impairments in physical function and an associated physical and psychological fatigue that made them unable or unwilling to either perform their work or activities of daily living. This loss of independence and greater reliance on family members for support was the most challenging aspect of recovery for many patients, who described a feeling of helplessness as they transitioned from a provider role to a dependent role within their families.

Other research has confirmed the negative effect of extremity injury on self-perception. The 2014 Chauvet report noted that double amputees tended to have greater distortion of body image than single amputees, suggesting that the extent of injury correlated with increasingly negative perception of self [57]. Patients with recent trauma leading to deformity also reported a more distorted body image than those with congenital deformities, likely due to a greater opportunity by those born with extremity defects to incorporate such anatomic differences into their body image [58].

Given the psychological distress experienced by these patients, it is evident that trauma providers must play a greater role in identifying and addressing post-injury issues of identity and self-perception. The change in a patient's identity and resultant feelings of helplessness may be exacerbated by a lack of agency in their initial care. Given that mangled extremity injuries are often life-threatening, treatment teams follow a "life over limb" paradigm, where a portion or entirety of the non-viable limb may be amputated in the interest of saving patient's life, often on extremely short notice [59]. Patients are not always fully informed with regard to such time-sensitive and important decisions (i.e., amputation versus salvage of a mangled extremity) and may be confused, sedated, or even unconscious in the immediate hours following trauma and thus unable to accurately process information given by treatment teams [56]. Such patients may wake up following surgery surprised with the resultant deformity or loss and may be frustrated that they have had little or no input on such a life-changing decision.

Whenever possible, depending on the extent of injuries, treatment teams should attempt to fully inform and counsel the patient and include him or her in the decision-making process. This can mitigate confusion, allow the patient to process the impending loss or deformity, and may aid in post-injury adaptive coping.

Psychiatric Comorbidities

Depression (Situational/Major)

Depression is perhaps the most common psychiatric comorbidity associated with chronic pain from upper extremity injury. To discern, two simple questions can be effective:

- Over the past 2 weeks, have you ever felt down, depressed, or hopeless?
- Over the past 2 weeks, have you felt little interest or pleasure in doing things?

DSM V notes that symptoms must be present for longer than 2 weeks, represent a change from previous functioning, and must cause significant decreased ability in most areas of functioning. These symptoms cannot be attributable to another psychiatric disorder (e.g., bipolar disorder) or to the effects of a substance or another medical condition. [60]

In a study involving men with lower extremity amputation, 34.7% of traumatic amputees and 51.4% of surgical amputees were identified as suffering from depression [61]. Developing depression was associated with patient age, educational level, marital and economic status, time since amputation, and access to rehabilitation with prosthesis [61]. Another study highlighted perceived social stigma, negative body image, and poor social support as risk factors for post-injury depression [17].

Pre-existing cognitive beliefs can impact whether a patient develops depression. Two cognitive beliefs in particular, catastrophic thinking and cognitive fusion, can significantly influence a patient's long-term mental health following a traumatic event [62]. Catastrophic thinking involves the tendency to respond to actual or expected pain with negative thoughts, whereas cognitive fusion occurs when behaviors are overly regulated and influenced by cognition, such that a person acts on imagined thoughts as if they were truth [62]. Both catastrophic thinking and cognitive fusion are examples of modifiable psychological factors that influence pain response and subsequent disability. Individuals exhibiting both catastrophic thinking and cognitive fusion have been shown to have the highest levels of pain intensity relative to individuals with neither cognitive distortion.

As these cognitive distortions are modifiable, there exists a possible role for cognitive behavioral therapy (CBT) for patients in whom these maladaptive traits are identified. Acceptance and commitment therapy (ACT) along with a tailored psychosocial intervention may help to alleviate patient-specific cognitive distortions and reduce depressive symptoms with subsequent improvement of chronic pain management [62].

Social Consequences

Social considerations following extremity injury include the implications of chronic pain on interpersonal relationships, employment, and financial stability. Wounded individuals needing surgery and a prolonged rehabilitation may require an extensive amount of time off of work.

This often results in loss of income, the burden of which is compounded by medical costs incurred (in addition to baseline bills and financial obligations) [63]. The financial cost of recovery is greater in those patients suffering from comorbid psychiatric illness following their injury. An analysis of lower-limb amputees by the Department of Veterans Affairs found that PTSD was associated with approximately a 3.42-fold increase in psychiatric costs and with a greater than 2-fold increase in total pharmaceutical costs [64]. According to the Department of Veterans Affairs, while amputation status was the main driver of prosthetic costs, a diagnosis of PTSD resulted in a 5.04-fold increase in prosthetics costs, as these individuals had prolonged recovery time with lower levels of functional rehab [64].

A systematic review of early predictors of return to work after extremity trauma revealed little consideration of the role of pain across studies [24]. Yet pain intensity at 3 months post major extremity trauma was identified as a significant predictor of return to work at 84 months (relative rate ratio (RRR) = 0.98, $p < 0.01$) [65]. In this study ($n = 423$), only 42% of injured individuals returned to work at 84 months and, of those who were working, 25% were limited in their ability to perform the demands of their job. Pain was recognized to be a significant determinant (gender adjusted RRR = 0.47, $p = 0.008$) of return to work after nonlife-threatening extremity trauma ($n = 168$) where 32% of patients were still not working at 6 months post-injury and 56% had returned to modified work [24]. These data further show the disparity between acute and chronic pain and again highlight the outsized role chronic pain plays in delaying or limiting recovery.

People with chronic pain have a tendency to self-isolate, withdraw from work and social interactions, and thereby experience magnified disability. [66] A downward spiral of unrelieved pain and loss of social functioning results in emotional stress and may amplify the perception of pain and loss. Recognizing this detrimental positive feedback loop is a necessary first step toward restoring balance to the trauma victim.

Anxiety

Anxiety is the feeling of apprehension or distress associated with a heightened condition of autonomic arousal [17]. Behaviors such as fear and avoidance are hallmarks of anxiety.

DSM V (2013) defines generalized anxiety disorder as excessive worry (in a fashion that is disproportionate to the actual risk) about an assortment of topics and life events and activities for at least 6 months. The anxiety is often difficult to control, can be associated with physical or cognitive symptoms, affects the patient's ability to function in a variety of settings, and cannot be otherwise attributable to a different medical, drug-induced, or psychiatric condition [60].

The anxiety can result in increased pain perception and/or the anticipation of personal harm. Patients with anxiety disorder often demonstrate behavioral changes to compensate for an anticipated stimulus.

Anxiety has a significant physiological component that includes the neuroendocrine secretion of catecholamines. These hormones increase cardiac output and alter sympathetic tone [17]. Anxiety can modify the response to pain and can result in symptoms of allodynia and hyperalgesia.

Post-traumatic Stress Disorder

Post-traumatic stress disorder is a psychiatric diagnosis long recognized but not included in the DSM until the third revision in 1980. One can develop PTSD when, after exposure to a significant life stressor, a patient manifests intrusive memories and reminders of the event despite attempts to avoid situational triggers. For patients with upper extremity trauma, this initial life stressor could either be the sudden loss of body integrity or fear of losing one's life.

Symptoms of PTSD include *recurrent and intrusive* symptoms which may include visual flashbacks, nightmares, anxiety, fear of reinjury, depression or disgust over physical disfigured appearance, irritability, hyperarousal, social withdrawal, or avoidance of stimuli associated with accidents [67].

DSM V (**2013**) notes that the diagnosis can only be applied to patients greater than 6 years old when symptoms have been present for at least 1 month and cannot be attributable to another cause or diagnosis [60].

Related diagnoses include acute stress disorder and adjustment disorder. Acute stress disorder (considered a precursor to PTSD) can also occur after a traumatic event and is characterized by the same symptoms of PTSD but is shorter in duration than PTSD (3 days to 4 weeks following a trauma). When symptoms persist for a month or greater, the diagnosis changes from acute stress disorder to PTSD.

Adjustment disorder can also occur as a result of a stressful event and results in an unexpected inability to cope with, or incorporate the event into the patient's life. The symptoms usually develop within a month, and do not last for more than 6 months. If adjustment disorder symptoms last longer than 6 weeks, another diagnosis should be considered.

Approximately 50% of workers with hand-related trauma have experienced some degree of PTSD [68]. Perhaps because of the difficult to conceal physical disfigurement associated with upper extremity trauma, PTSD occurs more commonly in upper limb amputations than lower-limb amputations (in work-related injuries) [17].

The treatment of PTSD can be challenging and begins with identifying the potential for illness. Failure to recognize symptoms of PTSD can result in delayed treatment. This can contribute to unnecessarily prolonged emotional stress, financial loss, and the downstream ramifications of such [67].

Currently, treatment of PTSD includes psychotherapy (cognitive behavior therapy), medications, or both.

Pre-existing Psychiatric Illness

Trauma patients with a known pre-existing psychiatric illness have lower rates of timely hospital discharge and lower rates of returning to work when compared to those without pre-existing psychopathology [69, 70].

While it is important for the treatment team to consider a patient's pre-existing psychiatric illness when determining a comprehensive plan of care, it appears that psychological impairments post-injury are better predictors of long-term recovery and rehabilitative potential than are pre-existing psychiatric disease [71].

Treatment Strategy

In addition to dysfunction and disfigurement, a mangling injury of the upper extremity imparts psychologic stress. This stress will be managed differently by different patients. Those patients with resilience and healthy coping strategies more easily adapt to their impairment and have a greater likelihood of optimal and timely recovery than those without. Unfortunately, the treating surgeon is often poorly equipped to know which patients carry what psychologic tools. It is therefore useful, at or around the time of presentation, to activate a multidisciplinary upper extremity trauma team and screen the patient for past or present psychopathology. This team should include a trauma/upper extremity surgeon, a pain medicine specialist, a psychologist or psychiatrist, occupational and physical therapist, prosthetist, and social worker. Each member of this team can offer physical and psychological comfort as well as counseling in different ways and, as such, minimize early psychological distress.

Of the team members, the psychologist (or psychiatrist) is in the unique position of recognizing and managing psychopathology as it arises. This is of paramount importance since it is well-known that greater early psychological distress leads to a worse prognosis later [71]. The mental health professional should be knowledgeable in the diagnosis and management of depression, acute stress disorders, and PTSD and should work closely with the therapists and prosthetists to devise a recovery program that allows for the early pursuit of personally valued activities and imparts a feeling of self-worth [72]. If depressed mood or poor coping strategies are identified at any point during the course of recovery, cognitive behavioral therapy can be of benefit [71, 73].

Following the patient over time with planned serial evaluations of disability, pain and psychologic distress can help identify problems de novo thus allowing for timely intervention [73].

Conclusions

The potential psychological implications of upper extremity trauma are as important as they are many. Pain, depression, anxiety, PTSD, and loss of identity are just some possible outcomes following upper extremity injury – with many patients experiencing multiple symptoms that blur the lines between these distinct categories. The *psychological* response to trauma can ultimately disrupt normal *physiologic* processes leading to injurious feedback loops, subjectively increased pain for any given stimulus, and the development of chronic pain. This, in turn, can derail the expected course of a patient's recovery.

To provide comprehensive and well-balanced care, the treatment team needs first to be aware of the burden of psychiatric illness in the trauma population and second the potential for the development of psychiatric illness in an individual patient. Only then can these issues be routinely assessed and adequately addressed allowing the drag on recovery be lifted.

This is not to say that there exists a definitive cure for the challenging problems discussed above. To the contrary, for many of these issues, treatment may be time-consuming and at most palliative. Without treatment however, an artificial ceiling on somatic recovery may exist which can frustrate provider and patient alike.

Management of the mangled upper extremity should be a multidisciplinary effort that includes surgeons, physical and occupational therapists, nurses, and mental health professionals.

Case Example

RH is a 61-year-old man who sustained an amputation of his dominant right hand when he made accidental contact with a meat grinder (Figs. 12.1, 12.2, and 12.3). This resulted in a

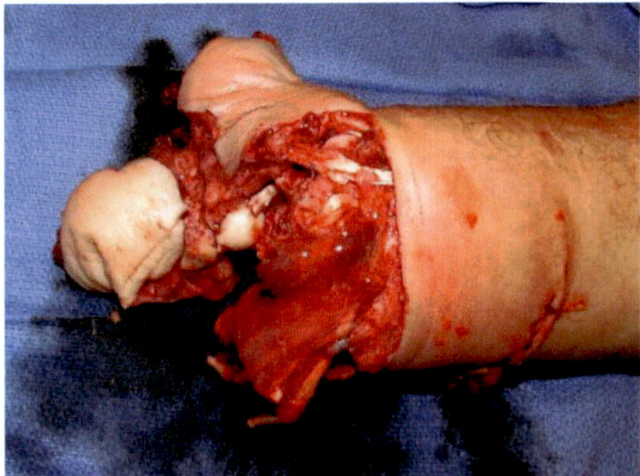

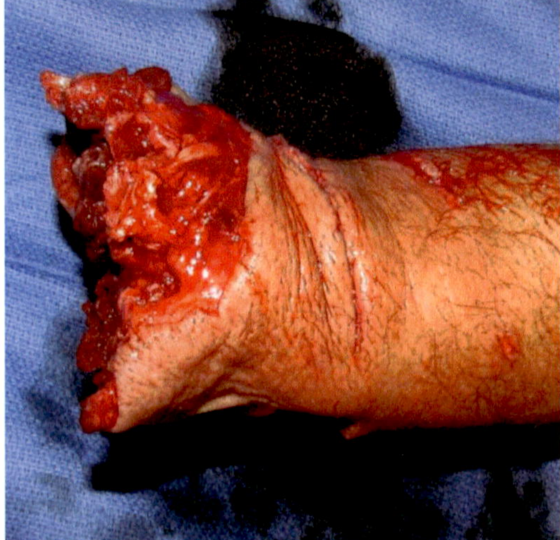

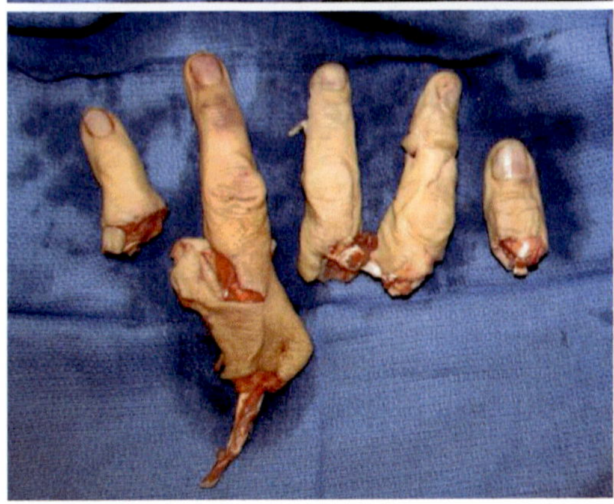

Figs. 12.1–12.3 A 61-year-old man who sustained an amputation of his dominant right hand when he made accidental contact with a meat grinder. One can appreciate a multilevel injury with loss of soft tissue and bone.

multilevel segmental injury to the hand with associated open dislocations of multiple carpal bones (Fig. 12.4). Initially, ectopic banking of two digits was performed on the contralateral

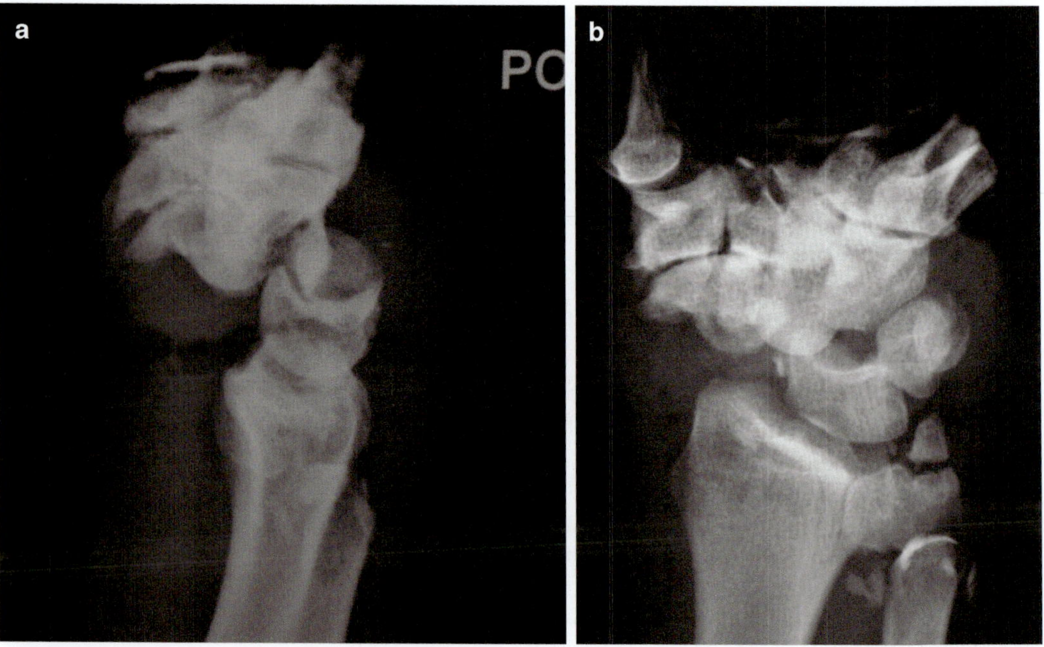

Fig. 12.4 An X-ray of the injury presented in Figs. 12.1, 12.2, and 12.3 is shown: a multilevel segmental injury to the hand with associated open dislocations of multiple carpal bones.

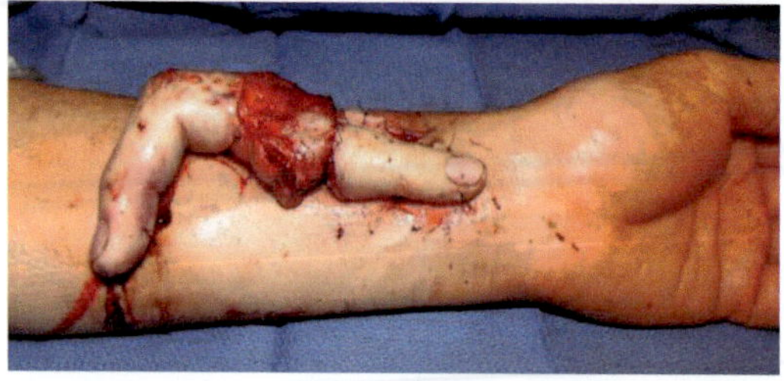

Fig. 12.5 For the patient in Figs. 12.1, 12.2, 12.3, and 12.4, ectopic banking of two digits was performed on the contralateral arm while reconstructive options were considered. Following surgery, psychology was called proactively to evaluate the patient early in their hospital stay.

arm, while reconstructive options were considered (Fig. 12.5). During this time, the patient was seen by a psychologist, and resilience and coping strategies were assessed. The patient, with guidance from the surgical team, ultimately elected to undergo a formal amputation. The patient's postoperative needs were discussed with the prosthetist prior to amputation, and it was felt that he would benefit from preservation of the distal radioulnar joint. The amputation was therefore performed at the radiocarpal level.

His soft tissue deficit was managed with a free anterolateral thigh flap (Fig. 12.6). Postoperatively, his pain was managed by a pain medicine specialist who helped with an early transition from narcotic to non-narcotic medications. A social worker aided in facilitating home accommodations and helped guide the patient through the intricacies of the hospital and insurance processes. An occupational therapist helped minimize edema in the amputation stump after the initial surgery and subsequent serial debulkings.

The patient was ultimately fitted for a body-powered prosthesis which he uses for most activities including hunting (Fig. 12.7). He also occasionally wears a myoelectric prosthesis though he feels it is less reliable than the body-powered (Fig. 12.8).

During his recovery, he was seen routinely for serial physical and mental health evaluations. He proved quite resilient with excellent coping skills and no catastrophizing. Despite initial mild depression, he came to accept his disability. This acceptance has allowed him to pursue activities that he finds satisfying, personally valuable, and

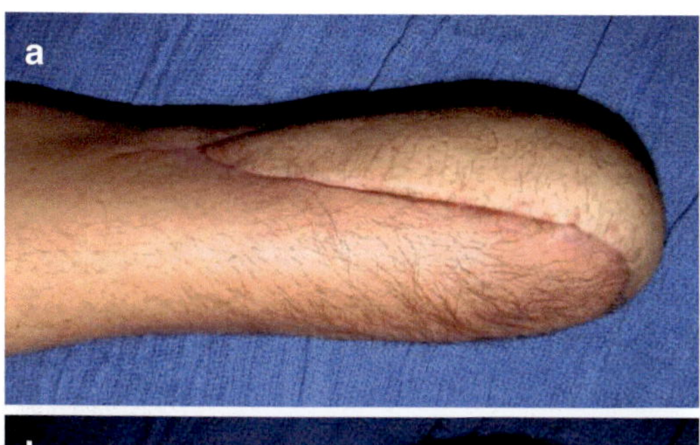

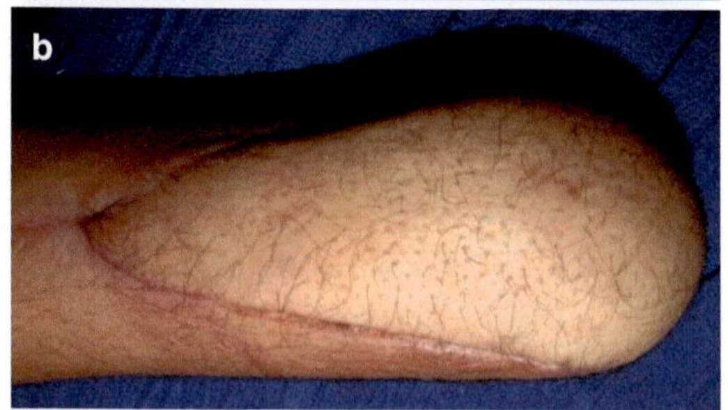

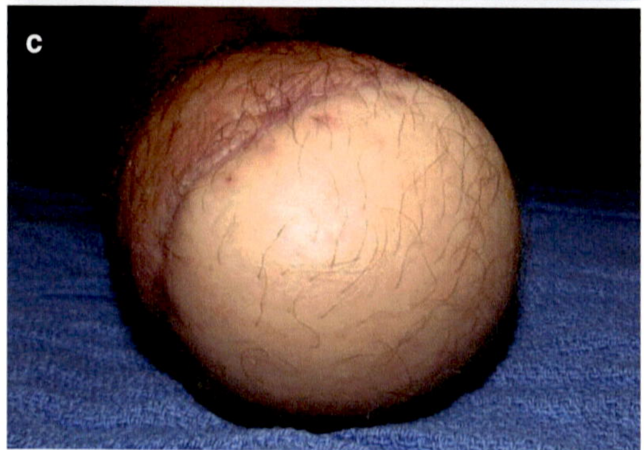

Fig. 12.6 Regarding the patient in Figs. 12.1, 12.2, 12.3, 12.4, and 12.5, the psychologist reviewed resilience and coping strategies with the patient, which supported the shared decision-making process. The patient, with guidance from the psychiatric and surgical teams, ultimately elected to undergo a formal amputation with preservation of the distal radio-ulnar joint. The amputation was therefore performed at the radiocarpal level. His soft tissue deficit was managed with a free anterolateral thigh flap.

pleasurable. Such re-engagement with life has minimized the potential devastating impact of dominant hand loss.

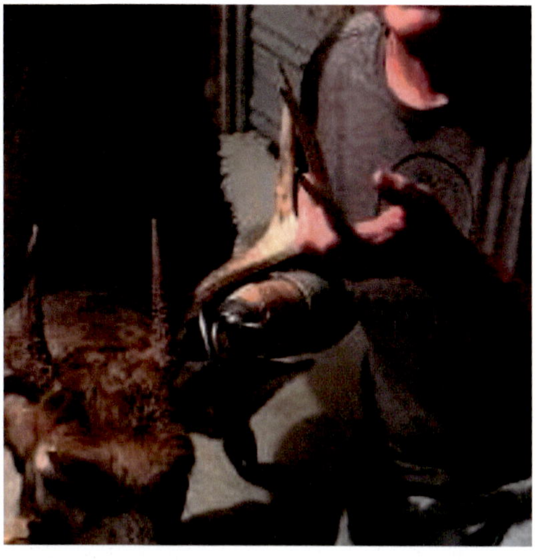

Fig. 12.7 Regarding the patient in Figs. 12.1, 12.2, 12.3, 12.4, 12.5, and 12.6, the patient was ultimately fitted for a body-powered prosthesis which he uses for most activities including hunting.

Clinical Pearls and Pitfalls
- The clinician must not overlook the psychological effects of trauma, which have a high likelihood of resulting in chronic pain and prolonged recovery.
- It is important to assemble a multidisciplinary team capable of screening for and treating the inevitable psychological sequelae of trauma.
- If maladaptive coping strategies are recognized or psychopathology diagnosed, early treatment can facilitate a return to personally valued pursuits, reintegration into society, weaning from pain medications, and a functionally meaningful recovery.
- As the patient progresses through recovery, the team should try to mini-

mize the risk of opioid abuse by responsibly using narcotics and weaning when appropriate. A pain medicine specialist on the treatment team can be a valuable resource.
- The physician should be wary of malingering and secondary gain issues which

could impede recovery. If identified, the physician should document all findings objectively, continue to show empathy and notify the practice manager or legal team for guidance.

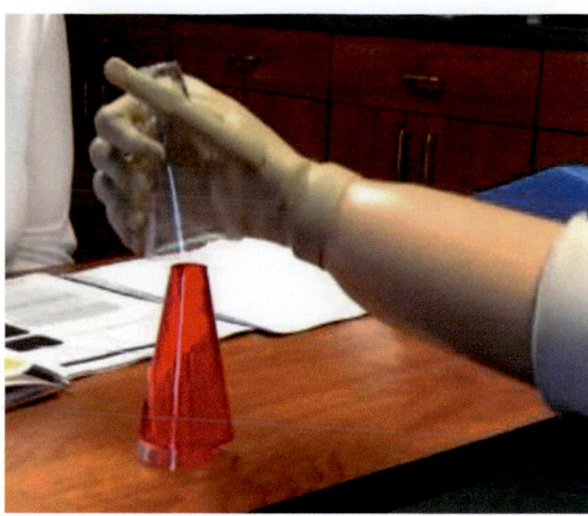
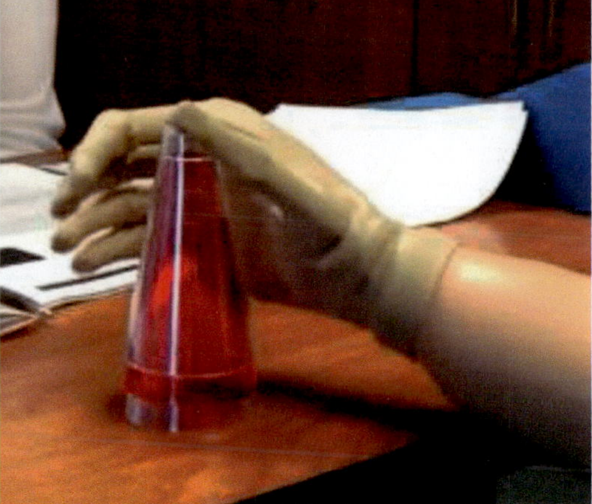

Fig. 12.8 Regarding the patient in Figs. 12.1, 12.2, 12.3, 12.4, 12.5, 12.6, and 12.7, he also occasionally wears a myoelectric prosthesis. During his recovery, he was seen routinely for serial physical and mental health evaluations. He proved quite resilient with excellent coping skills and no catastrophizing. Despite initial mild depression, he came to accept his disability. This acceptance has allowed him to pursue activities that he finds satisfying and personally valuable.

References

1. Williams AE, Newman JT, Ozer K, Juarros A, Morgan SJ, Smith WR. Posttraumatic stress disorder and depression negatively impact general health status after hand injury. J Hand Surg Am. 2009;34(3):515–22. https://doi.org/10.1016/j.jhsa.2008.11.008.
2. Starr AJ, Smith WR, Frawley WH, et al. Symptoms of posttraumatic stress disorder after orthopaedic trauma. J Bone Joint Surg Am. 2004;86-A(6):1115–21. http://www.ncbi.nlm.nih.gov/pubmed/15173282. Accessed 28 Apr 2018
3. Sutherland AG, Hutchinson JD, Alexander DA. The orthopaedic surgeon and post-traumatic psychopathology. J Bone Joint Surg Br. 2000;82(4):486–8. http://www.ncbi.nlm.nih.gov/pubmed/10855867. Accessed 28 Apr 2018.
4. Wiseman T, Foster K, Curtis K. Mental health following traumatic physical injury: an integrative literature review. Injury. 2013;44(11):1383–90. https://doi.org/10.1016/j.injury.2012.02.015.
5. Kretschmer T, Ihle S, Antoniadis G, et al. Patient satisfaction and disability after brachial plexus surgery. Neurosurgery. 2009;65(suppl_4):A189–96. https://doi.org/10.1227/01.NEU.0000335646.31980.33.
6. Gustafsson M, Amilon A, Ahlström G. Trauma-related distress and mood disorders in the early stage of an acute traumatic hand injury. J Hand Surg Br. 2003;28(4):332–8. http://www.ncbi.nlm.nih.gov/pubmed/12849944. Accessed 28 Apr 2018.
7. Gustafsson M, Ahlström G. Emotional distress and coping in the early stage of recovery following acute traumatic hand injury: a questionnaire survey. Int J Nurs Stud. 2006;43(5):557–65. https://doi.org/10.1016/j.ijnurstu.2005.07.006.

8. Franzblau L, Chung KC. Psychosocial outcomes and coping after complete avulsion traumatic brachial plexus injury. Disabil Rehabil. 2015;37(2):135–43. https://doi.org/10.3109/09638288.2014.911971.

9. Novak CB, Anastakis DJ, Beaton DE, Mackinnon SE, Katz J. Biomedical and psychosocial factors associated with disability after peripheral nerve injury. J Bone Joint Surg Am. 2011;93(10):929–36. https://doi.org/10.2106/JBJS.J.00110.

10. Shalev AY, Freedman S, Peri T, et al. Prospective study of posttraumatic stress disorder and depression following trauma. Am J Psychiatry. 1998;155(5):630–7. https://doi.org/10.1176/ajp.155.5.630.

11. Opsteegh L, Reinders-Messelink HA, Groothoff JW, Postema K, Dijkstra PU, van der Sluis CK. Symptoms of acute posttraumatic stress disorder in patients with acute hand injuries. J Hand Surg Am. 2010;35(6):961–7. https://doi.org/10.1016/j.jhsa.2010.03.024.

12. Himmelstein JS, Feuerstein M, Stanek EJ, et al. Work-related upper-extremity disorders and work disability: clinical and psychosocial presentation. J Occup Environ Med. 1995;37(11):1278–86. http://www.ncbi.nlm.nih.gov/sites/entrez?Db=pubmed&DbFrom=pubmed&Cmd=Link&LinkName=pubmed_pubmed&LinkReadableName=RelatedArticles&IdsFromResult=8595497&ordinalpos=3&itool=EntrezSystem2.PEntrez.Pubmed.Pubmed_ResultsPanel.Pubmed_RVDocSum.

13. Henderson M, Kidd BL, Pearson RM, White PD. Chronic upper limb pain: an exploration of the biopsychosocial model. J Rheumatol. 2005;32(1):118–22. http://www.ncbi.nlm.nih.gov/sites/entrez?Db=pubmed&DbFrom=pubmed&Cmd=Link&LinkName=pubmed_pubmed&LinkReadableName=RelatedArticles&IdsFromResult=15630736&ordinalpos=3&itool=EntrezSystem2.PEntrez.Pubmed.Pubmed_ResultsPanel.Pubmed_RVDocSum.

14. Scott DJ, Arthurs ZM, Stannard A, Monroe HM, Clouse WD, Rasmussen TE. Patient-based outcomes and quality of life after salvageable wartime extremity vascular injury. Surg e171. 2014;59(1 SRC-BaiduScholar FG-0):173–9.

15. Perkins ZB, Ath HD, Sharp G, Tai NR. De' Factors affecting outcome after traumatic limb amputation. Br 99 Suppl. 2012;1(SRC-B):75–86.

16. Berube M, Choiniere M, Laflamme YG, Gelinas C. Acute to chronic pain transition in extremity trauma: A narrative review for future preventive interventions (part 1). Int Trauma Nurs. 2016;23(SRC):47–59.

17. Koestler AJ. Psychological perspective on hand injury and pain. Ther quiz 211. 2010;23(2 SRC-BaiduScholar FG-0):199–210.

18. Merskey H, Bogduk N. Task Force on Taxonomy of the International Association for the Study of Pain. Lesions of the ear, nose, and oral cavity. http://www.researchgate.net/publication/286141091_Task_Force_on_Taxonomy_of_the_International_Association_for_the_Study_of_Pain_Lesions_of_the_ear_nose_and_oral_cavityLK-link%7C http://www.researchgate.net/publication/286141091_Task_Force_on_Taxonomy_o.

19. Melzack R, Wall PD. Pain mechanisms: a new theory. Science. 1965;150(3699):971–9. http://www.ncbi.nlm.nih.gov/sites/entrez?Db=pubmed&DbFrom=pubmed&Cmd=Link&LinkName=pubmed_pubmed&LinkReadableName=RelatedArticles&IdsFromResult=5320816&ordinalpos=3&itool=EntrezSystem2.PEntrez.Pubmed.Pubmed_ResultsPanel.Pubmed_RVDocSum.

20. Melzack R. From the gate to the neuromatrix. Pain. Suppl 1999;6:S121–6. http://www.ncbi.nlm.nih.gov/sites/entrez?Db=pubmed&DbFrom=pubmed&Cmd=Link&LinkName=pubmed_pubmed&LinkReadableName=RelatedArticles&IdsFromResult=10491980&ordinalpos=3&itool=EntrezSystem2.PEntrez.Pubmed.Pubmed_ResultsPanel.Pubmed_RVDocSum.

21. Engel GL. The clinical application of the biopsychosocial model. J Med Philos. 1981;6(2):101–23. http://www.ncbi.nlm.nih.gov/sites/entrez?Db=pubmed&DbFrom=pubmed&Cmd=Link&LinkName=pubmed_pubmed&LinkReadableName=RelatedArticles&IdsFromResult=7264472&ordinalpos=3&itool=EntrezSystem2.PEntrez.Pubmed.Pubmed_ResultsPanel.Pubmed_RVDocSum.

22. Gerbershagen HJ, Aduckathil S, van Wijck AJ, Peelen LM, Kalkman CJ, Meissner W. Pain intensity on the first day after surgery: a prospective cohort study comparing 179 surgical procedures. Anesthesiology. 2013;118(4 SRC-BaiduScholar FG-0):934–44.

23. Williamson OD, Epi GD, Gabbe BJ. Predictors of moderate or severe pain 6 months after orthopaedic injury: a prospective cohort study. Trauma. 2009;23(2 SRC-BaiduScholar FG-0):139–44.

24. Clay FJ, Watson WL, Newstead SV, McClure RJ. A systematic review of early prognostic factors for persisting pain following acute orthopedic trauma. Pain Res Manag. 2012;17(1):35–44. http://www.ncbi.nlm.nih.gov/sites/entrez?Db=pubmed&DbFrom=pubmed&Cmd=Link&LinkName=pubmed_pubmed&LinkReadableName=RelatedArticles&IdsFromResult=22518366&ordinalpos=3&itool=EntrezSystem2.PEntrez.Pubmed.Pubmed_ResultsPanel.Pubmed_RVDocSum.

25. Castillo RC, MacKenzie EJ, Wegener ST, Bosse MJ, Group LS. Prevalence of chronic pain seven years following limb threatening lower extremity trauma. Pain. 2006;124(3 SRC-BaiduScholar FG-0):321–9.

26. Donnell ML, Varker T, Holmes AC. O' Disability after injury: the cumulative burden of physical and mental health. Psychiatry. 2013;74(2):e137–43.

27. Stewart WF, Ricci JA, Chee E, Morganstein D, Lipton R. Lost productive time and cost due to common pain conditions in the US workforce. JAMA. 2003;290(18):2443–54.

28. Shivarathre DG, Howard N, Krishna S, Cowan C, Platt SR. Psychological factors and personality traits associated with patients in chronic foot and ankle pain. Foot Ankle Int. 2014;35(11):1103–7.

29. Castillo RC, Wegener ST, Heins SE, Haythornthwaite JA, Mackenzie EJ. Longitudinal relationships between anxiety, depression, and pain: results from a two-year

lower). EPM and EAM are key in facilitating tendon gliding to prevent adhesions [19]. Within postoperative protocols (both early passive and active) for repaired tendons, care must be taken to limit range when specified by the surgeon. For example, a repaired distal bicep EPM protocol would typically include full passive elbow flexion to 90° active elbow extension and gradually increase until full extension is achieved over a course of several weeks. Flexor and extensor tendon repairs in the hand and/or wrist are placed in a custom-fabricated splint/orthosis to protect the tendon from full stretch and either an EPM or EAM protocol initiated per the surgeon's order. Both protocols are based on a graduated progression of ROM to slowly stretch the tendon during the healing process [19–21]. By initiating EPM of the repaired structure, this allows tendon gliding to occur during the initial phases of wound healing, therefore making it difficult for any adhesions to form between the tendon and the surrounding soft tissue layers. The same concept applies for massive rotator cuff repairs where a specific amount of ROM is allowed for therapy and then is gradually increased to achieve a full and/or functional arc. Not only is EPM a key factor in preventing tendon adhesions, it is also important to emphasize the frequency of performance. It is not uncommon for a patient to be seen twice a day for treatment sessions during inpatient admissions following upper extremity tendon repairs. This high frequency must also be maintained post discharge and throughout outpatient therapy in order to have non-adhered functional ROM.

Tendon gliding is an important part of both passive and active motion protocols and, when performed according to therapist's recommended frequency, can prevent adhesions [16, 18] (Fig. 13.5). Joint blocking is yet another tool used by therapists to gain increased motion and prevent adhesions [17]. Both tendon gliding and blocking are used to elicit a particular muscle to activate in isolation, specifically addressing the tendon in question. Blocking can also be used once adhesions are present [16], but must be performed under supervision of a skilled therapist due to the risk of rupture if done with too much force. Both tendon gliding and joint blocking are

aimed at "lengthening adhesions to allow greater glide" rather than ripping the adhesions, as this would restart the body's inflammatory process, leading to more scar tissue [16]. Joint mobilization (joint mobs) is a technique used once all skeletal, tendinous, and ligamentous structures are well-healed due to the stress put on the joint, but when necessary, can be quite effective at increasing ROM in a stiff joint [15, 22]. There are several grades of joint mobilizations, ranging from small to large amplitude. When deciding which grade to perform (grade I through grade V), the therapist must consider many factors including end-range feel, degree of stiffness, and timeframe of injury and healing process, among others [22]. Due to these many factors, joint mobs should only be performed by a skilled therapist, as mentioned above, who is quite familiar with all repaired structures and surrounding anatomy, as well as the involved kinematics of the particular body part [10].

Despite early ROM protocols, scar formation and adhesion can sometimes be so robust that joint contracture occurs, limiting the patient's functionality [19]. In these situations, the surgeon may offer contracture releases (i.e., capsulotomies and potentially tenolyses) to remove the scarred tissues and allow improved mobility in the joint. Knee and elbow releases are the most common surgical procedures required after complicated injuries due to the nature of these hinged joints. Tenolysis to increase tendon glide is common after extensive soft tissue damage when involving a mangled limb [18]. Therapy becomes a top priority for postoperative care of capsulotomies and tenolyses and is often best to have appointments scheduled before the surgeon performs the operation. Without post-op therapy, the intraoperative increases in ROM (i.e., the purpose of the surgical intervention) significantly decrease due to the body's natural healing response of scar tissue creation from this most recent surgery. To preserve as much ROM as possible post-op, therapy begins on postoperative day 1, with a frequency goal of 5–7 days per week. The patient is also highly encouraged to perform a home exercise program 2–3 times a day in addition to the attended therapy sessions.

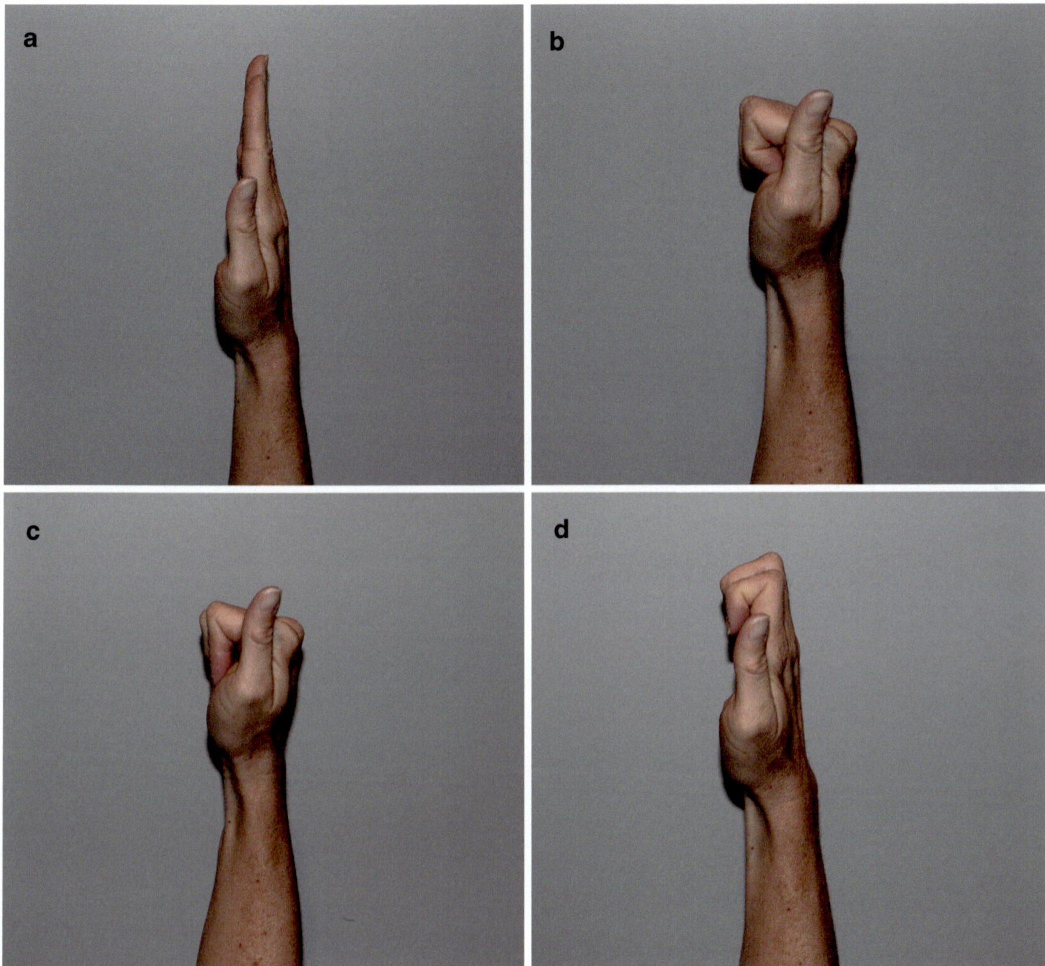

Fig. 13.5 Tendon gliding

Splints/Orthoses

Splints (orthoses) often have a role in therapy when there is extensive soft tissue damage in addition to fractures and tendon injuries. These splints are typically static in nature to provide protection and soft tissue rest during the early days of wound healing and progress to dynamic splints if the patient develops joint stiffness and/or tendon/soft tissue tightening. Following elbow releases, for example, a common treatment is the use of an anterior extension splint/orthosis to allow the shortened muscles a sustained low-load stretch and have a typical wearing schedule of all hours in between therapy sessions and HEP sessions, as well as at night for several weeks after the surgery. In the case of a free or rotational muscle flap, a patient may be placed in a protective orthosis that has been custom fabricated with extra space along flap perimeter, therefore not putting any pressure on the flap (Figs. 13.6 and 13.7).

If the patient then developed extrinsic tendon tightening from early immobilization to allow the flap time to integrate, a dynamic splint may be required to provide low-load, long-duration stretch [23]. Figure 13.8 demonstrates a dynamic thumb abduction splint fabricated to correct an adductor policies contraction.

After major trauma, it is not uncommon for portions of non-viable muscles and tendons to be debrided in surgery, therefore leaving a weak-

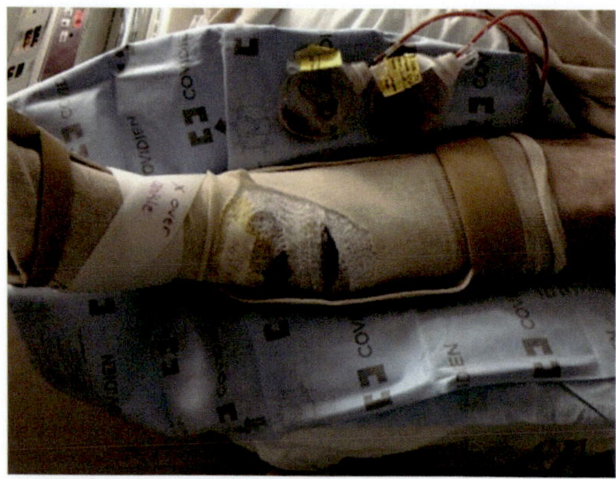

Fig. 13.6 Foot splint molded around free flap, leaving gap to avoid pressure on flap

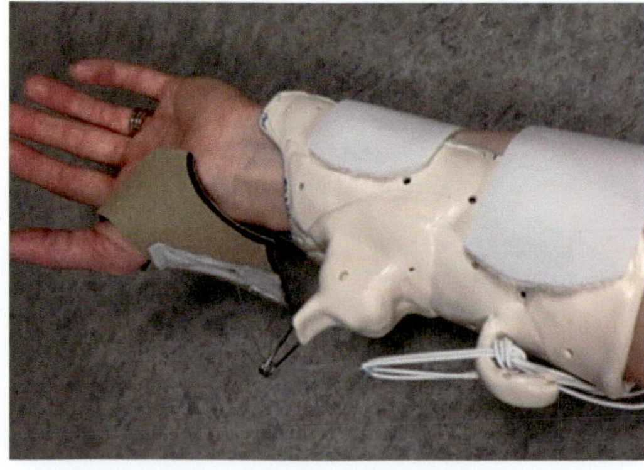

Fig. 13.8 Dynamic thumb abduction splint for low-load long-duration stretch of the first webspace

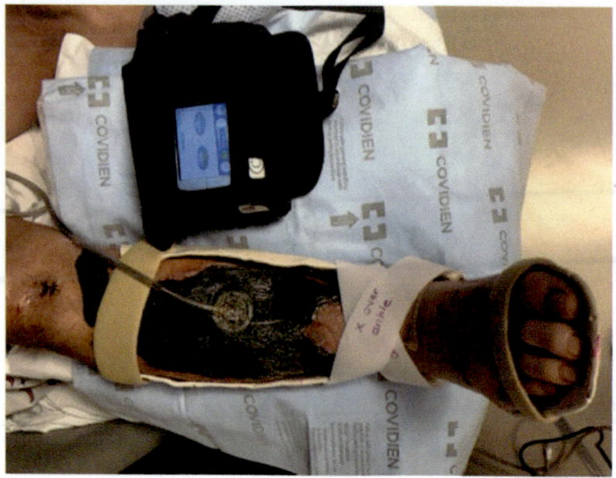

Fig. 13.7 Foot splint molded around VAC with straps placed around flap to avoid pressure on flap

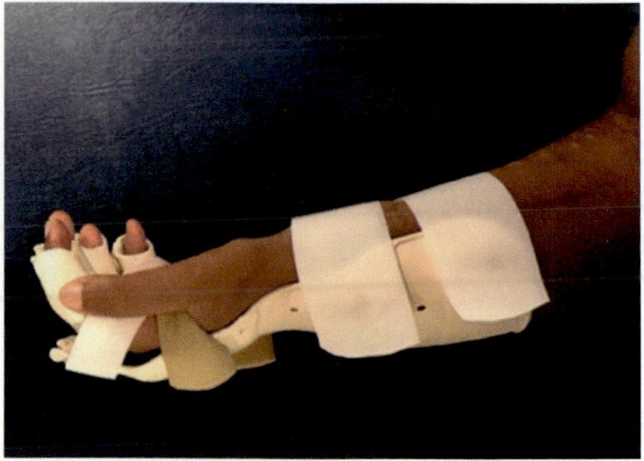

Fig. 13.9 "Exercise splint" to isolate the FDP

ened muscle and/or tendon. Weakened muscle action can also be the case after a tendon transfer. Splints can be fabricated for the purpose of holding certain joints in an immobile position while performing an exercise to target a specific muscle during ROM and strengthening. For example, when the patient pictured below (Fig. 13.9) had weakness of the flexor digitorum profundus (FDP), an "exercise splint" was made to isolate the FDP and therefore held the metacarpal phalangeal (MCP) and proximal interphalangeal (PIP) joints as well as the wrist immobile, so when the flexor tendons attempted activation, all of the excursion would be firing the FDP.

When incorporating a splint/orthosis into a patient treatment program, it is important to perform splint checks. Specifically, the splint fit must be monitored over a several-day (or possibly week(s)) period to ensure proper skin integrity is maintained. This is especially true with a mangled limb because of the already fragile skin from the nature of the injury, as well as any nerve damage sustained, in which case the patient may not feel any pressure areas, making the visual skin checks that much more important. The patient requires education on splint wear and skin checks, and this should be part of the home exercise program. Extra consideration must be given when the patient has further reconstructive surgery on the limb and thus will require a longer splint monitoring process. Splints/orthoses, when used in conjunction with ROM, scar management, edema control, and a home exercise program, can often provide the missing piece of the puzzle in achieving a level of independence for a patient not otherwise obtained.

Patient and Family Education

Patient and therapist rapport is an essential piece of the therapy foundation and is required for a good outcome. Often, the patient and therapist have the most time-intensive relationship, ranging several months to 1 or 2 years, depending on the severity of the injury and any subsequent reconstructive surgeries. During this timeframe, the therapist must educate the patient to take ownership of their limb in order for a successful outcome to be achieved. It is important for a patient to "buy-in" to the therapy goals and thereby be more willing to participate. Therapy does not finish once the patient leaves the clinic, but rather it continues at home where the patient completes the home exercise program. Family can also be encouraged to assist at home both physically through passive ROM and emotionally through verbal support and reminders to perform the exercises. In the case of a mangled limb, the patient may have sustained additional injuries and due to the overall medical condition may not be able to take an active role in their own care. For these patients' therapy to succeed, the family/friends must be involved.

One major part of education of the patient with a mangled limb must center on lack of sensation. Typically, when dealing with a massive trauma to a limb, sensation is compromised either directly through injury to one or multiple nerves or indirectly through subsequent pressure on nerve(s) from persistent swelling. In either case, impaired sensation requires the patient to make a lifestyle change to include constant visual awareness of where the limb is in space as well as daily skin checks to ensure that any defect to the skin (as "minor" as a small abrasion or papercut to as severe as a burn) is noted and attended to immediately to prevent further soft tissue damage.

Patient education occurs throughout the longevity of therapy as the patient's needs change with achieved motion and strength and will require several updates over the course of treatment; however, the two main staples of the home exercise program should be scar management and range of motion, both of which have been addressed above. Through thorough patient education, the big picture can truly be painted for the patient who can impart the importance of therapy to achieve the best possible function of the involved limb. It will also assist in preparation for future surgeries or even elimination of the need for them (i.e., preventing joint contractures and therefore no need for capsulotomies or tenolyses).

Case Example

Sarah[*], a left-hand dominant 17-year-old female, was involved in a rollover motor vehicle collision and sustained a mangled left upper extremity (near-complete amputation) that extended from the elbow joint to just proximal to the wrist (Fig. 13.10). Her injuries included complete loss of forearm wrist and digit flexors, severe degloving of the forearm soft tissue, open both-bone forearm fracture (BBFF) (with severe comminution of the ulna), and transections of the ulnar nerve, ulnar artery, and anterior interosseous system. She underwent 19 reparative surgeries and a reconstructive surgery over the course of 22 months to salvage the extremity. The reparative surgeries included repairs of ulnar nerve, ulnar artery, and cephalic vein using lower extremity vein graft, open reduction with internal fixation (ORIF) of the BBFF, multiple irrigation and debridements (I&Ds), periscapular free flap (Fig. 13.10b) and multiple split-thickness skin grafts for coverage of volar forearm, placement of antibiotic beads, thrombectomy secondary to blockage in periscapular flap, and revision ORIF. Free flap failure ensued and Sarah, along with her family, decided no further free flaps. This led to Sarah undergoing a bipedicled thoracoabdominal fasciocutaneous flap where her forearm was inserted into the flap to allow volar forearm tissue granulation. Prior to the flap being able to take place, she had soft tissue expanders placed in the abdomen (Fig. 13.10c) to stretch the skin enough that once divided, there would be enough skin to cover the large forearm defect. The thoracoabdominal flap was then divided in two stages to ensure the flap had taken to the forearm before dissecting in entirety (Fig. 13.10d). Once the flap was 100% dissected,

____

[*]name has been changed to protect patient privacy.

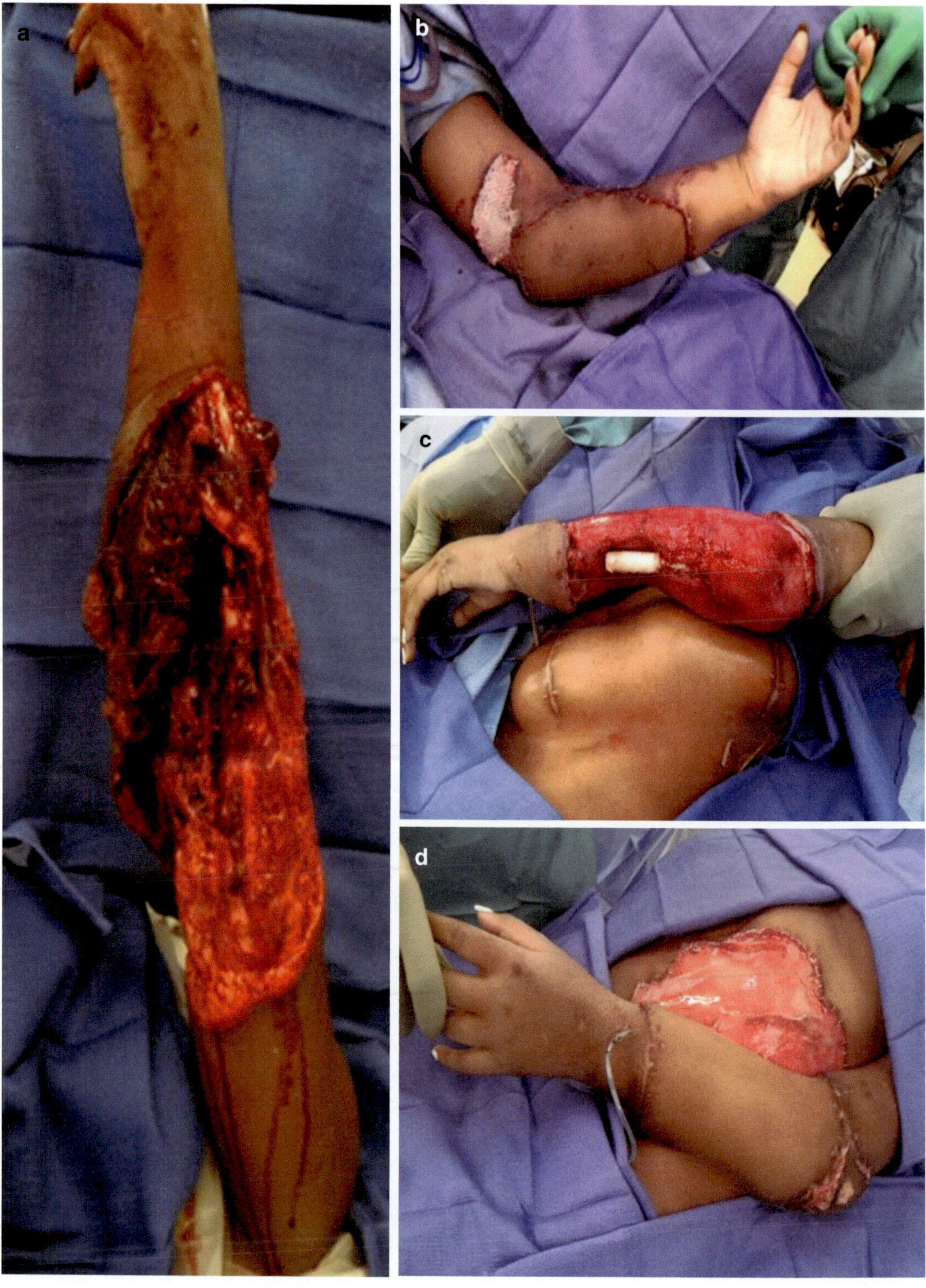

Fig. 13.10 (**a**) Mangled LUE prepped for surgery s/p rollover MVC. (**b**) periscapular free flap and BBFF ORIF. (**c**) Intra-abdominal soft tissue expanders after 6 weeks of gradual inflation. (**d**) thoracoabdominal bipedicled flap after two-stage division

the flap had taken to the forearm, and infection was cleared (through multiple I&Ds and antibiotic beads), discussions could then begin for how to make the extremity functional due to the missing wrist/digit flexors that were lost in the initial injury.

Many factors are involved when making a decision to salvage an arm versus amputation which will be discussed in Chap. 16. For Sarah's case, those factors were her age, prior functional status including overall health, and level and severity of injury when she arrived at the trauma center, among others. Most importantly for her case was the decision to use a parascapular and subsequent fasciocutaneous thoracoabdominal flap for soft tissue coverage rather than a full- or splint-thickness skin graft (FTSG, STSG). This decision was made in the very early stages of her care but would go on to set the stage for possible future functional tendon transfers to allow her active wrist and digit flexion. Prior to this injury, Sarah was an active teenager, competed in cheerleading tournaments and led a very productive life. Providing the chance for future functional use of her dominant hand would prove to have a major impact on her quality of life. The orthopedic surgeon had this fact, and future therapy, in mind when choosing the flap for soft tissue coverage, specifically due to the fact that less scar adhesions would form with use of a flap than either a FTSG or STSG. Less scar adhesions during wound healing would allow for better tendon and soft tissue mobility and lay the groundwork necessary for a successful flexor tendon transfer. Nine and half months after the initial injury, Sarah underwent a left extensor carpi radialis longus (ECRL) transfer to flexor digitorum superficialis (FDS) of the index finger (IF), long finger (LF), ring finger (RF), and small finger (SF). It was decided to only transfer to the FDS due to the limited eligible donor tendons and the surgeon's knowledge that her final outcome wasn't expected to have a full active composite grip with fine motor capability, but rather to have a functional gross grasp to assist with activities such as holding a cup or other light object to assist with basic activities of daily living (ADLs).

Occupational therapy (OT) was initiated several days postoperative during Sarah's inpatient admission to include ROM to uninvolved joints (shoulder and digits) and edema control (utilizing elevation and ace wrap, no compression sleeves at that time). As noted above, it is crucial to preserve motion of all uninvolved joints to prevent stiffness that could lead to contracture. Her restrictions for the left upper extremity (LUE) were non-weight bearing (NWB) and no strengthening. The patient and family were both educated on ROM of the shoulder and digits that could be safely performed, and they were encouraged to engage Sarah in these activities whenever OT was not occurring. This was a way for her to become acclimated to her new extremity and be an active participant in the long road to recovery in addition to keeping focus on the need for joint mobility throughout the recovery process. Throughout the many operations, OT's top concern was to keep all joints supple and therefore consisted primarily of ROM (active, active-assisted, and passive within surgeon's specifications). Due to the loss of wrist and hand flexors, passive range of motion (PROM) only could be performed; however, active and active-assisted range of motions (AROM, AAROM) were also addressed at the elbow and forearm status post the periscapular flap and bony fixation. OT would begin a gradual elbow flexion program to 45° with 15° increases in flexion each week to slowly regain full elbow ROM over 3–4 months post-op. Once Sarah underwent the fasciocutaneous abdominal flap, the shoulder, elbow, and forearm were no longer in a capacity for ROM now that they were attached via flap, but the digits (although close in proximity to the abdomen) remained unattached and therefore PROM continued to all digits despite the flap in place. Strengthening and weight-bearing continued to be restricted. At this time, OT was also addressing goals of self-care utilizing only Sarah's right upper extremity for activities such as dressing, bathing, and feeding with her nondominant hand. Therapy continued in this respect throughout her inpatient hospital stay that spanned 1 month and 19 surgeries. After the abdominal flap was divided, ROM to her shoulder, elbow, forearm, and wrist resumed (Fig. 13.11). Sarah was discharged from the hospital and seen on an outpa-

Conclusion

Therapy is typically one of the last components of the treatment team to become involved with a patient with a mangled limb. The patient has already endured the injury, been admitted to the hospital, undergone surgery(ies), and received nursing care during their stay before ever seeing the therapist. Although therapy cannot begin until these other events have occurred, it is by no means less important. The patient's goal after a major trauma is to return to life as normal as possible, and this is where therapy has the most impact. Realistic goals are established, with patient input, and although the end result won't be the same as prior to the trauma, the patient can attain a meaningful, well-rounded life with a functional limb.

References

1. Facs.org. (2016). National Trauma Data Bank 2016 Annual Report. [online] Available at: https://www.facs.org/~media/files/quality%20programs/trauma/ntdb/ntdb%20annual%20report%202016.a.shx.
2. Htcc.org. (2017). Hand Therapy Certification Commission - Definition of Hand Therapy. [online] Available at: https://www.htcc.org/consumer-information/the-cht-credential/definition-of-hand-therapy.
3. Occupational therapy practice framework: domain and process (3rd Edition). Am J Occup Ther. 2014;68(Supplement_1):S1–S48.
4. Apta.org. (2017). The physical therapist scope of practice. [online] Available at: http://www.apta.org/ScopeOfPractice/. Accessed 30 Aug 2017.
5. TheFreeDictionary.com. (2009). Therapeutic use of self. [online] Available at: http://medical-dictionary.thefreedictionary.com/therapeutic+use+of+self. Accessed 20 Jun 2017.
6. Pettengill K. Therapist's management of the complex injury. In: Skirven TM, Osterman AL, Fedorczyk JM, Amadio PC, editors. Rehabilitation of the hand and upper extremity. 6th ed. Philadelphia: Elsevier Mosby; 2011. p. 1238–51.
7. Miller J (2017). How does kinesiology tape reduce swelling?. [online] Physioworks.com.au. Available at: http://physioworks.com.au/FAQRetrieve.aspx?ID=38758. Accessed 30 Aug 2017.
8. Wolkenberg A, McDuffie M, Terrazas J, Salisbury C, editors. KT1: fundamental concepts of the Kinesio taping method, vol. 25. Albuquerque: Kinesio IP, LLC; 2011. p. 34.
9. Kase K, Wallis J, Kase T. Clinical therapeutic applications of the Kinesio taping method; 2003. p. 80.
10. Ezerins SA, Harm CJ, Kempton SJ, Salyapongse AN. Rehabilitation following replantation in the upper extremity. In: Salyapongse AN, et al., editors. Extremity replantation: a comprehensive clinical guide. New York: Springer Science+Business; 2015. p. 191–206.
11. von der Heyde R, Evans R. Wound classification and management. In: Skirven TM, Osterman AL, Fedorczyk JM, Amadio PC, editors. Rehabilitation of the hand and upper extremity. 6th ed. Philadelphia: Elsevier Mosby;pp; 2011. p. 219–32.
12. Hardy M. The biology of healing: connective tissue. In: Surgery and rehabilitation of the hand with emphasis on the elbow. Philadelphia: Hand Rehabilitation Foundation; 2008. p. 377–80.
13. Bracciano AG, Constantine G, McPhee SD. Physical agent modalities credentialing course: for the occupational therapy practitioner. Franklin: PAMPA, LLC; 2007. p. 50, 53,75, 78–81.
14. McVeigh K, Herman M. Wound healing. In: American Society of Hand Therapists, editor. Test prep for the CHT exam. 3rd ed. USA: ASHT; 2012. p. 65–89.
15. Davila SA. Therapist's management of fractures and dislocations of the elbow. In: Skirven TM, Osterman AL, Fedorczyk JM, Amadio PC, editors. Rehabilitation of the hand and upper extremity. 6th ed. Philadelphia: Elsevier Mosby;pp; 2011. p. 1061–74.
16. Pettengill K, Van Strien G. Postoperative management of flexor tendon injuries. In: Skirven TM, Osterman AL, Fedorczyk JM, Amadio PC, editors. Rehabilitation of the hand and upper extremity. 6th ed. Philadelphia: Elsevier Mosby; 2011. p. 457–78.
17. Reiffel RS. Prevention of hypertrophic scars by long term paper tape application. Plast Reconstr Surg. 1995;96:1715–8.
18. Sturm SM, Oxley SB, Van Zant RS. Rehabilitation of a patient following hand replantation after near-complete distal forearm amputation. J Hand Ther. 2014;27(3):217–24.
19. Evans RB. Managing the injured tendon: current concepts. J Hand Ther. 2012;25(2):173–90.
20. von der Heyde R. Flexor tendon rehabilitation. In: ASHT comprehensive hand therapy review course. USA: ASHT; 2013.
21. Taras JS, Martyak GG, Steelman PJ. Primary care of flexor tendon injuries. In: Skirven TM, Osterman AL, Fedorczyk JM, Amadio PC, editors. Rehabilitation of the hand and upper extremity. 6th ed. Philadelphia: Elsevier Mosby; 2011. p. 445–56.
22. Fedorczyk F. Manual therapy in the management of upper extremity musculoskeletal disorders. In: Skirven TM, Osterman AL, Fedorczyk JM, Amadio PC, editors. Rehabilitation of the hand and upper extremity. 6th ed. Philadelphia: Elsevier Mosby; 2011. p. 1539–47.
23. Veltman ES, Doornberg JN, Eygendaal D, van den Bekerom MPJ. Static progressive versus dynamic splinting for posttraumatic elbow stiffness: a systematic review of 232 patients. Arch Orthop Trauma Surg. 2015;135:613–7.

Renan C. Castillo and Anna McGinnis

The Need to Responsibly Manage Opioid Use

Consequences of Inadequate Pain Management (Fig. 14.1)

Poorly controlled postoperative pain in orthopedic trauma patients leads to increased length of hospital stays, repeat hospitalizations, psychological distress, delayed functional recovery, and failure to return to work. In longitudinal studies with trauma patients, elevated pain intensity early in the recovery process predicts chronic pain, poor functional outcomes, low satisfaction with healthcare, and failure to participate in physical therapy. Despite the importance of controlling postoperative pain, pain management for orthopedic trauma patients remains inconsistent and often inadequate. Studies continue to show patients experience moderate to severe pain in acute care settings and report insufficient pain relief postoperatively.

Considerable evidence exists that uncontrolled postoperative pain, especially in orthopedic trauma patients, is a major risk factor for the development of chronic pain, psychosocial problems, and physical disability. This is a particular problem for military care, as soldiers increasingly survive high-energy blasts but experience long-term pain and post-traumatic stress disorder (PTSD) [1]. At the same time, poor postoperative pain management has substantial negative consequences for orthopedic injuries of all severities, with isolated and closed fractures still constituting the bulk of orthopedic injuries in both the civilian and military settings. The benefit to civilian and military patients of even small reductions in pain intensity may be substantial. As an example, results from one study suggest that if one-half standard deviation decrease in postsurgical pain could be achieved, this would result in dramatic reductions in the risk of PTSD [2]. The use of multimodal perioperative pain management has the potential to reduce pain intensity by this amount. Many other potential benefits may be attainable as well, including reduced opioid consumption, improved functional outcomes, and decreased healthcare resource utilization.

Pain is a common consequence of orthopedic trauma, and poor postoperative pain control predicts physical disability, delayed return to work, psychological distress, low satisfaction with healthcare, and failure to participate in physical therapy [3–5]. Despite increased awareness of the negative consequences of poor pain control, pain care among hospitalized patients remains inconsistent and inadequate [6, 7]. Studies continue to reveal that 50–70% of patients experience moderate to severe pain in acute care

R. C. Castillo (✉) · A. McGinnis
Health Policy and Management, Johns Hopkins
Bloomberg School of Public Health,
Baltimore, MD, USA
e-mail: rcastill@jhsph.edu; rcastil1@jhu.edu

© Springer Nature Switzerland AG 2021
R. A. Pensy, J. V. Ingari (eds.), *The Mangled Extremity*, https://doi.org/10.1007/978-3-319-56648-1_14

216

R. C. Castillo and A. McGinnis

Table 14.1 Pain management intervention opportunities for orthopedic trauma patients

	Pre-surgery	Surgery	Post-surgery	Discharge	Acute period (0–6 weeks)	Post acute (6 + weeks)
Education class	X					
Acupuncture	X	X	X			
Music		X	X			
Multimodal analgesia		X	X			
Pain medications	X		X	X	X	X
Therapy dogs			X			
Physical therapy			X		X	X
Wakefulness aids			X	X	X	X
Transfer intervention				X		
Specialist referral				X		
Post-discharge phone calls					X	
Appointment with specialist					X	X
Comprehensive pain rehabilitation program						X
Opioid tapering						X

higher satisfaction with the hospital and had lower narcotics usage [23]. PAIs are the Ranawat Center's multimodal analgesic of choice as well; the Ranawat Center specializes in orthopedic surgeries, specifically TKAs and THAs, and is working to minimize perioperative pain and with the technology available now supports PAIs as the way to minimize pain and decrease parental narcotics use [24]. The purpose of multimodal analgesia is to move away from risky narcotics usage without sacrificing the patients' well-being, and that appears to be achieved in these studies.

Another method of multimodal analgesia is a peripheral nerve block (PNB), where the anesthetic is injected close to a nerve to anesthetize the nerve and block pain. One study done at Mayo Clinic compared patients receiving a new protocol, Total Joint Regional Anesthesia (TJRA) protocol, to historical matches who had received more opioid-centric pain management protocol. The study found that through the use of PNB, part of TJRA, while stopping intravenous opioid administration, patients reported improvements in pain relief, adverse effects, recovery, and decreased opioid use [25]. Multiple factors changed in this study between the historical matches and those who received the multimodal treatment, so one limitation is the inability to isolate one factor responsible for these improve-

ments, but the PNB likely played a role and continued to be used in other studies. PNB is very effective for eliminating pain, but it also poses risks and can increase mobilization time and thus the length of stay [22].

One study compared PAIs to a standard treatment of femoral nerve blocks, a specific kind of PNB, and PCA for TKA recovery and found no difference in pain scores to be found between treatments [23]. When comparing just PNB to PAI for pain treatment of both THA and TKA, no significant difference was found in pain scores suggesting that the two methods of multimodal analgesia are comparable in their effects, yet since PAIs pose a lower risk and cost to the patient, perhaps they are preferred; more research needs to be done on the topic and for a wider range of procedures to support this claim [22].

Perioperative Pain Medicine

Perioperative pain management using nonsteroidal anti-inflammatory drugs (NSAIDs) such as ketorolac (*Toradol*), and anticonvulsants such as pregabalin (*Lyrica*), has been found to substantially improve postsurgical pain control in numerous clinical settings. However, multimodal perioperative pain management has not been widely used in orthopedics due to conflicting data about the increased risk of nonunion, wound closure, and bleeding complications.

NSAIDs are used extensively, most often as a component of a multimodal analgesic regimen, to treat the pain and swelling that accompanies orthopedic injury, and as a component of perioperative analgesic regimens following orthopedic surgery. Current data leave little doubt that perioperative NSAIDs can reduce postoperative pain and opioid consumption for many types of surgery in addition to orthopedic surgery, though the same structured review identified substantial gaps related to methodology, study size, study population, nature of the intervention, and choice of outcomes [26]. Further, concerns about renal impairment, gastrointestinal irritation, and platelet inhibition constrain usage and limit the dose and duration of ketorolac administration. More directly relevant to orthopedics, in animal models, NSAIDs in general and ketorolac in particular are known to impair osteogenesis [27, 28]. Similarly, animal studies with chronic ketorolac administration raise concern with respect to the strength of healed wounds, with variable results for muscle and ligamentous injury [29, 30]. In human studies of spinal fusion, 48 hours of ketorolac therapy for a total dose of 240 mg appears not to affect the fusion rate, but longer duration therapy, even at lower doses, may be problematic [31, 32]. However, in a fracture model with young mice, a variety of COX antagonists did not affect long-term tibial healing, consistent with a similar observation in young patients undergoing scoliosis surgery [33, 34]. A recent meta-analysis of 13 randomized trials confirmed prior findings that perioperative ketorolac is effective at reducing both pain and opioid consumption. However, the evidence was stronger for 16 mg per day as opposed to 30 mg per day doses [35]. Importantly, however, a meta-analysis of 27 studies found no evidence of perioperative bleeding following multimodal ketorolac use among surgical patients [36].

Gabapentin, developed as an anticonvulsant drug, has been FDA-approved for the treatment of postherpetic neuralgia and recommended as a first-line drug for neuropathic pain. A newer analog, pregabalin, has also been shown to be effective in the management of many chronic pain states and approved in the USA for use in postherpetic neuralgia, painful diabetic neuropathy, and fibromyalgia [37]. Over that last decade, 22 RCTs have investigated the potential benefits of gabapentin in postoperative pain management in over 1900 patients, and eight studies have also examined the effects of pregabalin in about 700 surgical patients. Meta-analysis and critical reviews conclude that gabapentin and pregabalin provide better postoperative analgesia than placebo [38]. In addition, gabapentin and pregabalin reduced opioid consumption in the first 24 hours post-surgery by 20–62% or by 25–30 mg of morphine. However, most of these studies include a small number of primarily non-orthopedic surgical patients who were followed during the immediate postoperative period (up to 7 days). In only half of the studies was pain evaluated with movement, and only seven gabapentin studies followed patients from 1 to 3 months post-surgery. Only two RCTs with pregabalin included patients undergoing elective orthopedic surgeries. Two more recent combined systematic review and meta-analysis of 33 clinical trials demonstrated once again that perioperative gabapentinoids are effective in reducing the incidence of chronic and acute postsurgical pain [39, 40]. Further, a meta-analysis of 12 perioperative pregabalin randomized trials identified 225–300 mg/day as the lowest effective dose, though prior meta-analyses and systematic reviews have shown substantial dosing variation ranging between 300 and 1200 mg per day [41]. Interestingly, another small randomized trial found no such effect among elective ankle surgery patients [42]. Similarly, in another small randomized trial, the same group found no effect for perioperative pregabalin among total knee arthroplasty patients though it is unclear if both of these studies were sufficiently powered [43]. A more recent review of 17 randomized trials of pregabalin alone found improved analgesia but also significant side effects, though not with severe clinical consequence [44]. A handful of recent randomized trials in the elective orthopedic literature also suggest a similar pattern. A small randomized trial of lumbar discectomy patients showed improvements in both pain and functional outcome among patients receiving perioperative gabapentinoids [45].

Acetaminophen can be administered intravenously as an alternative to opioids for treating pain postoperatively. Acetaminophen is a pain reliever that, when administered following surgery, can supplement and thus decrease opioid requirement while also limiting patients' pain following orthopedic surgery [46].

Capsaicin is a naturally occurring TRPV-1 agonist that is used in cream or injection form to control pain, and as a topical cream, it can be applied to the area of pain while the injection is used for postoperative pain control. Both forms are methods of pain control that can combat opioid use by providing an alternative form of pain relief [47]. One study of patients' pain following total knee replacement surgery found that participants that received capsaicin used fewer opioids postoperatively and had a better range of motion [48].

Antidepressants, specifically tricyclic or serotonergic-noradrenergic antidepressants, have been shown to have antinociceptive properties for neuropathic pain at lower dosage levels than required for the antidepressive effects to be seen [49, 50]. The analgesic effect of antidepressant medications is separate from their effect on mood; however, the mechanism of action is unknown. Antidepressants have not been used to treat acute pain due to their delayed effects but can be used as a form of non-opioid pain treatment in chronic pain patients [51].

Other Medical Interventions

Spinal cord stimulation (SCS) is an effective form of pain management for chronic pain and other related conditions that utilizes an electrical implant that alleviates pain by blocking nerve signals to the brain [52]. Although not used for acute pain or trauma conditions, it offers a unique method of relieving pain through nerve stimulation and, though invasive, helps identify biological areas that could be targets for acute pain as well, such as the dorsal root ganglion [53]. Pulsed radiofrequency lesioning utilizes the dorsal root ganglion to reduce pain [55]. This method works in a similar way that SCS does by obstructing the pain signal in the nerves to reduce the sensation of pain by interrupting the pathways to the brain [54].

Referral to physical therapy following orthopedic trauma results in beneficial outcome to patients, although orthopedic surgeons are better at making referrals than primary care physicians. Physical therapists, who have kinesiology expertise, are even better at identifying patients who could use physical therapy to improve their pain and recovery, which calls for physical therapists to visit orthopedic trauma patients in hospitals prior to discharge [55]. Additionally, those patients identified for physical therapy referral who did not received it had lower levels of improvement than those whose needs were met, supporting the role of physical therapy in pain management of orthopedic trauma [53].

One additional method of traditional pain management treatment is through the use of wakefulness aids, which, contrary to their name, actually help patients sleep better. When patients are sedentary and/or in a half-sleep stage due to injury and medication, giving them a wakefulness aid will help them sleep better because they will feel more awake during the day and be able to sleep better at night. A sedentary lifestyle with poor sleep can contribute to pain and the encouragement of a full night's sleep is an important part of managing pain because a lack of sleep independent of other ailments can cause pain [56, 57].

Traditional perioperative pain management treatments help patients control their pain but are not always safe or extremely effective. In order to better treat patients' pain, it is necessary to look outside of the traditional treatments to find methods that can manage pain more completely without limitations or serious adverse effects. Comprehensive interdisciplinary pain care combines traditional and alternative pain treatments to maximize pain relief while minimizing patients' risks.

Comprehensive Interdisciplinary Pain Care

Various methods of alternative treatment are on the rise to treat patients' pain without introducing a risky pharmacological agent, providing little risk with large reward potential. These methods, summarized below, are widely used, but most are supported mostly by anecdotal evidence, demonstrating the need to build the evidence base.

Pain is a result of biological and psychosocial factors, but most treatment plans focus solely on biomedical treatments. A need exists to integrate treatment of psychosocial factors that contribute to pain by increasing knowledge of pain psychology, emphasizing it in physicians', "especially physiatrists'", education and creating specific APA certifications for pain psychology as learning incentives [58, 59]. If medical professionals had an increased understanding of pain psychology, they could help patients come up with strategies to more effectively deal with their pain instead of catastrophizing, which can make their pain feel more intense [60]. One study found, through literature searches and analysis, that chronic pain and psychiatric disorders are comorbid, yet patients suffering from pain are not given adequate psychiatric treatment that could help ease their pain if they received it [61].

When a patient prepares to have surgery, they may not understand all the complications they will face after surgery. One way to prepare patients for their surgery is to have them attend an education class with other patients. This class helps ease patients' anxiety about the surgery, set expectations for the surgery and recovery, and emphasizes the importance of creating a discharge plan [22, 24, 25]. Another way is to implement a discharge-transfer intervention that engages the patient, inpatient care team, and the primary care physician's office. One study conducted at Somerville Hospital in MA implemented such an intervention and found that the intervention group, when compared to both concurrent and historical controls, had increased rates of follow-up and recommended workshop completion. The intervention was four-pronged, and it included a discharge form filled out by the patient, electronic transfer of this form to the patient's primary care physician, a telephone call from a nurse at the primary care physician's office, and a review of the discharge plan by the primary care physician [62]. The intervention played on the concept of redundancy to reinforce the discharge procedures in patients' minds as well as ensuring no steps were missed in the transition.

Acupuncture is used to relieve pain in certain areas through the stimulation of corresponding pressure points. One study found that THA patients in Germany who received auricular acupuncture during surgery required less piritramide than their counterparts who received sham acupuncture [63]. Another study found that patients who elected to receive acupuncture following joint replacement surgery experienced clinically meaningful pain reduction; acupuncture brought patients' pain to levels below the threshold for intravenous narcotic administration [64]. Both studies credited acupuncture with benefiting patients not only through pain reduction but also by reducing narcotic exposure and thus the adverse effects related to narcotics.

Music has been explored in Sweden as another form of complementary pain management. Patients that underwent outpatient surgeries while listening to music either during surgery or immediately after (while still unconscious) reported lower pain scores in the first 2 hours post-surgery [65]. Although not backed by numerous studies exposing patients to music during procedures poses little to no risk, this study illustrates that it can reduce patients' subsequent pain.

Therapy dog exposure following total knee or hip replacement for 15 minutes preceding physical therapy sessions for 3 days post-op was shown to result in decreased pain scores [66]. The mechanism behind this observed pain reduction is unknown but is hypothesized to be related to the neuroendocrine effect, which acts as an analgesic, or to the decreased depression and anxiety symptoms that have been linked to therapy dog exposure in other populations.

Massage is a non-medicinal form of therapy that can reduce patients' pain. One study collected pain scores of hospital inpatients before and after massage and found that massage reduced VAS pain scores and that the majority of patients felt the pain reducing effects for 1–4 hours post-massage [67].

Another approach focusing on the psychological factors of pain is hypnosis, which has been shown to relieve both acute and chronic pain although the mechanism is unknown and can only be hypothesized. Additionally, there is high variability between individuals in response to hypnosis; further research is needed to gain insight into the mechanism of hypnosis and factors that may make an individual more likely to respond to it as part of a pain treatment plan [68].

Mindfulness-based meditation is another psychological method of treatment that has been shown to alleviate pain and decrease pain sensitivity in both experimentally induced and chronic pain patients [69, 70]. Meditation is not a new practice, but it has not been extensively studied and therefore incorporated into the evidence base for pain management. One study looked at the effects of meditation on areas of the brain and found that pain is likely reduced through multiple brain mechanisms including the anterior cingulate cortex, anterior insula, orbitofrontal cortex, and thalamus [71]. More research about the connection between mindfulness and brain areas is needed to further support these claims and learn more about psychophysical pain.

Comprehensive pain rehabilitation programs are used to help patients experiencing chronic pain through the utilization of various types of therapeutic techniques, and some of the same ideas could be applied to trauma patients post-discharge. A study was conducted at Mayo Clinic examining the relationship between pain catastrophizing and pain treatment outcomes in an intensive outpatient comprehensive pain rehabilitation program [72]. Questionnaires were given to the patients at admission and discharge from the program, which met for 8 hours a day, 5 days a week. These questionnaires were analyzed and revealed that pain catastrophizing was positively correlated with adverse functioning factors such as depressed mood, decreased quality of life, life interference, and higher pain severity. A significant relationship was found between program participation and decreased pain catastrophizing. This study, while supporting comprehensive pain rehabilitation improving pain catastrophizing, had some limitations such as the inability to isolate the portions of the program (CBT, education, self-management, mood management, relaxation training, occupational therapy, and physical therapy) to see which, if any, had the greatest effect on mitigating catastrophizing. Additionally, there was no long-term assessment beyond the completion of the program to determine the lasting effects of pain rehabilitation.

The legalization of medical marijuana offers a potential substitution for opioids in pain management settings [73]. Due to limited research on marijuana, as it is classified as a schedule 1 drug, the evidence base is sparse and focuses primarily on the relationship between cancer pain and marijuana use where pain relief is supported. A number of policy studies have also been released recently that suggest medical marijuana policies may be associated with a reduction in opioid overdoses (ref, ref). However, the causal pathway for this effect is unclear as of yet and may be simply the result of confounding. Cannabinoids could have an opioid-sparing effect by offering pain relief, either on their own or in combination with COX-2 inhibitors, but more research needs to be done in additional populations, such as orthopedic trauma, to more accurately assess the analgesic properties of medical marijuana [74].

Kratom is a controversial drug that comes from a tree native to Southeast Asia and has been marketed as an herbal remedy for diarrhea, pain, hypertension, and cough; it has also been used for chronic pain treatment and to aid in opioid withdrawal symptoms although no research has been done on its pharmacological effects [75]. Currently, kratom is not an illegal drug in the USA, but other countries, including Australia, have regulated it. Kratom works to alleviate pain by binding to opioid receptors, which is why it is popular for treating opioid withdrawal since it mimics opiate effects and why there is concern about its use [76]. There is a lot of discussion by the FDA and the NIDA about kratom's potential for abuse and addiction, but more research on the pharmacokinetics of the substance is needed before any claims can be made [77].

Comprehensive interdisciplinary pain care offers a promise of better pain management treatment for patients across the board but especially those suffering from traumatic orthopedic injuries. In order to better understand alternative pain management methods and their interactions with traditional treatments, more research needs to be done on various populations to build the evidence base and increase knowledge.

Conclusion

The opioid epidemic plagues the USA, where overdoses increased to 30% between July 2016 and September 2017 in 45 states [78]. In order to effectively manage pain while reducing the use of opioids, alternative methods should be looked to as treatment options, and in order for them to be viable treatment options, more research and thus more funding are needed to build the evidence base. The Orthopaedic Trauma Association Musculoskeletal Pain Task Force recently published its "Clinical Practice Guidelines for Pain Management in Acute Musculoskeletal Injury." The group endorsed a number of the practices described above, including (1) judicious use of opioids, (2) the use of multimodal analgesia, (3) regional anesthesia, (4) psychosocial and anxiety reduction interventions, and (4) physical strategies (ice, elevation, and transcutaneous electrical stimulation) (ref JOT).

References

1. Clark ME, Bair MJ, Buckenmajer CC 3rd, Gironda RJ, Walker RL. Pain and combat injuries in soldiers returning from Operations Enduring Freedom and Iraqi Freedom: implications for research and practice. J Rehabil Res Dev. 2007;44(2):179–94.
2. Norman SB, Stein MB, Dimsdale JE, Hoyt DB. Pain in the aftermath of trauma is a risk factor for post-traumatic stress disorder. Psychol Med. 2008;38(4):533–42.
3. Bosse MJ, MacKenzie EJ, Kellam JF, Burgess AR, Webb LX, Swiontkowski MF, Sanders RW, Jones AL, McAndrew MP, Patterson BM, McCarthy ML, Travison TG, Castillo RC. An analysis of outcomes of reconstruction or amputation after leg-threatening injuries. N Engl J Med. 2002;347(24):1924–31.
4. O'Toole RV, Castillo RC, Pollak AN, MacKenzie EJ, Bosse MJ, LEAP Study Group. Determinants of patient satisfaction after severe lower-extremity injuries. J Bone Joint Surg Am. 2008;90(6):1206–11.
5. Castillo RC, MacKenzie EJ, Webb LX, Bosse M, Avery J, LEAP Study Group. Use and perceived need of physical therapy following severe lower-extremity trauma. Arch Phys Med Rehabil. 2005;86(9):1722–8.
6. Sherwood GD, McNeill JA, Starck PL, Disnard G. Changing acute pain management outcomes in surgical patients. AORN J. 2003;77(2):374. 377-380, 384-390
7. Warfield CA, Kahn CH. Acute pain management. Programs in U.S. hospitals and experiences and attitudes among U.S. adults. Anesthesiology. 1995;83(5):1090–4.
8. Apfelbaum JL, Chen C, Mehta SS, Gan TJ. Postoperative pain experience: results from a national survey suggest postoperative pain continues to be undermanaged. Anesth Analg. 2003;97(2):534–40.
9. Pavlin DJ, Chen C, Penaloza DA, Polissar NL, Buckley FP. Pain as a factor complicating recovery and discharge after ambulatory surgery. Anesth Analg. 2002;95(3):627–34.
10. Tang R, Evans H, Chaput A, Kim C. Multimodal analgesia for hip arthroplasty. Orthop Clin North Am. 2009;40(3):377–87.
11. Gottschalk A, Raja SN. Severing the link between acute and chronic pain: the anesthesiologist's role in preventive medicine. Anesthesiology. 2004;101(5):1063–5.
12. Kehlet H, Jensen TS, Woolf CJ. Persistent post-surgical pain: risk factors and prevention. Lancet. 2006;367(9522):1618–25.
13. Perkins FM, Kehlet H. Chronic pain as an outcome of surgery. A review of predictive factors. Anesthesiology. 2000;93(4):1123–33.
14. Haythornthwaite JA, Raja SN, Fisher B, Frank SM, Brendler CB, Shir Y. Pain and quality of life following radical retropubic prostatectomy. J Urol. 1998;160(5):1761–4.
15. Bay-Nielsen M, Perkins FM, Kehlet H, Danish Hernia Database. Pain and functional impairment 1 year after inguinal herniorrhaphy: a nationwide questionnaire study. Ann Surg. 2001;233(1):1–7.
16. Ochroch EA, Mardini IA, Gottschalk A. What is the role of NSAIDs in pre-emptive analgesia? Drugs. 2003;63(24):2709–23.
17. Von Korff M, Simon G. The relationship between pain and depression. Br J Psychiatry. 1996;30:101–8.
18. Castillo RC, MacKenzie EJ, Wegener ST, Bosse MJ, LEAP Study Group. Prevalence of chronic pain seven years following limb threatening lower extremity trauma. Pain. 2006;124(3):321–9.
19. Woolf CJ, Salter MW. Neuronal plasticity: increasing the gain in pain. Science. 2000;288(5472):1765–9.
20. Han B, Compton WM, Blanco C, et al. Prescription opioid use, misuse, and use disorders in U.S. adults: 2015 national survey on drug use and health. Ann Intern Med. 2017;167(5):293–301.
21. Srivastava AB, Gold MS. Beyond supply: how we must tackle the opioid epidemic. Mayo Clin Proc. 2018;93(3):269.
22. Spangehl MJ, Clarke HD, Hentz JG, Misra L, Blocher JL, Seamans DP. Periarticular injections and femoral & sciatic blocks provide similar pain relief after TKA:

Salvage v Amputation: Lower Extremity and Upper Extremity

Michael J. Bosse and Chris Langhammer

Lower Extremity

Advances in the treatment of extremity trauma have significantly improved the orthopedic surgeon's ability to salvage the high-energy lower extremity trauma (HELET) injuries (Fig. 15.1a, b). The recognition of the need for aggressive and repeated zone-of-injury debridement and immediate fracture stabilization by tissue-friendly techniques coupled with the introduction of third-generation antibiotics advanced bone defect reconstruction options, and the development and reliability of microsurgical free tissue transfers have made limb salvage "feasible" in the majority of HELET cases. At present, and perhaps unfortunately, it appears that we are approaching a point where the only absolute contraindication to limb salvage in a candidate limb might be the inability to obtain or maintain limb perfusion. Continued comparative outcomes research is required to refresh the treatment recommendations as new treatment strategies are introduced.

There are specific patient conditions that require treatment decisions outside of the typical isolated HELET injury in a healthy patient. Trauma patients in extremis, in multiple organ failure or with severe head trauma or complete spinal cord injuries, are typically not candidates for aggressive limb salvage. On the contrary, morbidly obese patients who will be unable to fit a prosthesis or patients without access to lifelong prosthetics are typically not good candidates for amputation, if limb salvage is a possibility.

Prior to 2002, most evidence related to treatment decision-making and outcomes from the care of HELET injuries was anecdotal or based on small retrospective series without modern patient-reported outcome assessments. The amputation treatment decisions were often influenced by senior surgeon practice bias, by unvalidated "limb salvage scores" and by the belief that the absence of plantar sensation favored amputation. Limb salvage was selected when the injury and the patient were agreeable to the application of the advanced surgical techniques. Limbs that were once amputated became candidates for complex and prolonged limb reconstruction pathways as surgical techniques evolved. As the limb salvage experience enlarged and disappointing long-term results mounted, a debate began related to "the feasibility versus the advisability" of limb salvage for some of the HELET injuries. Parallel improvement in lower extremity prosthetics – low weight, improved socket fit and comfort, and energy return components – raised the speculation that the amputee was "enabled" and could

M. J. Bosse
Atrium Health – Carolinas Medical Center,
Charlotte, NC, USA
e-mail: Michael.Bosse@atriumhealth.org

C. Langhammer (✉)
University of Maryland, Department of Orthopaedics,
Baltimore, MD, USA
e-mail: clanghammer@som.umaryland.edu

© Springer Nature Switzerland AG 2021
R. A. Pensy, J. V. Ingari (eds.), *The Mangled Extremity*, https://doi.org/10.1007/978-3-319-56648-1_15

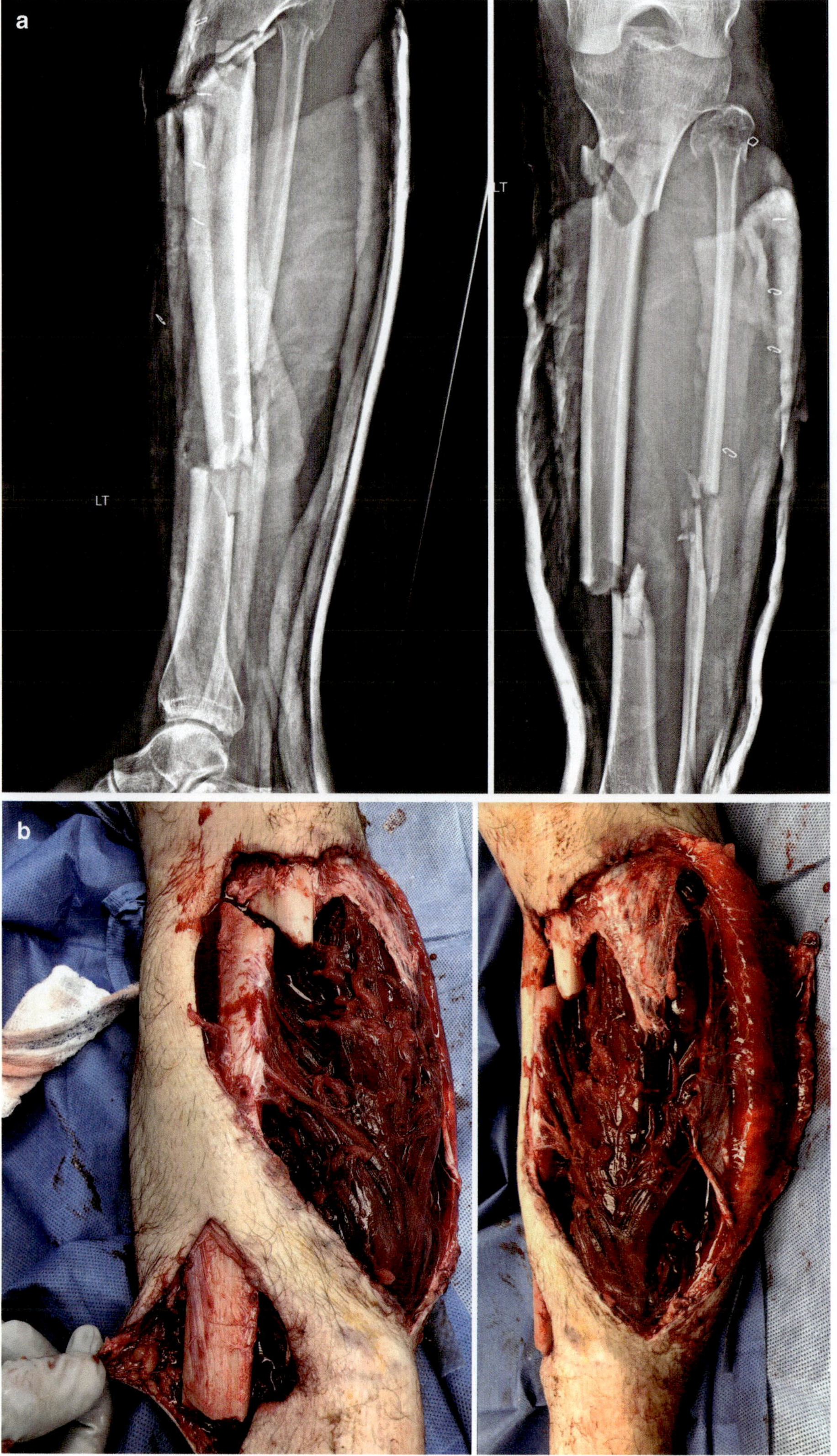

Fig. 15.1 (**a**) Is the initial radiograph and (**b**) the presenting soft tissue injury appearance of a type IIIB segmental tibia fracture associated with significant degloving, muscle crush, and heavy environmental contamination

have an outcome better than those possible with a heroic limb salvage effort. The concern that the aggressive placement of patients with HELET injuries into the limb salvage pathway because of the enhanced feasibility of salvage was possibly detrimental to the long-term outcome of the patient compared to those treated with early amputation prompted the development of the "Lower Extremity Assessment Project" (*LEAP*) in the early 1990s [1].

The *LEAP* study was a multicenter, prospective, longitudinal observational study of 569 patients with severe HELET injuries distal to the femur. The study incorporated modern validated patient-reported functional outcomes as well as basic physical performance and return-to-work assessments and hypothesized that after adjustment for injury and patient and environmental characteristics, those patients treated with early amputations would have better outcomes than those patients treated by limb reconstruction. The study was designed to capture detailed injury, treatment, patient, and environmental factors that might impact the final patient outcome and also captured the discreet factors that influenced the patient's and surgeon's decision to select either limb salvage or amputation.

LEAP Study: Results

Contrary to the study hypothesis, *LEAP* found that at 2 and 7 years, patients with limb reconstruction had outcomes that were equivalent to those who underwent amputation. Both groups were disabled – 40% of the patients severely. Only half of the patients in each group returned to work. Both cohorts demonstrated long-term psychosocial dysfunction (42%) that was likely related to unrecognized and untreated PTSD [2].

The functional outcomes of the selected HELET injuries were not affected by the severity of the fracture and/or soft tissue injury or the presence of associated injuries. The factors that were found to be predictors of poor outcome, regardless of the treatment provided, are listed in Table 15.1. The study concluded that *patients with HELET injuries at high risk for amputation*

Table 15.1 Factors associated with poor outcome

Rehospitalization for a major complication
Having less than a high school education
Having a household income less than the federal poverty level
Being non-white
Having no insurance or having Medicaid
Having a poor social support network
Having a low level of self-efficacy
Smoking
Involving the legal system for injury compensation

could be advised that reconstruction typically results in outcomes equivalent to those of amputation. The reconstruction effort was associated with a higher risk of complications, additional surgeries, and rehospitalizations [3]. At 2 years, however, the cost of care for the amputee was much higher than the cost of care for the reconstruction patient, driven by the expense of the prosthetics. The projected lifetime cost for the amputation patient was three times higher than for the limb reconstruction patient [4]. Busse et al. reported a meta-analysis of HELET limb salvage vs. early amputation observational studies in 2007 and emphasized that research was needed to optimize early limb triage decisions to avoid failed limb salvage [5].

In efforts to direct the limb salvage vs. amputation decision in patients with HELET injuries, multiple groups worked to produce injury scoring systems – the "limb salvage scores." These scores stratified the severity of injury in the tissue and patient domains thought to influence limb outcome. The Mangled Extremity Salvage Score (MESS) was employed in the USA after its introduction in 1990 [6]. The MESS provided numerical scores for the degree of injury in two extremity injury domains – skeletal/soft tissue injury and limb ischemia – and in two physiology domains, shock and patient age (Table 15.2). The threshold score for amputation was 7 points. The selected scoring domains appear arbitrary and do not correlate with patient reserve or physiology. What was the difference between the 29 year old (*0 points*) or the 31 yo (*1 points*)? Similarly, a systolic blood pressure transiently

Table 15.2 Extremity injury scoring systems

	HFS – 1982	MESI – 1985	PSI – 1987	MESS – 1990	LSI – 1991	NISSA – 1994	GHOISS – 2006	OTA-OFC – 2010
Demographic		40–50 – 1 50–60 – 2 60–70 – 3 Comorbidities – 1 Shock – 2		<30 – 0 <50 – 1 >50 – 2		<30 – 0 <50 – 1 >50 – 2	>65 – 2	
Systemic (shock)		ISS 0–25 – 1 ISS 25–50 – 2 ISS >50 – 3		Normotensive – 0 Responsive – 1 Prolonged – 2		Normotensive – 0 Responsive – 1 Prolonged- 2	ISS >25 – 2 Shock on presentation – 2	
Timing	<6 – 0 <12 – 1 >12 – 3	+1 for each hour >6	<6 – 1 <12 – 2 >12 – 3	<6 – 0 >6 – 2	<6 – 0 <9 – 1 <12 – 2 <15 – 3 >15 – 4	<6 – 0 >6 – 2	Injury to debridement >12H – 2	
Contamination/other	None – 0 Single foreign body – 1 Multiple foreign bodies – 1 Massive contamination – 10 Single bacteria – 2 Polymicrobial – 3 Mixed flora – 4 Amputation – 20 Crush – 30						Farm/industrial contamination – 2	Superficial contamination – 2 Imbedded/high risk contamination – 3
Bone	Type A – 1 Type B – 2 Type C – 3 Bone loss <2cm – 1 Bone loss >2cm – 2	Simple – 1 segmental – 2 Comminuted – 3 Bone loss >6 cm – 4 Intraarticular – 5 Intraarticular bone loss – 6	Mild – 1 Moderate – 2 Severe – 3	Low – 1 Medium – 2 High – 3 Extreme – 4	closed or Gustilo 1 – 0 Gustilo 2 – 1 Gustilo 3 – 2	Low energy (spiral/oblique) – 1 Medium (transverse) – 2 High (comminution) – 3 Extreme (segmental) – 4	Simple – 1 Butterfly – 2 segmental/comminuted – 3 Bone loss < 4cm – 4 Bone loss > 4cm – 5	No bone loss – 1 Partial bone loss – 2 Segmental bone loss – 3

	HFS – 1982	MESI – 1985	PSI – 1987	MESS – 1990	LSI – 1991	NISSA – 1994	GHOISS – 2006	OTA-OFC – 2010
Skin	None – 0 <1/4 circumference – 1 >3/4 – 4 <1/2 – 2 <3/4 – 3	Sharp laceration – 1 Crush/burn – 2 Avulsion – 3			Primary repair – 0 Secondary closure – 1	Gustilo 1 – 0 Gustilo 2 – 1 Gustilo 3A – 2 Gustilo 3B – 3	No skin loss – 1 No skin loss + exposed fracture – 2 Skin loss – 3 Skin loss over fracture – 4	Can approximate – 1 Cannot approximate – 2 Extensive degloving – 3
Muscle	None – 0 <1/4 circumference – 1 >3/4 – 4 <1/2 – 2 <3/4 – 3		Mild – 1 Moderate – 2 Severe – 3		Single compartment – 0 Multiple compartments – 1 Crush – 2		Partial injury – 1 Reparable injury – 2 Irreparable/partial compartment – 3 Irreparable/full compartment – 4 Loss of 2+compartments – 5	Minimal injury with intact function – 1 Partial loss with intact muscle-tendon unit – 2 Necrosis/disruption of muscle-tendon unit – 3
Nerve	Useful sensation (plantar/palmer) – 0 No sensation (plantar/palmar) – 8 Yes finger/toe motion – 0 No finger/toe motion – 8	Contusion – 1 Transection – 2 Avulsion – 3			In continuity – 0 Transection of some major nerves – 1 Transection of all major nerves – 2	Sensate – 1 Minor distribution insensate – 2 Major distribution insensate – 3 All distributions insensate – 4		
Vessel	None – 0 Incomplete – 10 Complete <4 hr – 15 >4 hr – 20 >8 – 25	Vein only – 1 Transection – 1 Thrombosis – 2 Avulsion – 3	Suprapop – 1 Pop – 2 Infrapop – 3	Normal – 0 Mild (diminished pulses) – 1 Moderate (ischemic changes/paresthesias) – 2 Severe (cold/numb) – 3	Contusion – 0 Pulseless (multiple vessels) – 1 No run-off (all vessels) – 2 (+1 if no veinous return)	No change – 0 Diminished pulses – 1 Pulses by Doppler – 2 Pulseless/cold – 3		No injury – 1 Arterial injury without ischemia – 2 Arterial injury with ischemia – 3
Amputation threshold	≥11	≥20	≥8	≥7	≥6	≥11	≥14	≥10

below 90 mm Hg blood pressure *wins a point.* A hypothetical 51 yo (*2 points*) with a contaminated type IIIA open tibia fracture (*4 points*) associated with reduced pulses but normal perfusion (*1 point*) and a transient systolic pressures <90 mm Hg (*1 point*) totals 8 points and is above the MESS amputation threshold! These injuries are rarely, if ever, amputated.

The LEAP study design embedded all of the components of five limb salvage scores into the initial patient data capture. Analysis of the limb salvage scores failed to validate the clinical utility of any of the lower extremity limb salvage scores as their low sensitivity did not support the score's employment as predictors of amputation [7]. A recent vascular injury study validated the LEAP findings [8]. An analysis of the ability of limb salvage scores to predict the functional outcome of the salvaged limb found that the scores did not identify the final outcome of the salvaged patient [9].

The absence of plantar sensation was once used as a critical factor to decide on amputation and was included as a key component of many of the limb salvage scores. Swiontkowski et al. examined the factors that influenced the decision to amputate or reconstruct the HELET patients in the LEAP study and found that the severity of the soft tissue injury and the *absence of plantar sensation* were critical factors driving the decision [10]. The LEAP study found that absent plantar sensation at the time of patient presentation did not adversely impact the outcome of those patients treated with limb salvage and advised that plantar sensation should not be a component of the limb salvage decision assessment [11]. Over half of the patients who presented with absent plantar regained sensation by two years. Orthopedic surgeons treat many other conditions that result in loss of plantar sensation – complete and incomplete spinal cord injuries and peripheral neuropathies as examples. Barring major complications from foot ulcerations and infection, leg amputation is not a go-to treatment in these conditions. It made little sense that a HELET injury with absent plantar sensation would be treated differently.

Interpreting the LEAP Results and "What LEAP Didn't Say"

As a prospective randomized trial was considered to be unethical, LEAP was designed as a longitudinal observational study. Experienced orthopedic trauma surgeons at high-volume academic level 1 trauma centers employed contemporary decision-making strategies – including limb salvage scores, the absence of plantar sensation, and their personal gestalt/common sense as to the expected eventual treatment of the extremity if treated by limb salvage – and their surgical skill set, to balance the feasibility v advisability equation. *At the time of the LEAP study patient enrollment, surgeons typically advised for amputation if they were concerned that the reconstruction effort would be too risky or would result in an outcome worse than a transtibial amputation.*

The results of the LEAP study, unfortunately, were stated without sufficient qualification. While the LEAP conclusion that "patients with limbs at high risk for amputation can be advised that reconstruction typically results in two-year outcomes equivalent to those of amputation" is true, it required better context. It was never implied that all HELET injuries should undergo reconstruction if salvage was possible. A better stated conclusion might have been *that patients with severe HELET that were capable of limb salvage (it's feasible) and had anticipated functional level at or better than a transtibial amputation (it's likely advisable) should be advised to pursue limb reconstruction.*

LEAP Observations and "Lessons Learned"

There were significant observations and lessons learned from the design, conduct, and analysis of the LEAP study. While the study did capture the design and cost of the prosthetics provided to the amputation patients, it recognized that amputation outcomes were likely influenced by factors associated with device alignment, fit, and comfort. At present, there are no standardized "best practice windows" to capture or account for these critical prosthetic cofactors. Current efforts are underway to standardize the evaluation of fit, alignment, and comfort of the prosthesis in an attempt to better understand the impact on functional outcomes related to the amputation. Is the functional and performance outcome from an amputation the result of the stress of the amputation and the residual limb limitations, or is the amputation outcome further downgraded by a tissue-prosthetic interface mismatch? Poor outcomes related to the prosthesis need to be accounted for to better understand extremity trauma limb salvage vs. amputation research and to identify critical prosthetic-related factors that can be modified.

Research comparing the outcomes of HELET patients is still hampered by an injury classification technique that is too encompassing. Figure 15.2a, b demonstrates the difficulties when the Gustilo/Anderson fracture grading scheme is employed to drive patient selection and to stratify for the analysis of results. Both patients are classified as type IIIB injuries. Patient 2B has significant soft tissue loss including skin and volumetric muscle loss, segmental bone loss, and heavy wound contamination. Patient 2A has a small pretibial defect at the fracture site that requires a local tissue transfer and has no bone loss, minimal contamination, and no major muscle damage. *Both patients are type IIIB!* Patient 2B is clearly more severely injured and at higher risk for injection, nonunion, and possible amputation.

The AO/OTA fracture classification is well validated and routinely used to identify the critical differences in bone segment injury patterns. The LEAP investigators included all of the critical extremity injury elements into their data collection strategy but recognized the clear need for a unified open fracture soft tissue injury classification that could better stratify the critical components of the associated soft tissue injury. The LEAP investigators requested that the OTA consider assigning a task group to study and resolve the classification deficiency. The OTA Open Fracture classification was published in 2010. The new classification system was designed to address two critical needs – provide better stratification of extremity injury severity and to optimize communication for both clinical care and research [12]. The Major Extremity Trauma and Rehabilitation Research Consortium (metrc.org) has included the OTA-OFC in all of their open fracture studies.

Another critical lesson learned from the LEAP study was the importance of including the high-end performance test into the final outcomes assessment. The LEAP study used the self-selected walking speed as the major performance outcome discriminator. In the final analysis, LEAP recognized that a battery of tests was probably required in order to assess both high-end and

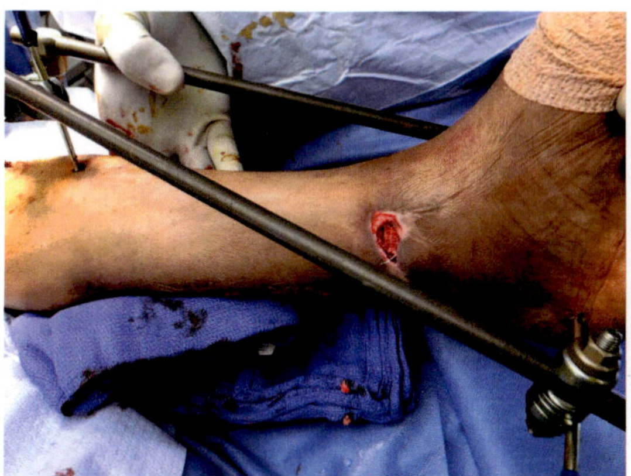

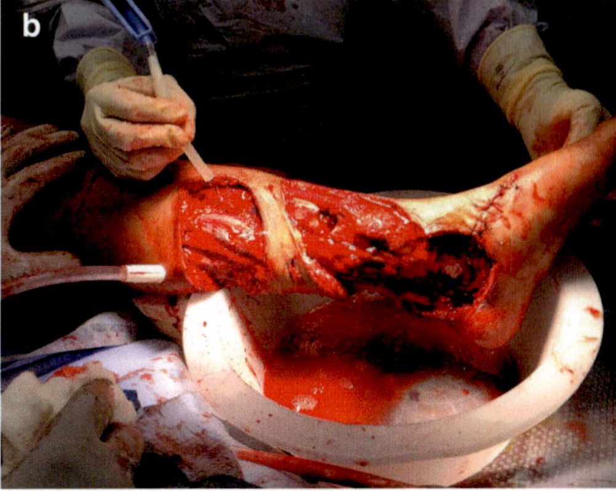

Fig. 15.2 (**a**) Patient with a type IIIB injury needing small tissue coverage and associated with minimal bone and muscle loss. (**b**) Represents the other extreme of the type IIIB spectrum with significant bone and muscle loss and heavy wound contamination

Table 15.3 HELET performance test battery

Agility	Four square step test
	Illinois agility test
Strength/power	Sit to stand
	Timed stair ascent
Speed	Self-selected walking speed
	10 meter shuttle run
Postural stability	Single leg stance test

low-end functions following HELET in order to identify patients that managed only ADLs from those engaged in vigorous activities. In current METRC studies, a patient's physical performance and overall activity are objectively evaluated for agility, strength/power, speed, and postural stability [13] (Table 15.3). The battery of test were selected by an expert panel of physical therapists and orthopedic surgeons with the requirement that the tests had to be able to be conducted in a typical outpatient office setting.

The final most important lesson from the LEAP study was that resources and research were needed to focus on factors that impact the outcomes that are modifiable. Surgeons can work to minimize major complications (infection and nonunions as examples) and engage the patient in smoking cessation programs. The identification and treatment of the modifiable psychosocial recovering stressors (PTSD and low self-efficacy) are resource-intensive, and access varies by community and patient's insurance coverage.

The "LEAP Effect"

Prior to the publication of the LEAP study in 2002, single or combined factors including surgeon experience and training, site bias, plantar sensation, limb salvage scores, severity of the soft tissue injury, and patient cofactors and demands served as the drivers of the treatment salvage – amputation decision. No credible EBM was available to provide direction based on treatment outcomes. With the publication of the LEAP results, for the first time, surgeons were able to employ the findings of a large prospective multicenter outcomes study as a basis for the formulation of a treatment strategy and "inform-

ing the patient." *Unfortunately, many surgeons interpreted the LEAP findings that there was no difference in the outcomes of patients treated by amputation or limb salvage as a blanket endorsement that if feasible, limb salvage should be pursued.* Failure to acknowledge the context of the study and recognize that experienced surgeons at high-volume level 1 trauma centers were making the treatment decision during the study recruitment based on the factors mentioned above possibly resulted in more heroic efforts to retain severely mangled extremities and create a new cycle of decision-making challenges (Fig. 15.1). Employing the results of the LEAP study out of proper context when engaging the patient in a "shared-decision-making" discussion could provide the patient with assurance that salvage of a hopelessly injured extremity will provide them with an outcome comparable to amputation (Fig. 15.3). This, simply, is not true.

Better stated, the LEAP conclusion should be that when limb salvage is considered in cases where the expected functional outcomes are expected to be no worse than a best level amputation, then limb salvage pursuit is advisable.

HELET Studies Following LEAP

Casualty care from the Global War on Terrorism (GWOT) challenged the surgical team's limb salvage selection and advanced limb reconstruction capability. The DoD orthopedic teams provided exceptional injury documentation and outcomes data that focused on the gaps in our current care strategies and highlighted the possible misinterpretation of the LEAP paper results. The METALS study was published in 2013 [14]. It was a retrospective study of 324 combat injured service members with lower extremity trauma requiring either amputation or complex reconstruction procedures. After adjusting for many covariates, the amputees had better SMFA scores in all domains compared to the reconstruction patients. The results of the study need to be interpreted with some caution, however. This was a retrospective study with a 59% response rate. The

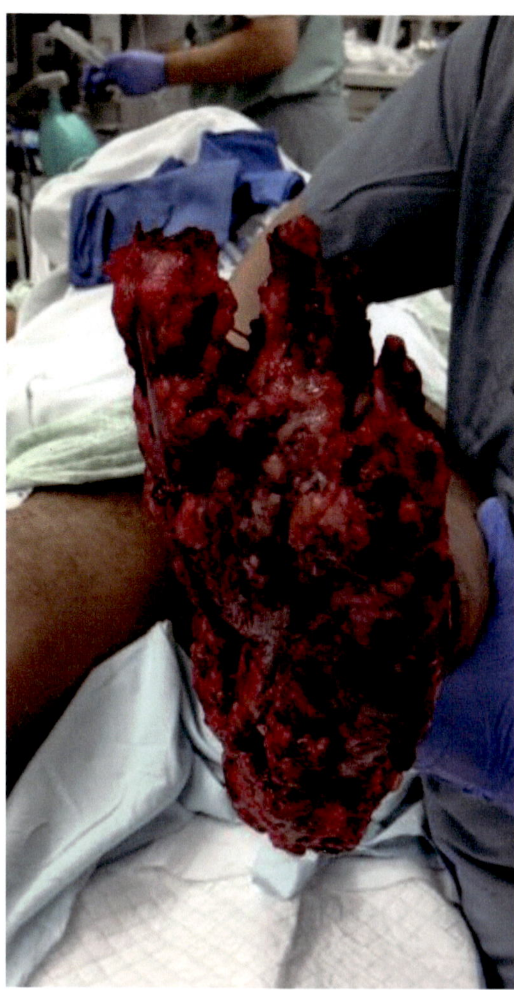

Fig. 15.3 This is a clinical photo of an example patient who was not included in the LEAP salvage cohort. This more recent patient "selected limb salvage." The foot, from the ankle to the toes, is completely degloved

injury mechanism (typically blast) was much different than in the LEAP study, and the patients were younger, fitter, and with access to better post-injury resources. The amputees had access to the best prosthetics available and received significantly more rehabilitation than the limb salvage cohort. Of note, almost half of the patient had injuries to the distal tibia, ankle, and/or foot, as might be expected from a dismounted battle injury/IED blast. Was the improvement found in the amputee cohort related to a change in care or related to the employment of the findings of the

LEAP study that might have encouraged a more heroic approach to the salvage of the extremities in the HELET patients?

In an attempt to provide clarity to the foot and ankle injuries, a subgroup of 174 patients with severe foot trauma included in the LEAP study were separately evaluated in an effort to determine the impact of a mangled foot and ankle on patient outcomes. The study found that patients with severe injuries to the foot and ankle who required free tissue transfers for wound coverage and/or ankle arthrodesis were significantly worse than those with transtibial amputations. The data suggested that additional research was needed to clarify the regional injury impact of severe soft tissue and ankle trauma [15].

Results from the care of military patients with severe distal tibia and foot and ankle trauma were reported at the same time from multiple centers, all suggesting that, perhaps, the limb salvage effort in many patients was too aggressive.

Dickens et al. reported on 89 patients with 102 open calcaneus fractures. Forty-three limbs (42%) were amputated (35% delayed) [16]. A blast injury, plantar wound location, large wounds, and high-grade fractures were predictive of eventual amputation. Amputation patients exhibited improved pain and activity levels compared to those still in the salvage cohort. The UK military reported their outcomes on 114 patients (134 fractures) with severe hindfoot injuries. At 5 years, they found that the patients with hindfoot reconstructions had outcomes that were inferior to patients treated with a delayed amputation [17]. Ramasamy et al. reported on patient with IED foot and ankle blast injuries and reported similar poor outcomes [18]. Penn-Barwell et al. challenged surgeons with the "could" and the "should" of reconstructing severe hindfoot injuries [19].

The US Department of Defense, recognizing the need for large prospective clinical studies to help guide development of or refine future extremity trauma care, funded the Major Extremity Trauma Research Consortium (metrc. org) in 2009. One of METRC's major studies is focused on the injuries to the distal tibia and

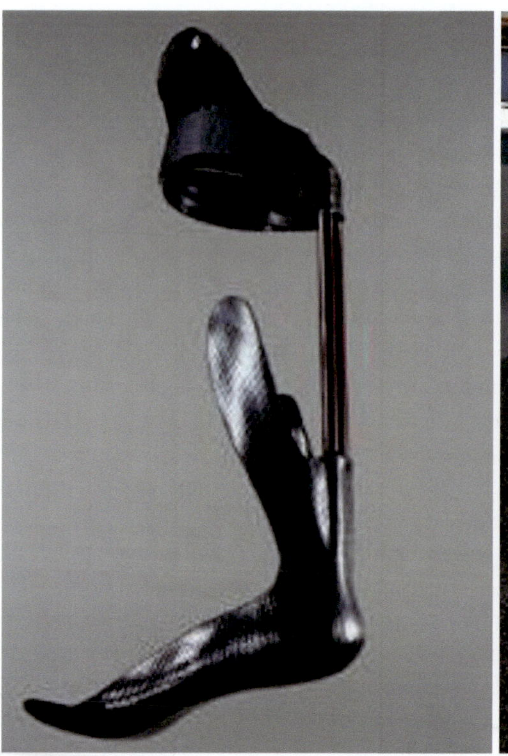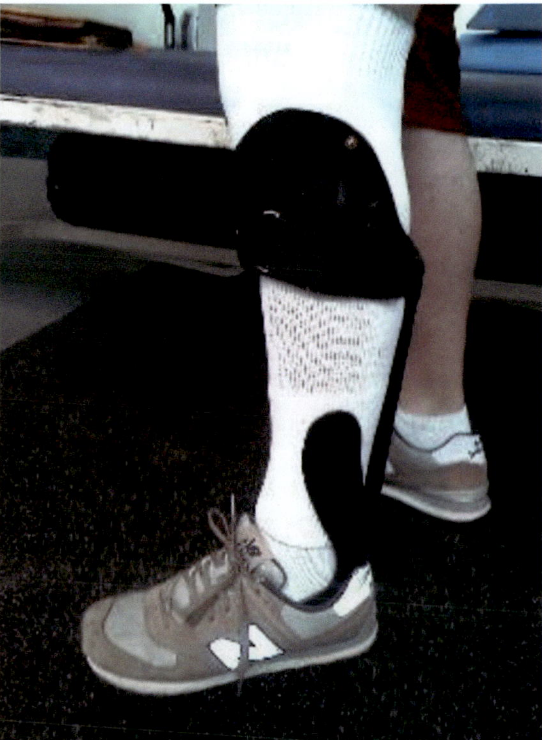

Fig. 15.4 IDEO brace

hindfoot in an attempt to provide better data to assist the surgical team and the patient with complex treatment decisions [13]. The Short Form Musculoskeletal Assessment (SMFA) tool was used to assess functional outcomes of the limb salvage and the amputation patients at 18 months. Data from this study was published in 2020.

Adjunctive Therapy to Improve Outcomes of the Limb Salvage Patient

Limb salvage patients are challenged with friable tissue coverage at the foot and ankle, volumetric muscle loss, nerve injury, ankle arthrodesis, or post-traumatic arthritis. Many are provided with standard foot orthotics or ankle-foot orthosis. The need to couple the technology of the modern amputation prosthesis with the bracing needs of the limb salvage patient has been recognized [20, 21]. The Center for the Intrepid at Brooke Army Medical Center developed a custom dynamic off-loading carbon fiber ankle-foot orthosis (IDEO) specifically for the extremity trauma patient (Fig. 15.4). The bracing was coupled with an intense run-focused rehabilitation program. Results have demonstrated device satisfaction and improved function [22].

Ongoing Challenges

The care of patients with HELET injuries continues to challenge the surgical and rehabilitation teams. Long-term success appears to be coupled to the initial triage of the patient to a limb salvage or an amputation pathway. It is critical to refine the "contraindications" for limb salvage and to develop schemes that can appropriately educate the patient to the point where their participation in a shared decision-making intervention moves beyond the "doc, just save my leg" response. What should we tell a patient or do for a patient with the injury shown in Fig. 15.3?

In cases where I truly have equipoise related to the outcome and feel comfortable offering either reconstruction or amputation based on patients' needs and expectations, I engage the plastic surgeons, rehabilitation team, prosthetist, and amputation and salvage peer counselors to provide insight and education that informs the patients' treatment selection. In cases where I do not think that the reconstruction outcome will be at least as good as a best level amputation, I still employ the approach that I used during the LEAP study recruitment – I give my opinion and request that the patient strongly consider an amputation and I often suggest that the patient obtain a second opinion. I also engage my rehabilitation and peer amputation counselors, the true "shared decision-making" process emphasized in elective medical care might not be the best approach in the care of a trauma patient. Additional work is required to refine our patient engagement process.

The care of the HELET and the limb salvage decision-making remains dynamic. Better guidance is needed for the care of the severe foot and ankle injuries. The development of the IDEO-brace might be the signature orthopedic contribution to patient care that resulted from the GWOT and the long-term outcomes game changer for patients with residual lower extremity deficits after limb salvage care. This technology needs to be rapidly transferred to the civilian trauma patients and subjected to prospective comparative effectiveness research to clearly define the clinical impact.

Upper Extremity

Regrettably, less concrete progress has been made in providing guidance regarding early amputation versus limb salvage in the upper extremity than in the lower extremity. The reasons are in large part driven by the difference in incidence of these injury types, HELET injuries occurring with greater frequency than mutilating upper extremity injuries. Recent studies of a US civilian population using the National Trauma Data Bank have demonstrated that only 18% of major limb amputations occur in the upper extremity (~180 lower extremity vs. ~40 upper extremity per 100,000 trauma admissions) [23, 24], while recent military data indicates a similar figure of 14% [25]. Because of this sixfold increase in incidence, analysis of the injury patterns driving lower extremity amputation has largely informed the development and characterization of the most commonly used limb injury grading systems. The availability of HELET patients for study and the improved characterization of their injuries have facilitated the completion of gold-standard prospective longitudinal observational studies such as LEAP and METALS that direct treatment decisions, while no upper extremity analog exists.

Upper Extremity Injury Classification

Historically, limb salvage treatment decision-making has been clouded by difficulty in classifying injury patterns in a way that is prognostically meaningful. A variety of injury severity scores have been devised including the HFS [26], MESI [27], PSI [28], AO [29], MESS [30], LSI [31], NISSA [32], GHOISS [33], and OTA-OFC [34] and were described briefly in Table 15.2, and references have been provided should you wish to learn more about the development of each score. In-depth review of each scale is available [35, 36] but is outside the scope of this chapter.

A critical barrier to the application of these scoring systems to the upper extremity is that they were developed and validated on data sets primarily consisting of lower extremity injuries. The upper extremity tolerates reconstruction better than the lower extremity for a variety of physiologic reasons primarily driven by the improved recoverability of soft tissue injuries and lower incidence of infection. As a result, scoring thresholds developed from mixed data sets and lower extremity data sets generalize poorly to the upper extremity. Additionally, many of the scoring systems were developed between 20 and 30 years ago, and advances in trauma care and reconstructive techniques have changed what is considered a salvageable injury [37].

For example, early assessment demonstrated utility of the MESS (the most widely characterized scoring system) score in predicting successful limb salvage in both upper and lower extremities [38, 39]. However, in much the same way that subsequent testing over the LEAP data set demonstrated specificity and sensitivity for these scores that was felt to be unacceptably low [40], more recent re-examination of the MESS on upper extremity limb salvage populations has shown that limbs with scores over the recommended injury threshold are now routinely salvaged [41–46]. This has generated skepticism regarding the use of quantitative scores in predicting upper extremity amputation.

Finally, it is important to consider the method by which these scores were developed, which was through retrospective chart review using the ultimate performance of an amputation as the clinical endpoint. The architecture of these scores is, therefore, designed to answer the question "which of these extremities *received* an amputation?" When applied prospectively to a group of patients, this means they answer the question "which of these extremities *will* receive an amputation?" As the development of these scores did not incorporate cost or outcomes measures, it is important to re-emphasize that none of them are capable of answering the question "which of these extremities *should* receive an amputation?"

Additional upper extremity-specific literature revolves around "mutilating hand injuries," which include a wide variety of injury patterns to the hand. Systems-based approaches similar to the major limb injury scoring systems, in which the skeletal system, soft tissue, vessels, and nerves are independently considered, have subsequently been developed for the upper extremity and hand specifically. The "tic-tac-toe" injury classification system integrates a systems-based approach with a location-based approach in order to account for the different functions the radial and ulnar column of the hand, or volar and dorsal structures, have on upper extremity function [47]. Special attention should be given to the Hand Injury Severity Scoring System, which also includes consideration of integument, skeletal,

motor, and sensory systems in a location-specific fashion [48], and has been durably shown to correlate with functional outcomes including return to work [49–52]. A subsequent modification of this scale has been developed including injuries of the forearm and wrist [49]. While these upper extremity-specific classification systems have failed to gain clinical traction, they are instructive regarding one of the fundamental differences between the upper and lower extremities which is lost in the application of lower extremity-based injury scales to the upper extremity: *the importance of anatomic location to function.*

Benefits of Salvage over Amputation

Literature informing the "salvage vs. amputation" dialogue in the upper extremity is based on retrospective case series of major upper extremity replants, which necessarily suffer from non-standardized injury descriptions and disproportionally draw from injury patterns at one very extreme end of the spectrum. Historically, this literature has overwhelmingly supported reconstruction (in this case replantation) over amputation. As early as 1980, large case series demonstrated the feasibility of both upper and lower extremity replants after traumatic amputation and endorse a number of very forward-thinking concepts such as the development of regional centers of excellence and that the superiority of replantation in the upper extremity over the lower extremity was due in large part to the poor restorative capacity of upper extremity prostheses relative to lower extremity prostheses [53]. Two decades later in 1998, matched cohorts of replant versus revision amputation/prosthetic users demonstrated the superiority of upper extremity salvage over amputation using quantitative functional outcomes [54]. Another two decades later in 2016, a multi-institution retrospective review demonstrated the superiority of replantation at the forearm level using patient-reported outcomes [55]. These examples have been selected specifically because the outcome instruments evolve from "feasibility," to "functionality," to "preference," mirroring a similar trend in orthopedic literature more globally. A contemporary systematic review of replantation versus prosthetic fitting for major upper extremity injuries fails to draw direct comparisons between the two treatment modalities given the diversity of the outcomes reporting in the literature, but emphasizes the overall high levels of patient satisfaction and good/excellent outcomes following replantation and the persistent barriers to prosthetic usage faced by upper extremity amputees, and that outcomes become worse at more proximal levels of injury for both treatment modalities [56].

However, more recent studies based on the METALS study group have characterized outcomes for mangling injuries to the upper extremity not requiring strict replant relative to amputation in a prospectively collected military cohort. While upper limb amputation is a cause of substantial disability [57], it may coexist with other modifiable psychological factors impeding recovery, and overall disability may not be reduced substantially through limb salvage [58].

Primary and Secondary Costs of Upper Extremity Salvage

The costs of limb salvage attempts may be underappreciated when secondary costs including the emotional drain and time commitment are considered. Secondary procedures in the case of mutilating hand reconstruction are frequent, involving reconstitution of both bony and soft tissue structures, may be delayed for 3–6 months while awaiting soft tissue stability, and may occur serially during a prolonged reconstructive effort [59, 60]. More proximal limb salvage may require delayed reconstruction of even greater magnitude, including free functional muscle transfer, tendon transfers, and nonunion surgeries, burdening patients with risk of late morbidity and requiring dedication of significant time to rehabilitation starting at a time which is likely to be 6 months or more from their initial injury [61]. This recurrent disability occurs at a time when the patient is likely to be readjusting from their initial injury and comes at the expense of other processes associated with returning to normal activity.

Furthermore, in the context of heroic limb salvage attempts, the possible outcomes to be considered must include not only early amputation and successful limb salvage but also late amputation following failed salvage. Secondary upper extremity amputation during the acute hospitalization after at least one surgical salvage attempt may occur in as many as 35% of cases in one recent study [62]. In this study, the patients undergoing early salvage failure demonstrated a trend toward having more extensive injury patterns in younger individuals, for whom salvage was likely attempted despite the high probability of failure due to many of the reasons stated above regarding the superiority of replant. A study in a military population demonstrated the existence of a tail of delayed upper extremity amputation (more than 90 days after injury), which was the case in 3% of their upper extremity amputee population [63].

Considering the toll associated with the sustained efforts associated with limb salvage, new evidence suggests early amputation may be superior to delayed amputation. While a UK military cohort undergoing delayed below-knee amputation for failed limb salvage appreciated functional improvement to a level comparable to an early amputation cohort [64], a similar US military cohort experienced persistently elevated dissatisfaction and disability after a delayed amputation [65]. Similarly, delayed amputation in the upper extremity is not necessarily associated with functional improvement, possibly due to the prolonged period of disability leading up to the amputation [63]. There may, therefore, be a meaningful clinical benefit to the patient to correct and early identification of extremities that will ultimately go on to delayed amputation and counseling patients appropriately.

Value-Based Decision-Making

Clinicians are left to triangulate from imperfect data what treatment is most appropriate for their patient. Considering the question of limb salvage versus early amputation in the light of a "value-based" decision can help provide a meaningful framework for evaluating treatment options as we increasingly appreciate the resource constraints faced by many healthcare systems and the effects of secondary treatment costs on patients and their families. Value is generally described as a measure of the benefit resulting from an intervention relative to the cost of that intervention. The complexity in making this calculation comes from the nuance in how benefit and cost are conceptualized.

The relative certainty with which we recommend upper extremity salvage versus lower extremity salvage is driven by two historical beliefs: (1) the cost of salvage is lower because the physiology of the upper extremity makes salvage attempts more likely to succeed, and (2) the costs of amputation are higher in part due to the inability of prosthetics to adequately supplement upper extremity function. Both of these assumptions are still largely true. The overall success rate of complex upper extremity salvage is traditionally of 80–90% [42, 43, 46, 66], which is noticeably higher than that of lower extremity salvage, and is higher than in the lower extremity when the two are included in the same study [45, 53]. Similarly, the rate of upper extremity prosthetic adoption is only around 50–60% [67–69] in the upper extremity versus 80–90% in the lower extremity [70].

Future Directions

This is a rare injury pattern for which prospective studies will continue to be exceptionally challenging. Meaningful advances in our understanding of limb-threatening upper extremity injuries can still be made in helping patients and physicians conceptualize the expected return on the investment they are about to make in a limb salvage attempt. Clarifying the value in limb salvage will mean (1) improving our understanding of the outcomes of limb salvage to the society and to the patient, (2) improving our understanding of the costs to the healthcare system associated with administering this care, and (3)

developing techniques to supplement the rich set of tools already available to help patients with limb-threatening injuries or with amputations of the upper extremity.

Exploring Costs and Benefits

Ongoing adoption of patient-centered instruments in outcomes research will continue to help physicians identify the priorities of patients. Historically, orthopedic research has focused on feasibility and functionality of an intervention, and only within the last decade has the focus shifted to include the patient experience, and we are still working as a community to develop guidelines regarding their use [71–73]. The development of new patient-centered instruments such as discrete choice experiments is now making it possible to evaluate patient values [74, 75] in the hopes that developing treatment strategies that meet these expectations will result in better outcomes [76, 77]. The incorporation of targeted outcomes instruments specifically designed for upper extremity deficits and amputees into future research will additionally help identify the effects of intervention on long-term function [78, 79].

Examining the systems-level response to these injuries will also continue to be important in designing patient management strategies and developing complimentary infrastructure. Multiple studies have demonstrated differences in treatment modalities for mangling upper extremity injuries based on noninjury-related factors such as geography, treatment environment, and ethnicity [23, 80] and have endorsed the formation of treatment centers of excellence for catastrophic upper extremity injury [81–84]. Similarly, there is a growing appreciation of the multidisciplinary approach required to care for these patients, including what infrastructure may be required to effectively use an "orthoplastics" approach to limb salvage [85, 86] and how this care burden is distributed across multidisciplinary teams [62]. This combined approach as applied in the lower extremity appears to improve surgical care including reducing the duration of disability experienced by patients [87, 88], and may be of even greater advantage in the long-term care of upper extremity injuries, where late functional reconstructions including tendon and nerve transfers are more frequent.

Advancement in Reconstructive Techniques

The ongoing development of extra-anatomic reconstructive techniques will continue to shift practice patterns and improve patient outcomes. Two notable areas of ongoing research are in targeted muscle reinnervation and osseointegration, both of which are technologies for amputees which may change the cost-benefit calculation by improving the outcome of amputation.

TMR is taking residual proximal nerve stumps at an amputation site and performing nerve transfers to residual muscle bellies with no remaining distal insertion. In cases where this is performed to assist with myoelectric prosthesis control, EMG-based signal acquisition from the reinnervated muscles is then used to translate muscle contraction into an electrical signal driving a powered prosthetic device. Recent work has demonstrated the utility of this technique in restoring dexterous volitional motor control over a powered prosthetic device in both proximal [89, 90] and distal [91] injury patters. In other cases, TMR is performed for pain control. In this capacity, it has demonstrated efficacy in reducing phantom limb pain and residual limb pain when performed in a delayed fashion for patients with chronic pain [92] and may be even more effective when performed in the acute setting [93].

Transcutaneous osseointegration is a technique meant to reduce the burden of socket-associated prosthetic wear problems, thereby improving the utility of the prosthetic device. Implants which are anchored in bone extend through the skin and mechanically link with the terminal device, providing a stable transcutaneous connection between the prosthetic device and the skeleton [94, 95]. Through careful surgical technique to create a stable transcutaneous implant, low rates of deep infection [96], and long-term implant survival >80% at 5 years have

been recorded, with notable improvement in patient-reported functional scores relative to preoperative levels [97, 98]. The combination of myoelectric control with transcutaneous osseointegrated implants has demonstrated tremendous restorative potential, restoring volitional motor control, sensation, and overhead range of motion not possible with traditional socket-based prosthetic interfaces [99], but is not available for widespread use.

Bibliography

1. Bosse MJ, MacKenzie EJ, Kellam JF, et al. An analysis of the outcomes of reconstruction or amputation of leg threatening injuries. N Engl J Med. 2002;347(24):1924–31.
2. McCarthy ML, MacKenzie EJ, Edwin D, et al. Psychological distress associated with severe lower-limb injury. J Bone Joint Surg. 2003;85 A(9):1689–97.
3. Harris AM, Althausen PL, Kellam JF, et al. Complications following limb-threatening lower extremity trauma. J Orthop Trauma. 2009;23(1):1–6.
4. MacKenzie EJ, Jones AS, Bosse MJ, et al. Health-care costs associated with amputation or reconstruction of a limb-threatening injury. J Bone Joint Surg. 2007;89 A(8):1685–92.
5. Busse JH, Jacobs CL, Swiontkowski MF, et al. Complex limb salvage or early amputation for severe lower-limb injury: a meta-analysis of observational studies. J Orthop Trauma. 2007;21(1):70–6.
6. Johansen K, Daines M, Howey T, et al. Objective criteria accurately predict amputation following lower extremity trauma. J Trauma. 1990;30:568–73.
7. Bosse MJ, MacKenzie EJ, Kellam JF, et al. A prospective evaluation of the clinical utility of the lower-extremity injury severity scores. J Bone Joint Surg. 2001;83A(1):3–14.
8. Loja MN, Sammann A, DuBose J, et al. The Mangled Extremity Score and amputation: time for a revision. J Trauma Acute Care Surg. 2017;82(3):518–23.
9. Ly TV, Travison TG, Castillo RC, et al. Ability of lower-extremity injury severity scores to predict functional outcome after limb salvage. J Bone Joint Surg. 2008;90 A(8):1738–43.
10. Swiontkowski MF, MacKenzie EJ, Bosse MJ, et al. Factors influencing the DEcision to amputate or reconstruct after high-energy lower extremity trauma. J Trauma. 2002;52(4):641–9.
11. Bosse MJ, McCarthy ML, Jones AL, et al. The insensate foot following severe lower extremity trauma: an indication for amputation? J Bone Joint Surg. 2005;87A(12):2601–8.
12. Evans AR, Agel J, DeSilva GL, et al., Orthopaedic Trauma Association: Open Fracture Study Group. A

new classification scheme for open fractures. J Orthop Trauma. 2010;24:457–65.

13. Bosse MJ, Teague D, Rider L, et al. Outcomes after severe distal tibia, ankle, and/or foot trauma: comparison of limb salvage versus transtibial amputation (OUTLET). J Orthop Trauma. 2017;31(4 Supplement):S48–55.

14. Doukas WC, Hayda RA, Frisch M, et al. The military extremity trauma amputation/limb salvage (METALS) study. J Bone Joint Surg. 2013;95 A(2):138–45.

15. Ellington JK, Bosse MJ, Castillo RC, et al. The mangled foot and ankle: results from a 2-year prospective study. J Orthop Trauma. 2013;27(1):43–8.

16. Dickens JF, Kilcoyne KG, Kluk MW, et al. Risk factors for infection and amputation following open, combat-related calcaneal fractures. J Bone Joint Surg. 2013;95 A(5):1–8.

17. Bennett PM, Stevenson T, Sargeant ID, et al. Outcomes following limb salvage after combat hindfoot injury are inferior to delayed amputation at five years. Bone Joint Res. 2018;7(2):1–8.

18. Ramasamy MA, Hill AM, Masouros S, et al. Outcomes of IED foot and ankle blast injuries. J Bone Joint Surg Am. 2013;95 A(5):1–7.

19. Penn-Barwell JG, Bennett PM, Gray AC. The "could" and the "should" of reconstructing severe hind-foot injuries. Injury. 2018;49(2):147–8.

20. Kinner B, Tietz S, Muller F, et al. Outcome after complex trauma of the foot. J Trauma. 2011;70(1):159–68.

21. Blair JA, Patzkowski JC, Blanck RV, et al. Return to duty after integrated orthotic and rehabilitation initiative. J Orthop Trauma. 2014;28(4):e70–4.

22. Potter BK, Sheu RG, Stinner D, et al. Multisite evaluation of a custom energy-storing carbon fiber orthosis for patients with residual disability after lower-limb trauma. J Bone Joint Surg Am. 2018;100A(20):1781–9.

23. Inkellis E, et al. Incidence and characterization of major upper-extremity amputations in the National Trauma Data Bank. JB JS Open Access. 2018;3(2):e0038.

24. Low EE, Inkellis E, Morshed S. Complications and revision amputation following trauma-related lower limb loss. Injury. 2017;48(2):364–70.

25. Krueger CA, Wenke JC, Ficke JR. Ten years at war: comprehensive analysis of amputation trends. J Trauma Acute Care Surg. 2012;73(6 Suppl 5):S438–44.

26. Tscherne H, Oestern HJ. [A new classification of soft-tissue damage in open and closed fractures (author's transl)]. Unfallheilkunde. 1982;85(3):111–5.

27. Gregory RT, et al. The mangled extremity syndrome (M.E.S.): a severity grading system for multisystem injury of the extremity. J Trauma. 1985;25(12):1147–50.

28. Howe HR Jr, et al. Salvage of lower extremities following combined orthopedic and vascular trauma. A predictive salvage index. Am Surg. 1987;53(4):205–8.

29. Muller M, et al. The comprehensive classification of fractures of long bones. Springer, New York, NY; 1990.

30. Johansen K, et al. Objective criteria accurately predict amputation following lower extremity trauma. J Trauma. 1990;30(5):568–72; discussion 572–3.

31. Russell WL, et al. Limb salvage versus traumatic amputation. A decision based on a seven-part predictive index. Ann Surg. 1991;213(5):473–80; discussion 480–1.

32. McNamara MG, Heckman JD, Corley FG. Severe open fractures of the lower extremity: a retrospective evaluation of the Mangled Extremity Severity Score (MESS). J Orthop Trauma. 1994;8(2):81–7.

33. Rajasekaran S, et al. A score for predicting salvage and outcome in Gustilo type-IIIA and type-IIIB open tibial fractures. J Bone Joint Surg Br. 2006;88(10):1351–60.

34. Orthopaedic Trauma Association: Open Fracture Study, G. A new classification scheme for open fractures. J Orthop Trauma. 2010;24(8):457–64.

35. Durrant CA, Mackey SP. Orthoplastic classification systems: the good, the bad, and the ungainly. Ann Plast Surg. 2011;66(1):9–12.

36. Schiro GR, et al. Primary amputation vs limb salvage in mangled extremity: a systematic review of the current scoring system. BMC Musculoskelet Disord. 2015;16:372.

37. Loja MN, et al. The mangled extremity score and amputation: time for a revision. J Trauma Acute Care Surg. 2017;82(3):518–23.

38. Durham RM, et al. Outcome and utility of scoring systems in the management of the mangled extremity. Am J Surg. 1996;172(5):569–73; discussion 573–4.

39. Slauterbeck JR, et al. Mangled extremity severity score: an accurate guide to treatment of the severely injured upper extremity. J Orthop Trauma. 1994;8(4):282–5.

40. Bosse MJ, et al. A prospective evaluation of the clinical utility of the lower-extremity injury-severity scores. J Bone Joint Surg Am. 2001;83(1):3–14.

41. Kumar RS, Singhi PK, Chidambaram M. Are we justified doing salvage or amputation procedure based on mangled extremity severity score in mangled upper extremity injury. J Orthop Case Rep. 2017;7(1):3–8.

42. Ege T, et al. Reliability of the mangled extremity severity score in combat-related upper and lower extremity injuries. Indian J Orthop. 2015;49(6):656–60.

43. Fochtmann A, et al. Third degree open fractures and traumatic sub-/total amputations of the upper extremity: outcome and relevance of the Mangled Extremity Severity Score. Orthop Traumatol Surg Res. 2016;102(6):785–90.

44. Togawa S, et al. The validity of the mangled extremity severity score in the assessment of upper limb injuries. J Bone Joint Surg Br. 2005;87(11):1516–9.

45. Hohenberger GM, et al. The mangled extremity severity score fails to be a good predictor for secondary limb amputation after trauma with vascular injury in Central Europe. World J Surg. 2020;44(3):773–9.

46. Prichayudh S, et al. Management of upper extremity vascular injury: outcome related to the

Mangled Extremity Severity Score. World J Surg. 2009;33(4):857–63.

47. Weinzweig J, Weinzweig N. The "Tic-Tac-Toe" classification system for mutilating injuries of the hand. Plast Reconstr Surg. 1997;100(5):1200–11.

48. Campbell DA, Kay SP. The hand injury severity scoring system. J Hand Surg Br. 1996;21(3):295–8.

49. Urso-Baiarda F, et al. A prospective evaluation of the Modified Hand Injury Severity Score in predicting return to work. Int J Surg. 2008;6(1):45–50.

50. Lee CL, et al. Prediction of hand function after occupational hand injury by evaluation of initial anatomical severity. Disabil Rehabil. 2008;30(11):848–54.

51. Saxena P, Cutler L, Feldberg L. Assessment of the severity of hand injuries using 'hand injury severity score', and its correlation with the functional outcome. Injury. 2004;35(5):511–6.

52. Matsuzaki H, et al. Predicting functional recovery and return to work after mutilating hand injuries: usefulness of Campbell's Hand Injury Severity Score. J Hand Surg Am. 2009;34(5):880–5.

53. Kleinert HE, Jablon M, Tsai TM. An overview of replantation and results of 347 replants in 245 patients. J Trauma. 1980;20(5):390–8.

54. Graham B, et al. Major replantation versus revision amputation and prosthetic fitting in the upper extremity: a late functional outcomes study. J Hand Surg Am. 1998;23(5):783–91.

55. Pet MA, et al. Comparison of patient-reported outcomes after traumatic upper extremity amputation: replantation versus prosthetic rehabilitation. Injury. 2016;47(12):2783–8.

56. Otto IA, et al. Replantation versus prosthetic fitting in traumatic arm amputations: a systematic review. PLoS One. 2015;10(9):e0137729.

57. Tennent DJ, et al. Characterisation and outcomes of upper extremity amputations. Injury. 2014;45(6):965–9.

58. Mitchell SL, et al. The military extremity trauma amputation/limb salvage (METALS) study: outcomes of amputation compared with limb salvage following major upper-extremity trauma. J Bone Joint Surg Am. 2019;101(16):1470–8.

59. Foo A, Sebastin SJ. Secondary interventions for mutilating hand injuries. Hand Clin. 2016;32(4):555–67.

60. Russell RC, Bueno RA, Wu T-YT. Secondary procedures following mutilating hand injuries. Hand Clin. 2003;19(1):149–63.

61. Fufa D, et al. Secondary reconstructive surgery following major upper extremity replantation. Plast Reconstr Surg. 2014;134(4):713–20.

62. Femke Nawijn B, et al. Factors associated with primary and secondary amputation following limb-threatening upper extremity trauma. Plast Reconstr Surg. 2020;145(4):987–99.

63. Krueger CA, et al. Common factors and outcome in late upper extremity amputations after military injury. J Orthop Trauma. 2014;28(4):227–31.

64. Ladlow P, et al. Influence of immediate and delayed lower-limb amputation compared with lower-limb salvage on functional and mental health outcomes post-rehabilitation in the U.K. military. J Bone Joint Surg Am. 2016;98(23):1996–2005.

65. Krueger CA, et al. Late amputation may not reduce complications or improve mental health in combat-related, lower extremity limb salvage patients. Injury. 2015;46(8):1527–32.

66. Paryavi E, et al. Salvage of upper extremities with humeral fracture and associated brachial artery injury. Injury. 2014;45(12):1870–5.

67. Dudkiewicz I, et al. Evaluation of prosthetic usage in upper limb amputees. Disabil Rehabil. 2004;26(1):60–3.

68. Wright TW, Hagen AD, Wood MB. Prosthetic usage in major upper extremity amputations. J Hand Surg Am. 1995;20(4):619–22.

69. Biddiss EA, Chau TT. Upper limb prosthesis use and abandonment: a survey of the last 25 years. Prosthetics Orthot Int. 2007;31(3):236–57.

70. Gailey R, et al. Unilateral lower-limb loss: prosthetic device use and functional outcomes in servicemembers from Vietnam war and OIF/OEF conflicts. J Rehabil Res Dev. 2010;47(4):317–31.

71. Gagnier JJ. Patient reported outcomes in orthopaedics. J Orthop Res. 2017;35(10):2098–108.

72. Group, M. Patient-reported outcomes in orthopaedics. J Bone Joint Surg Am. 2018;100(5):436–42.

73. Lubbeke A. Research methodology for orthopaedic surgeons, with a focus on outcome. EFORT Open Rev. 2018;3(5):160–7.

74. Helter TM, Boehler CE. Developing attributes for discrete choice experiments in health: a systematic literature review and case study of alcohol misuse interventions. J Subst Use. 2016;21(6):662–8.

75. Lancsar E, Louviere J. Conducting discrete choice experiments to inform healthcare decision making: a user's guide. PharmacoEconomics. 2008;26(8):661–77.

76. O'Hara LM, et al. What publicly available quality metrics do hip and knee arthroplasty patients care about most when selecting a hospital in Maryland: a discrete choice experiment. BMJ Open. 2019;9(5):e028202.

77. O'Hara NN, et al. Valuing the recovery priorities of orthopaedic trauma patients after injury: evidence from a discrete choice experiment within 6 weeks of injury. J Orthop Trauma. 2019;33 Suppl 7:S16–20.

78. Hill W, et al. Upper Limb Prosthetic Outcome Measures (ULPOM): a working group and their findings. J Prosthet Orthot. 2009;21:P69–82.

79. Wright V. Prosthetic outcome measures for use with upper limb amputees: a systematic review of the peer-reviewed literature, 1970 to 2009. J Prosthet Orthot. 2009;21:P3–P63.

80. Mahmoudi E, et al. Racial variation in treatment of traumatic finger/thumb amputation: a national comparative study of replantation and revision amputation. Plast Reconstr Surg. 2016;137(3):576e–85e.

81. Chung SY, Sood A, Granick MS. Disproportionate availability between emergency and elective hand coverage: a national trend? Eplasty. 2016;16:e28.

82. Maroukis BL, et al. Hand trauma care in the United States: a literature review. Plast Reconstr Surg. 2016;137(1):100e–11e.
83. Richards WT, et al. Hand injuries in the state of Florida, are centers of excellence needed? J Trauma. 2010;68(6):1480–90.
84. Rios-Diaz AJ, et al. Inequalities in specialist hand surgeon distribution across the United States. Plast Reconstr Surg. 2016;137(5):1516–22.
85. Fabricant PD, et al. Building bridges toward interdisciplinary surgical care. Plast Reconstr Surg. 2012;129(6):1025e.
86. Lerman OZ, Kovach SJ, Levin LS. The respective roles of plastic and orthopedic surgery in limb salvage. Plast Reconstr Surg. 2011;127 Suppl 1:215S–27S.
87. Boriani F, et al. Orthoplastic surgical collaboration is required to optimise the treatment of severe limb injuries: a multi-centre, prospective cohort study. J Plast Reconstr Aesthet Surg. 2017;70(6):715–22.
88. Toia F, et al. Microsurgery and external fixation in orthoplastic reconstruction of tibial injuries. Handchirurgie, Mikrochirurgie, plastische Chirurgie : Organ der Deutschsprachigen Arbeitsgemeinschaft fur Handchirurgie : Organ der Deutschsprachigen Arbeitsgemeinschaft fur Mikrochirurgie der Peripheren Nerven und Gefasse : Organ der V... 2019;51(6):484–91.
89. Kuiken TA, et al. Targeted muscle reinnervation for real-time myoelectric control of multifunction artificial arms. JAMA. 2009;301(6):619–28.
90. Gart MS, Souza JM, Dumanian GA. Targeted muscle reinnervation in the upper extremity amputee: a technical roadmap. J Hand Surg Am. 2015;40(9):1877–88.
91. Gaston RG, et al. A novel muscle transfer for independent digital control of a myoelectric prosthesis: the Starfish procedure. J Hand Surg Am. 2019;44(2):163 e1–5.
92. Dumanian GA, et al. Targeted muscle reinnervation treats neuroma and phantom pain in major limb amputees: a randomized clinical trial. Ann Surg. 2019;270(2):238–46.
93. Valerio IL, et al. Preemptive treatment of phantom and residual limb pain with targeted muscle reinnervation at the time of major limb amputation. J Am Coll Surg. 2019;228(3):217–26.
94. Tsikandylakis G, Berlin O, Branemark R. Implant survival, adverse events, and bone remodeling of osseointegrated percutaneous implants for transhumeral amputees. Clin Orthop Relat Res. 2014;472(10):2947–56.
95. Juhnke DL, Aschoff HH. [Endo-exo prostheses following limb-amputation]. Orthopade. 2015;44(6):419–25.
96. Tillander J, et al. Osseointegrated titanium implants for limb prostheses attachments: infectious complications. Clin Orthop Relat Res. 2010;468(10):2781–8.
97. Al Muderis M, Lu W, Li JJ. Osseointegrated Prosthetic Limb for the treatment of lower limb amputations: experience and outcomes. Unfallchirurg. 2017;120(4):306–11.
98. Matthews DJ, et al. UK trial of the osseointegrated prosthesis for the rehabilitation for amputees: 1995-2018. Prosthetics Orthot Int. 2019;43(1):112–22.
99. Ortiz-Catalan M, Hakansson B, Branemark R. An osseointegrated human-machine gateway for long-term sensory feedback and motor control of artificial limbs. Sci Transl Med. 2014;6(257):257re6.

Orthotic Management of the Mangled Extremity

Tyler Klenow and Phil Stevens

Introduction

Even after the successful surgical salvage of a mangled extremity, patients may be left with functional deficits which require an orthosis to help them return to their daily activities and work. Upper and lower extremity trauma patients often present with weakness, instability, contractures, fractures, and pain. Treatment objectives in such cases may include limiting the range of motion across targeted joint segments, positioning the joint in a desired alignment, mechanically assisting a desired motion, or unloading an injured part of the body. More recently, orthoses have been used to transfer dynamic forces across compromised lower extremity joints and tissues to restore loading moments during ambulation.

The successful design and application of an orthosis to a mangled extremity requires an understanding of each patient's history including deficits, mechanism of injury, potential for recovery, and comorbidities. Only then can design and materials be chosen by the rehab team which will allow an orthosis to act across the affected extremity to obtain the desired biomechanical effect and other treatment objectives.

Orthoses: General Principles

Orthoses have been described as "any externally applied device to an existing body part that improves function" [1]. Common goals for an orthosis applied to an extremity include the following:

- Stabilizing a weak, paralyzed, or fractured extremity segment or joint
- Limiting or augmenting motion across a joint
- Unloading a compromised body segment
- Reducing pain
- As an aid in rehabilitation

When referring to an orthosis, the terminology adopted by the International Organization for Standardization (ISO) is determined by the joints and body segments that are directly affected by the device. These are frequently referred to using acronyms for these body segments. In the management of a mangled extremity, these include:

- Shoulder orthosis (SO)
- Elbow orthosis (EO)
- Wrist hand orthosis (WHO)

T. Klenow (✉)
Martin Bionics Innovations, Clinical Care,
Tampa, FL, USA

P. Stevens
Department of Clinical and Scientific Affiars, Hanger
Inc., Salt Lake City, UT, USA
e-mail: pstevens@hanger.com

R. A. Pensy, J. V. Ingari (eds.), *The Mangled Extremity*, https://doi.org/10.1007/978-3-319-56648-1_16

- Hip orthosis (HO)
- Knee orthosis (KO)
- Ankle foot orthosis (AFO)

In addition, longer devices crossing multiple joint segments are also frequently encountered and include elbow-wrist-hand orthoses (EWHO) and knee-ankle-foot orthoses (KAFO). In the event that spinal injury has also occurred, a lumbar-sacral-orthosis (LSO) or thoracic-lumbar-sacral-orthosis (TLSO) may be indicated and, in extreme cases, upper or lower extremity devices may be attached to spinal orthoses.

Design and Materials

For many decades, orthoses were composed of a metal frame work inclusive of a pair of joints and uprights running the length of the involved body segments, joined by metal bands. This metal superstructure was occasionally supplemented by leather corsets that provided additional soft tissue containment proximal and distal to the targeted joint segment. Advances in technology have led to the wide spread adoption of thermoformable plastics, used both with and without articulating joint systems according to the needs of the individual. More recently, plastics have been supplemented by the use of light weight composite materials such as carbon fiber. Similarly, advances in technology have added to metal joint options with flexible urethane-based joints and, more recently, robust composite struts that deflect under dynamic load and then return to their original length, converting the potential energy of their deflected shape into propulsive kinetic energy. Shear and force absorbing materials such as foam and silicone make orthoses more comfortable and effective (Figs. 16.1 and 16.2).

Force Applications

The primary biomechanical principles incorporated into the design of the lower extremity orthosis are the three-point pressure system and proximal unloading of a distal limb segment or joint. These principles are paramount to developing a basic understanding of individual orthotic device application.

The three-point pressure system is the principle utilized to provide sagittal, coronal, or transverse plane stability to an affected limb and to limit or augment motion across a joint or direct force across a particular compartment of a joint space. These applications can be implemented independently or in combination in a single orthotic device. The three points of pressure constituting this system are two stabilizing forces at either end of the system and a corrective force applied between the two stabilizing forces [2–4]. The forces must be applied in this sequence to be effective and can be applied to nearly every joint in the human body.

When applying these stabilizing and corrective forces, it is important to recognize the concept of a lever arm. A basic principle of physics is that a moment is created when a force is applied to body around a fixed axis point [5]. A moment is the product of the force being applied and the

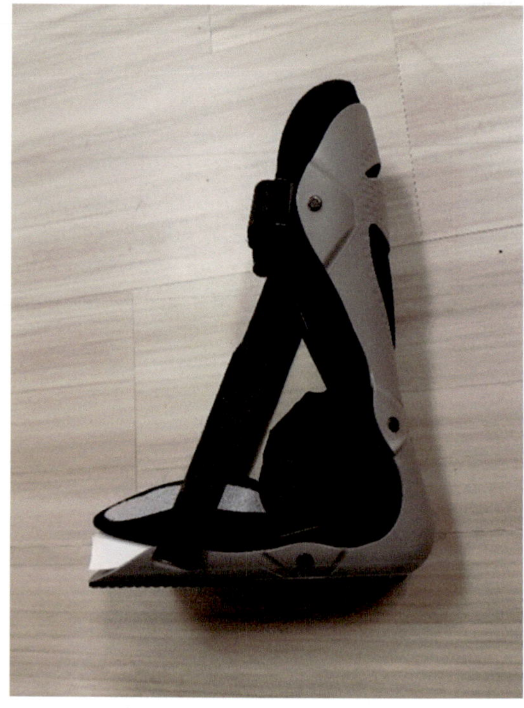

Fig. 16.1 Well-padded nocturnal AFO, worn to prevent loss of ankle mobility

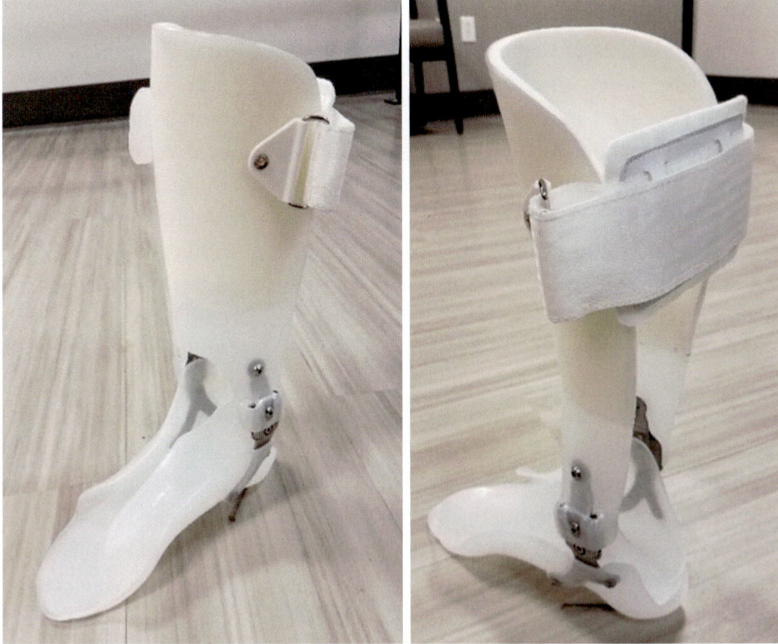

Fig. 16.2 Ground reaction AFO with foam padding to distribute forces over the dorsal surface of the tibia

distance from point of force application to the axis of rotation. The lever arm is the perpendicular distance between the point of force application and the axis. Therefore, in situations where the force being applied to the body is held constant, the moment created is directly proportional to the distance over which the force is being applied, this being the lever arm. In the case of the lower extremity orthotic intervention, the force being applied to the body is most commonly the ground reaction force created during the stance phase of gait and the body is a segment of the human body [5]. The lever arm then is length of the specific components of the orthosis itself.

The corrective and stabilizing forces in a three-point pressure system can be applied in a variety of ways including pads, straps, binders, or simply the trimlines (i.e., the terminal edges) of the orthosis [6]. Further, there may be a variety of intervention options to achieve a similar biomechanical function. When the mangled extremity is being treated, the device and application knowledge of the orthotist is critical to achieve the result desired by the physician. Greater biomechanical correction can be achieved and tolerated by the user when applied with medium durometer material compared to hard plastic [7, 8].

The expertise, judgment, and skills of an orthotist are required to optimize the fit and function of orthotic devices. Point pressures which may cause discomfort and skin breakdown can be reduced proactively in fabrication of the orthosis by creating reliefs for bony prominences and flaring or rounding trimlines. Material selection is critical to the prevention of point pressure development and various types of padding are often incorporated as an interface between the device and user. The majority of these methods can also be applied reactively if point pressures develop; however, the amount of interface modification and alteration of force application may be limited once an orthosis has been fabricated.

In the treatment of the mangled extremity, a variety of skin conditions and scarring often coexist and the orthotist must consider these when designing the orthotic intervention unique to each patient and specific joint segment being treated. Material selection and the location and method of force application become increasingly important when the skin or underlying anatomy have been altered, as some materials are designed to dissipate force and pressure or reduce impact, while other are designed to reduce shear forces. Materials can also be combined to compound the effects of multiple materials in a laminated fashion. Various types of socks and compression garments can also be used to reduce pressure and friction produced by orthosis use. In situations involving burns or grafted skin, silicone-infused material can be used to reduce skin breakdown and promote healing [9].

Unloading weight from a distal limb segment or joint is another commonly utilized principle in orthotic device design and application. In this application, force, typically axial force, is transferred from the proximal portion of the orthosis through uprights, struts, stays, or a typical orthosis configuration past the affected joint or segment to the distal portion of the orthosis. This unloading effect can be achieved through anatomical suspension [10, 11] or total contact [12] (Fig. 16.3). In these applications, the distracting or unweighting force can be total or partial and is applied in the static alignment of the device to reduce axial load. More recently, orthotic interventions have been developed to reduce unwanted forces dynamically through variable response to the motion of the orthosis itself [13].

In load-bearing applications, total contact compression is used to proximally unload a distal segment or joint through application of an infinite number of three point pressure systems [12]. This compression of soft tissue increases pressure within the limb segment, thereby supporting the addressed long bones by transferring axial force from those bones through the soft tissue to the surrounding orthosis. A similar effect has been noted using an alternating tissue compression and release technique in prosthetic sockets which may have application to orthotic interventions as well [14]. The uniform distribution of force using the total contact principle can be executed with lacers or ratchet closures which draw material together or through Velcro straps which hold together two or three rigid pieces in a bivalve or trivalve design. This method is thought to increase deep venous circulation similarly to a compression garment, which applies similar principles [15].

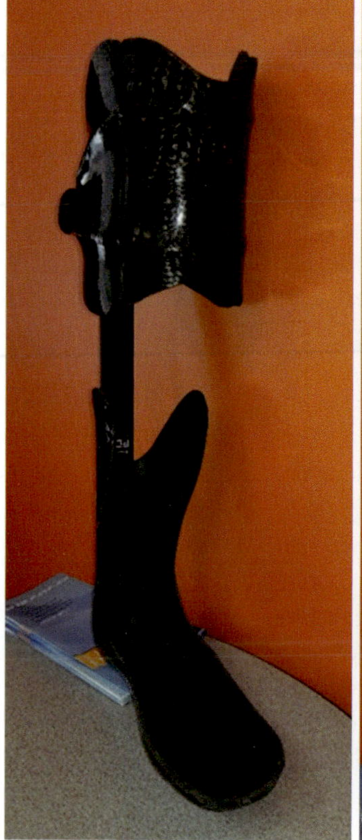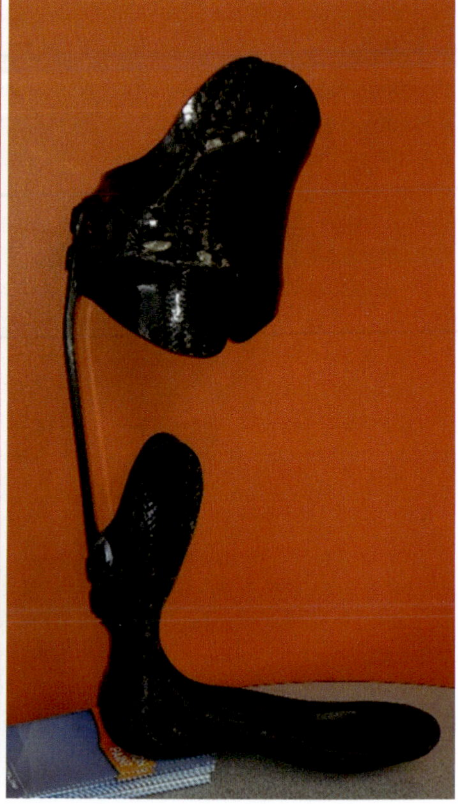

Fig. 16.3 Carbon AFO with posterior energy storing composite strut and proximal cuff used to off-load distal limb segments. (Photo courtesy of Mike Jenks, CPO, Hanger Clinic)

Orthotic Fracture Management

Additional applications of orthotic interventions include fracture management. Treatment of the mangled extremity will often include correction of multiple fractures. Fracture orthoses are typically modular or fully customized, and must include design elements to accommodate any surgical interventions present, such as fixation or incisions. The standard material selection is a thick layer of soft foam surrounded by a dense foam or plastic shell. Fracture orthoses typically utilize total contact compression to stabilize fractured bones and are applied in two or more pieces. Fracture location dictates required length of the orthosis in these cases. Mid-shaft fractures can often be stabilized by enclosing a single limb segment. Fractures in the proximal or distal third of the bone must cross the adjacent joint to reduce stress to the fracture site created by motion of the adjoining segments. Positioning of the particular limb segment must be complete prior to application of the fracture orthosis to ensure the bones and joints heal in optimal alignment. Potential migration of the orthosis is also an important factor in design. Upper extremity fracture orthoses can be anchored with shoulder caps, straps, or slings (Fig. 16.4). Lower extremity fracture orthoses can be secured by adding a footplate if intended for weight bearing or a belt if the patient is bed-ridden. These devices are available for each of the orthotic levels presented in this chapter.

Lower Limb Orthotic Interventions

Ankle-Foot Orthosis (AFO)

Perhaps the most common orthotic application to the mangled lower extremity is the ankle-foot orthosis (AFO). The AFO has multiple configurations and design elements which are uniquely designed and applied to each patient.

The overall height or length of an AFO may also vary within a particular design, which can further affect orthotic function. Generally, in accordance with the principle of the lever arm, longer lengths of orthosis segments provide more corrective moments or unwanted moment reduction. For example, the length of the footplate of an AFO determines the amount of foot joint movement. A full footplate reduces the most motion and can be used to influence initiation of tonal responses when present. Termination at the sulcus allows motion in the toes. Termination at the level of the metatarsal heads allow for motion of the toe and midfoot where a ¾ termination allows slightly more. Termination at the calcaneus allows complete motion of the midfoot and mostly influences hindfoot motion.

In general, orthotic interventions are meant to immobilize or augment the motion of a joint. In lower extremity applications, the orthotic devices can be either ambulatory to support the motions of gait, or non-ambulatory to maintain proper positioning. When seeking to immobilize the ankle joint in ambulation, the appropriate intervention is either the solid-ankle AFO or leather ankle gauntlet. It is important to note that in all ambulatory applications, changing shoes with differing heel heights will change the biomechanics and thus the effect of the device.

Solid AFO

When designing a solid-ankle AFO, which are typically thermoplastic and may also be lami-

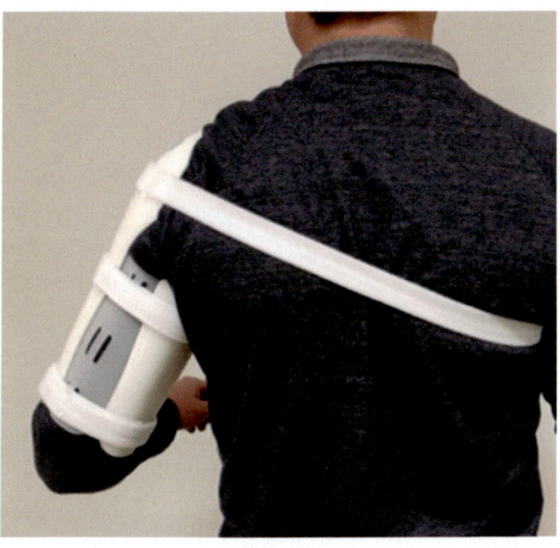

Fig. 16.4 Humeral Fracture Brace

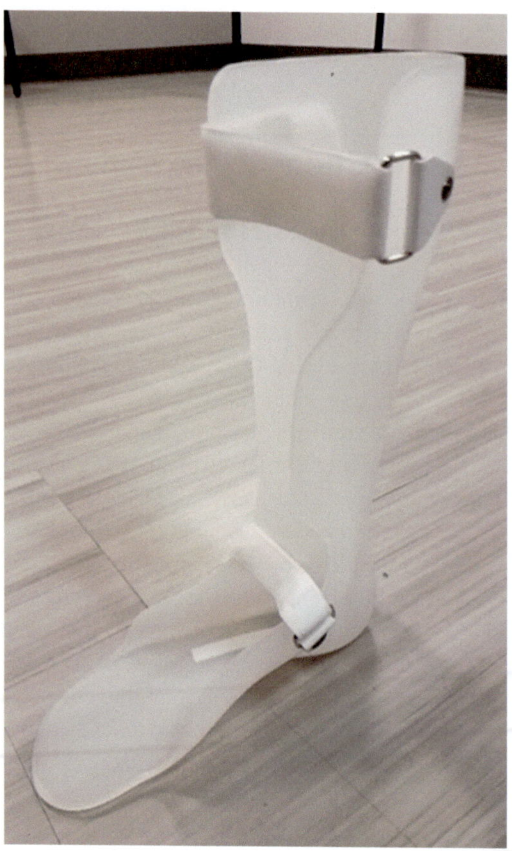

Fig. 16.5 Solid AFO

nated, the circumferential trimlines are directly related to stability (Fig. 16.5). As increasing amounts of material are left surrounding the shank, stability and support increase, and motion decreases. In practice, it is difficult to leave more than 2/3 of the total material surrounding the shank as this reduces ease of donning. Ease of donning can be improved, however, by implementing accessibility modifications to the orthosis which square the anterior trimlines to each other and can maximize the amount of material left in the orthosis.

Posterior Leaf Spring (PLS)

When the trimlines are reduced posteriorly to its minimally viable amount, the resulting design is referred to as the posterior leaf spring (PLS) AFO. While this design is of low profile and can be cosmetically appealing, it provides a reduced amount of triplanar control and increases allowed motion at the ankle compared to traditional solid-ankle designs. Increasingly rigid materials can reduce this motion and improve support, but these materials can be difficult to use, are more expensive, and are prone to failure at the base of the footplate.

Trimlines can be reduced on only one side to prevent motion toward the side which remains. This application is used mostly to prevent varus or valgus motion at the ankle and to influence tibial torsion. Such a configuration is referred to as a corrective tab or a Sabolich trimline, named after the clinician John Sabolich [6].

Leather Ankle Gauntlet

An additional application of the solid-ankle AFO is the leather ankle gauntlet originally fabricated by the Arizona AFO company. These gauntlets are simply solid-ankle AFOs skillfully wrapped in leather which utilize some form of anterior closure to implement the total contact principle (Fig. 16.6). Historically, gauntlets are made shorter than traditional AFOs, but they can be of full length if proximal unloading of the ankle is desired which may occur in long-term management of the mangled extremity. The leather interface reduces friction to the skin which may be necessary in mangled extremity cases as well.

Patellar-Tendon-Bearing AFO

In cases where aggressive proximal unloading of the foot, ankle, or shank is required, the patellar-tendon-bearing (PTB) AFO can be used. The PTB AFO utilizes an anatomical suspension principle commonly used in the below-knee prosthetic sockets where a bar is modified into a proximal cuff at the level of the patellar tendon opposed by a posterior wall in the popliteal fossa [10]. The patellar tendon is largely avascular, typically lacks coverage by fatty or soft tissue, and has a relatively low number of sensory nerves which all result in an ideal weight-bearing sur-

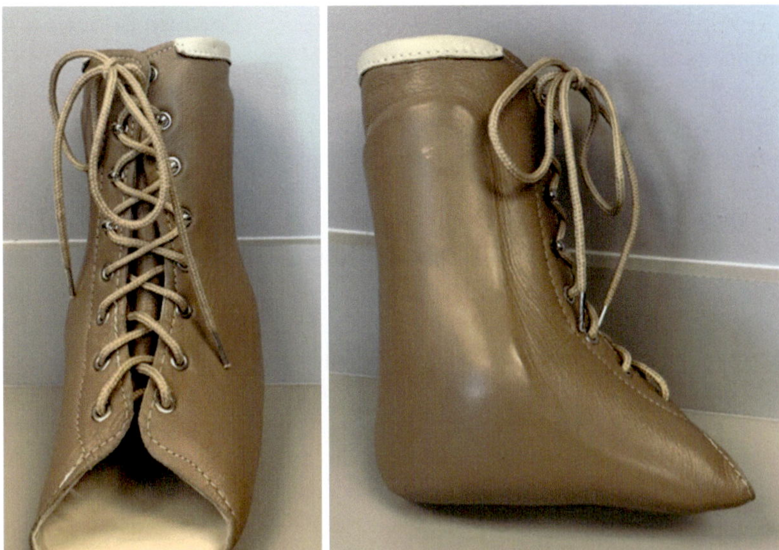

Fig. 16.6 Leather Ankle Gauntlet

face. The distance between the patellar bar and posterior wall is reduced compared to the anatomy of the patient which creates a suspending effect and, thus, the proximal unloading. In the case of the mangled lower extremity, PTB AFOs can be useful to reduce axial loading to healing tibial fractures or damage to the calcaneus, such as fracture, avascular necrosis, or absence. These orthoses must be adequately tightened by the patient in order to achieve distal unloading and even then it should be expected that some distal weight bearing will still occur. If complete non-weight bearing is required, the patient should be properly instructed and provided with an appropriate ambulatory aid.

Non-ambulatory AFOs

Non-ambulatory solid ankle AFOs are used in acute management scenarios. Additional position applications of solid-ankle AFOs are commonly used and include the pressure-relieving AFO (PRAFO), sometimes referred to as a multi-podus boot, and the night splint. PRAFOs were specifically designed to reduce pressure on the heel and subsequent sore development associated with prolonged bedrest, which may occur in patients with mangled extremities. Night splints are designed to prevent plantarflexion contracture

formation when sleeping or in periods of prolonged lying (Fig. 16.1). Night splints are also used to prevent tightening of skin grafts which cross the ankle. Splinting and casting may also be employed in these scenarios but are beyond the scope of this chapter.

Articulated AFO

There are several AFO designs which allow for supported motion in gait including the articulated AFO, ground reaction (GRAFO), and the dynamic AFO. Historically, articulated AFOs were fabricated around a schema or blueprint, based off a tracing, of the patient's limb in which one or two metal uprights are used to connect proximal leather cuffs to a shoe to reduce unwanted motion. These devices are often referred to as conventional AFOs. The joints used in these orthoses rotate around a single axis in which motion in the sagittal plane, either plantarflexion or dorsiflexion, can be resisted through the shape of the joint articulation. The dual-action joint or BiCAL allows for combinations of assistance and resistance in the same joint [16]. These actions are created through utilization and adjustment of metal pins or springs in chambers on either side of the joints. Further development of this design allows for specific assistance or resistance during particular phases of the gait cycle [17].

Indications for use of conventional AFOs include presence of edema and delicate skin considerations, both of which are commonly associated with the mangled lower extremity. The adjustability of the uprights used to connect the proximal cuff to the shoe also allow for elimination of contact in large portions of the orthosis or around a unique feature such as an external fixation frame or prominences created by internal fixation. Conventional AFOs also allow the use of T-straps which are fabricated pieces of material design to restrict motion in the coronal plane. The material is connected to one upright and loops around the user's limb to create a corrective force. In mangled extremity applications, T-straps can be useful when correction is needed, but available tissue purchase is limited due to skin integrity or other features.

Thermoplastic AFOs can be either solid-ankle or articulated designs. The articulated thermoplastic AFO is made possible through elastic polymer joints. These joints can be fabricated to allow free ankle motion or to assist motion in a particular direction and are formed directly into the shape of the orthosis in fabrication. "Stops", used to prevent motion in a particular direction can also be fabricated into the orthosis and the degree of articulation modified at the contact point the calf and footplate segments of the device.

Hybrid devices can also be created when indicated by patient anatomy and desired effect. Thermoplastic AFOs typically provide more correction than do conventional AFOs due to their intimacy with the user, but metal joints may be needed depending on forces traversing the articulation. Dual action joints may be preferred to polymer joints in progressive rehabilitation settings where the level or assistance or resistance to directional motion may need to be adjusted frequently with rapid changes or improvements in patient function. These hybrid designs can also be utilized when proximal unloading is desired with an articulating ankle joint.

Ground Reaction AFOs

The ground reaction AFO (GRAFO) or floor reaction AFO harnesses the forces being transferred through the ankle during the stance phase of gait to supplement limited or absent internal propulsive forces (Fig. 16.2). This presentation occurs when the gastrocnemius-soleus complex (*triceps surae*) or its innervating nerve pathways are damaged. Both conditions are common in the treatment of the mangled lower extremity. GRAFOs also provide stabilizing forces to the knee in stance phase [18].

These AFOs can be custom or prefabricated from thermoplastic or laminated and have either an anterior shell or posterior cuff in a spiral design. Anterior shells amplify the moments created about the ankle and knee in stance phase and are contraindicated when *genu recurvatum* is present. Anterior shell designs are commonly used to unload a damaged forefoot and offer an effective solution to partial foot amputees when used in conjunction with a toe-filler as it restores the absent anterior level arm. Prefabrication GRAFO designs typically utilize struts which allows for the use of T-straps. These combinations are commonly used in the chronic treatment of the mildly mangled lower extremity.

Energy Storage and Return AFOs

The energy storage and return AFO (ESR-AFO) utilizes one or more exoskeletal graphite struts to provide an exponentially greater energy return to increased moments at the ankle. The struts connect a reinforced, rigid carbon footplate, sometimes with medial and lateral wings to prevent excessive motion of the tibia, to a similarly rigid proximal cuff. The ESR-AFO was first introduced for application to the mangled or salvaged lower extremity through a US military application, the Intredpid Dynamic Exoskeletal Orthosis (IDEO™), in 2009 and later through a civilian application, the Exosym™ [19]. These custom-made orthoses were designed around principles first associated with prosthetic running blades to allow for high-impact activities following trauma (Fig. 16.3).

While meant to provide proximal unloading to the ankle joint similarly to the PTB AFO, the ESR-AFO accomplishes this principle by providing increasingly higher resistance to motion through deflection of the exoskeletal struts. Therefore, the orthosis provides more unloading in a loaded position created through user motion than it does in quiet standing. When used with an intense physical therapy program, ESR-AFOs have been shown to allow US Service members to return to duty and physical activity while decreasing pain [13]. A comparison of ESR-AFOs to traditional ambulatory AFOs is currently being conducted in the US Veterans Health Administration.

Knee-Ankle-Foot Orthosis (KAFO)

When correction or control of the knee cannot be accomplished by controlling the shank, the orthotic intervention must cross the joint and becomes a knee-ankle-foot orthosis (KAFO). KAFOs are fabricated in a similar fashion to AFOs and utilize similar material selection criteria. Carbon fiber laminations are more commonly used in custom applications of the KAFOs compared to AFOs, however, perhaps due to the commercially available selection of prefabricated AFOs. The KAFO utilizes multiple three or four-point pressure systems to stabilize the lower extremity in multiple planes. Drop locks are commonly utilized to immobilize the knee joint for ambulation or times of prolonged standing.

Joint motion assistance has become increasingly popular in KAFO applications in which externally mounted hydraulic systems are used to create external moments about the knee to assist the user. Nerve innervations are commonly damaged in the mangled lower extremity, so joint assistance can be critical to successful rehabilitation in these cases.

KAFO options can be fabricated with options for modification as the user progresses through therapy following an injured extremity. Combo KAFOs allow for the knee portion to be detached from the calf portion. While this option was originally created to remove the knee orthosis portion from an AFO, applications now exist where the two separated portions can both be usable ortho-

ses independent of one another [20]. This can be helpful in the acute rehabilitation of the mangled extremity as it is difficult to predict the amount of functional return any individual may have.

Stance Control KAFO

The stance control KAFO (SCO) allows for selective automatic locking and unlocking of a knee joint in stance. The SCO facilitates a more normal gait pattern compared to the drop-lock [21] and can be accomplished in multiple ways. Ankle-activated SCOs unlock the knee joint with dorsiflexion of the ankle as would be experienced in pre-swing. These devices are also useful when there is damage at the knee, but control is preserved at the ankle as the user is able to lock or unlock the knee when desired. Pendulum designs lock the knee when the orthosis reaches a certain angle and triggers a mechanical switch. Computerized control of knee joint motion in SCOs has greatly improved recently congruent with improvement in technology of the microprocessor-controlled prosthetic knee. These applications transfer data collected by multiple sensors throughout the orthosis to an on-board processor which controls the valves in a hydraulic cylinder which provides the user appropriate resistance to knee flexion.

Postoperative KAFO

Non-ambulatory KAFO options exist to control positioning following surgical repair of the mangled lower extremity. The most common application is the telescoping range of motion or T-ROM orthosis. This application often has a lock and range of motion limiters incorporated into the knee joint to prevent overuse or prevent contractures. These orthoses can be custom fabricated or assembled from modular parts. Contractures are common in the treatment of the mangled extremity due to extended bedrest, atrophy of oppositional muscle groups, and use of skin grafting. Further contracture management options are found in the static progressive and dynamic progressive KAFOs. These orthoses provide either increasing static positioning at select joint angles or a minimal continuous stretching force to the knee joint to prevent or reduce contractures. KAFOs are commonly used in fracture management of the femur and tibial plateau.

KO

While not commonly used in acute management of the lower extremity, the knee orthosis (KO) can be used in chronic treatment of mild cases. Configurations exist for support of particular ligaments such as the ACL or PCL with some spring-loaded joints reducing impact to particular motions of the knee. Medial and lateral compartment unloader knee orthoses can be used in the treatment of traumatic arthritis following reconstruction of the mangled lower extremity later in life.

HKAFO

Required stabilization of all three joints of the lower extremity is rare, but may present itself in the treatment of the mangled extremity. The hip-knee-ankle-foot orthosis (HKAFO) can be used in ambulatory and non-ambulatory applications. When ambulatory, the HKAFO incorporates many of the same principles and material selection criteria as the AFO and KAFO. Further options exist to provide assistance to joint motion at the hip or at multiple joints simultaneously, although the efficacy of these interventions is not readily available in the literature. Situations can occur where positioning of the hip joint is vital to the healing process in which the custom or modular hip abduction orthosis, a static version of the HKAFO, can be utilized.

Upper Limb Orthotic Interventions

WHO/WHFO

Wrist hand orthoses (WHO) are commonly used to stabilize the wrist joint and architecture of the hand. The wrist can be completely immobilized, permitted a desired range of flexion and extension, or assisted in a desired motion. A palmer segment is frequently used to support the architecture of the hand itself. When maintenance of a targeted finger position is desired, the palmer support can be made to extend distally, creating a wrist hand finger orthosis (WHFO).

EO

Elbow orthoses (EO) consist of a proximal humeral segment and distal forearm segment, frequently encompassing the ventral aspect of the limb. If elbow movement is desired, elbow joints connect the proximal and distal cuff. Applications include complete elbow immobilization, adjustable elbow joint stops to allow or restrict elbow motion as indicated by rehabilitation protocols, and adjustable locking joints that allow the elbow to be fixed at a targeted joint angle to preposition the hand in a desired position (Fig. 16.7). For example, in cases of targeted nerve damage to the elbow flexors, a locking EO would permit continued use of a functioning hand.

Prosthoses

In some applications, prosthetic and orthotic treatment principles may be coupled to create a prosthosis. In a common application, a WHO may be used to stabilize a non-functioning wrist-hand complex. If bimanual function remains a treatment objective, a prosthetic terminal device can be mounted to the palmer aspect of the WHO. This terminal device can be harnessed to the contralateral torso to permit actuation of the

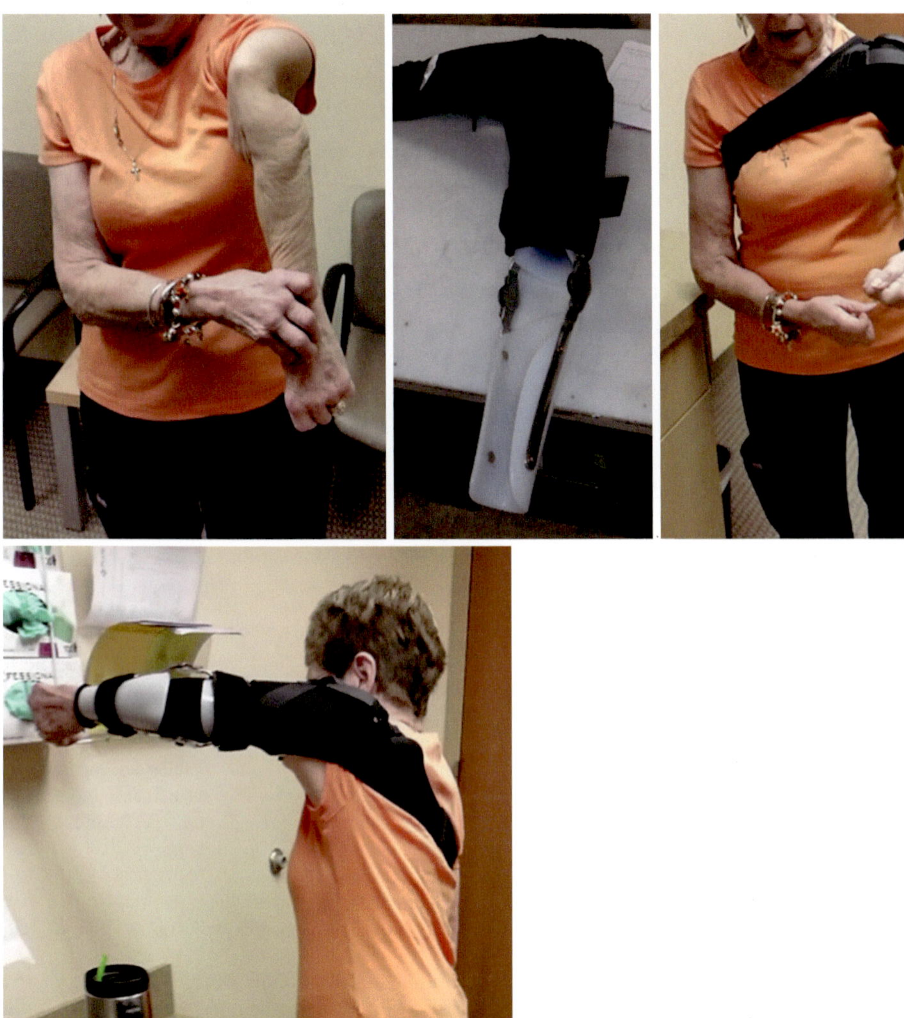

Fig. 16.7 Failed elbow replacement, elbow orthosis with mechanical lock used to preposition the functional hand in space. (Photo courtesy Kyle Rasmussen, CPO. Hanger Clinic)

hook using the conventional principles of body-powered prostheses. In a variant of this approach, the

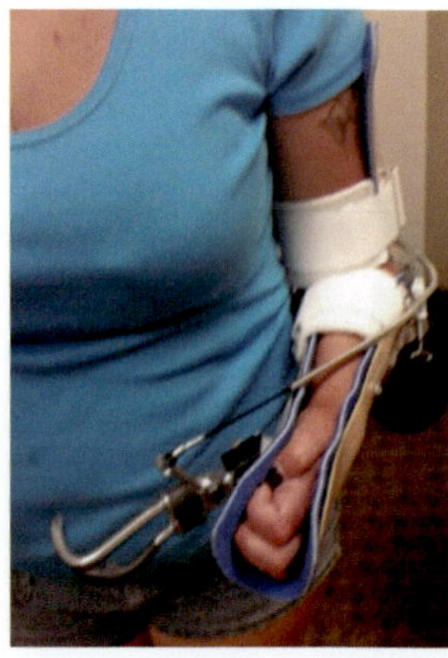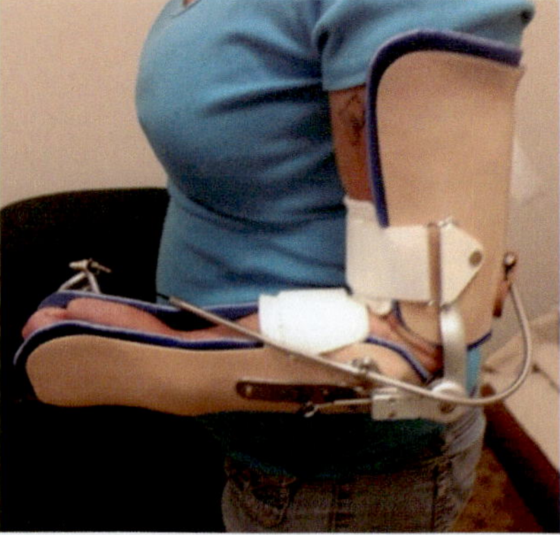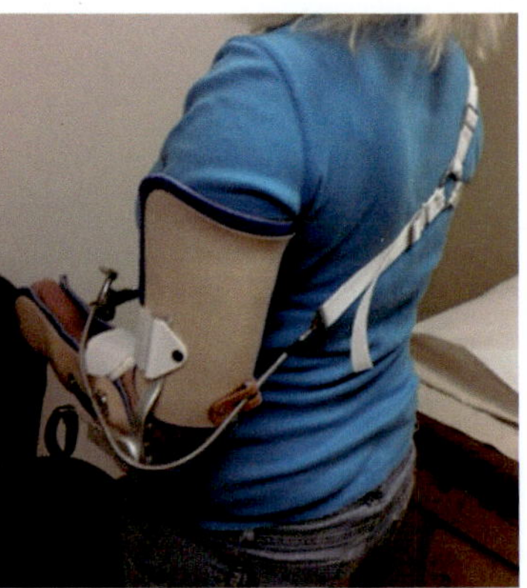

Fig. 16.8 Brachial Plexus injury, elbow orthosis with manual lock used to preposition the hand in space. However, the paralyzed hand has no function, so the orthosis acts as a mounting surface for a prosthetic hook which is activated using prosthetic harnessing principles

additional presentation of a flail elbow can be managed by the addition of locking elbow joints and a proximal humeral cuff. In such applications, a control harness can be integrated into the prosthosis to allow control of elbow position using the harnessing principles of transhumeral prostheses (Fig. 16.8).

Clinical Examples/Application

References

1. Uustal H. The orthotic prescription. In: Hsu JD, Michael JW, Fisk JR, editors. AAOS atlas of orthoses and assistive devices. 4th ed. Philadelphia: MOSBY; 2008. p. 9–14.
2. Esrafilian A, Karimi MT, Eshraghi A. Design and evaluation of a new type of knee orthosis to align the mediolateral angle of the knee joint with osteoarthritis. Adv Orthop. 2012;2012:6. https://doi.org/10.1155/2012/104927.
3. Neville C, Bucklin M, Ordway N, Lemley F. An ankle-foot orthosis with a lateral extension reduces forefoot abduction in subjects with stage II posterior tibial tendon dysfunction. J Orthop Sports Phys Ther. 2016;46(1):26–33. https://doi.org/10.2519/2Fjospt.2016.5618.
4. Chalmers DD, Hamer GP. Three point dynamic orthosis. Prosthetics Orthot Int. 1985;9:115–6.
   Retrieved from http://www.oandplibrary.org/poi/pdf/1985_02_115.pdf
5. Hinman RS, Bowles KA, Metcalf BB, Wrigley TV, Bennell KL. Lateral wedge insoles for medial knee arthritis: effects on lower limb frontal plane biomechanics. Clin Biomech. 2012;27(1):27–33. https://doi-org.portal.lib.fit.edu/10.1016/j.clinbiomech.2011.07.010/
6. Sabolich J. Modification of the posterior leaf-spring orthosis. Orthot Prosthet. 1976;30(3):35–6. Retrieved from http://www.oandplibrary.org/op/1976_03_035.asp
7. Su S, Zhongjun M, Guo J, Fan Y. The effect of arch height and material hardness of personalized insole on correction and tissues of flatfoot. J Healthcare Eng. 2017;2017:1. https://doi.org/10.1155/2F2017/2F8614341.
8. Birk JA, Foto JG, Pfiefer LA. Effect of orthosis material hardness on walking pressure in high-risk diabetes patients. J Prosthet Orthot. 1999;11(2):43–6. Retrieved from https://journals.lww.com/jpojournal/Abstract/1999/01120/Effect_of_Orthosis_Material_Hardness_on_Walking.7.aspx.
9. Perkins K, Davey RB, Wallis KA. Silincone gel: a new treatement for burn scars and contractures. Burns Incl Therm Inj. 1983;9(3):201–4. Retrieved from https://www.ncbi.nlm.nih.gov/pubmed/6831286.
10. Svend-Hansen H, Bremerskov V, Ostri P. Fracture-suspending effect of patellar-tendon-bearing cast. Acta Orthop Scand. 1978;50(2):237–9. https://doi.org/10.3109/17453677908989761.
11. May BJ, Lockard MA. Prosthetics & orthotics in clinical practice: a case study approach. 2nd ed. Philadelphia: F. A. Davis Company; 2011.
12. Sarmiento A. A functional below-the-knee cast for tibial fractures. 1967. J Bone Joint Surg Am.

2004;86A(12):2777. Retrieved from https://www.ncbi.nlm.nih.gov/pubmed/15590866.

13. Highsmith MJ, Nelson LM, Carbone NT, Klenow TD, Kahle JT, Hill OT, Maikos JT, Kartel MS, Randolph BJ. Outcomes associated with the Intrepid Dynamic Exoskeletal Orthosis (IDEO): a systematic review of the literature. Mil Med. 2016;181(S4):69–76. https://doi.org/10.7205/MILMED-D-16-00280.

14. Klenow TD, Highsmith MJ, Fedel FJ, Ropp J, Kahle JT. Comparative efficacy of transfemoral prosthetic interfaces: analysis of gait and perceived disability. J Prosthet Orthot. 2017;29(3):130–6. https://doi.org/10.1097/JPO.0000000000000135.

15. Styf JR, Nakhostine M, Gershuni DH. Functional knee braces increase intramuscular pressures in the anterior compartment of the leg. Am J Sports Med. 1992;20(1):46–9. https://doi.org/10.1177/036354659202000112.

16. Kobayaski T, Orendurff MS, Hunt G, Lincoln LS, Gao F, LeCursi N, Foreman KB. An articulated ankle-foot orthosis with adjustable plantarflexion resistance, dorsiflexion resistance and alignment: a pilot study on mechanical properties and effects on stroke hemiparetic gait. Med Eng Phy. 2017;44:94–101. https://doi.org/10.1016/j.medengphy.2017.02.012.

17. Campbell J, LeCursi N, Zalinski N. 2015. US20160361189A1. U. S. Patent and Trademark Office. Retrieved from https://patents.google.com/patent/US20160361189A1/en.

18. Aboutorabi A, Arazpour M, Bani MA, Saeedi H, Head JS. Efficacy of ankle foot orthoses types on walking in children with cerebral palsy: a systematic review. Ann Phys Rehabil Med. 2017;60:393–402. https://doi.org/10.1016/j.rehab.2017.05.004.

19. Blanck RV. 2011. US20120271214A1. U. S. Patent and Trademark Office. Retrieved from https://patents.google.com/patent/US20120271214A1/en.

20. Klenow TD, Kartel MS. A functional evaluation of a custom modular KAFO in a Veteran subject with TBI. In: 99th American Orthotic & Prosthetic Association 2016 National Assembly: Treatment Options in Lower Limb Orthotics. Boston; 2016.

21. Hebert JS, Liggins AB. Gait evaluation of an automatic stance-control knee orthosis in a patient with postpoliomyelitis. Arch Phys Med Rehabil. 2005;86(6):1676–80. https://doi.org/10.1016/j.apmr.2004.12.024.

Prosthetic Care for the Mangled Extremity

17

John Rheinstein, Kevin Carroll, and Phil Stevens

Despite the effective advances in treating mangled and diseased extremities, amputation may be the best or only option for a severely injured patient to regain mobility, function, or reduce pain [1] (Fig. 17.1). Prosthetic care for amputation [2] patients has evolved rapidly in recent years, with a wide array of available designs and technologies to help patients restore gait and hand function with comfort and to rebuild their lives. These advances allow amputations to be viewed and performed as reconstructive procedures rather than as failures. Just as a successful surgical repair results in limb salvage, an effective amputation can provide functional "gait salvage" or "grasp salvage." When regarded in a positive manner, it is also easier for both the patient and their physicians to accept an amputation, move forward, and achieve an optimal outcome, especially when it follows a series of unsuccessful limb salvage procedures. This chapter focuses on clinical knowledge and practices which restore function for patients to pursue their daily activities and reach their future goals and potential.

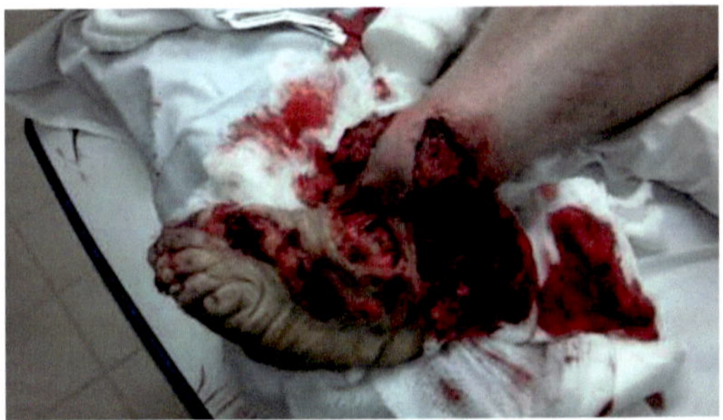

Fig. 17.1 Severely mangled extremity requiring amputation

General Demographics and Observations

Limb loss due to trauma constitutes a comparatively small percentage of the total amputations in the United States, with a greater percentage affecting the lower limbs [3, 4]. The majority of these life-changing injuries result from crush injuries secondary to workplace and motor vehicle accidents. A small percentage occurs as a result of military conflicts; however, battlefield injuries provide useful information regarding treatment [5–7]. In spite of the wide variety of physical presentations, there are a number of well-defined actions which should be taken to help patients recover from amputation, no matter what the cause, and become prosthetic users. A general timeline for prosthetic rehabilitation is presented

J. Rheinstein (✉)
Hanger Clinic, New York, NY, USA
e-mail: jrheinstein@hanger.com

K. Carroll
Hanger Clinic, Orlando, FL, USA
e-mail: kcarroll@hanger.com

P. Stevens
Department of Clinical and Scientific Affiars, Hanger Inc., Salt Lake City, UT, USA
e-mail: pstevens@hanger.com

© Springer Nature Switzerland AG 2021
R. A. Pensy, J. V. Ingari (eds.), *The Mangled Extremity*, https://doi.org/10.1007/978-3-319-56648-1_17

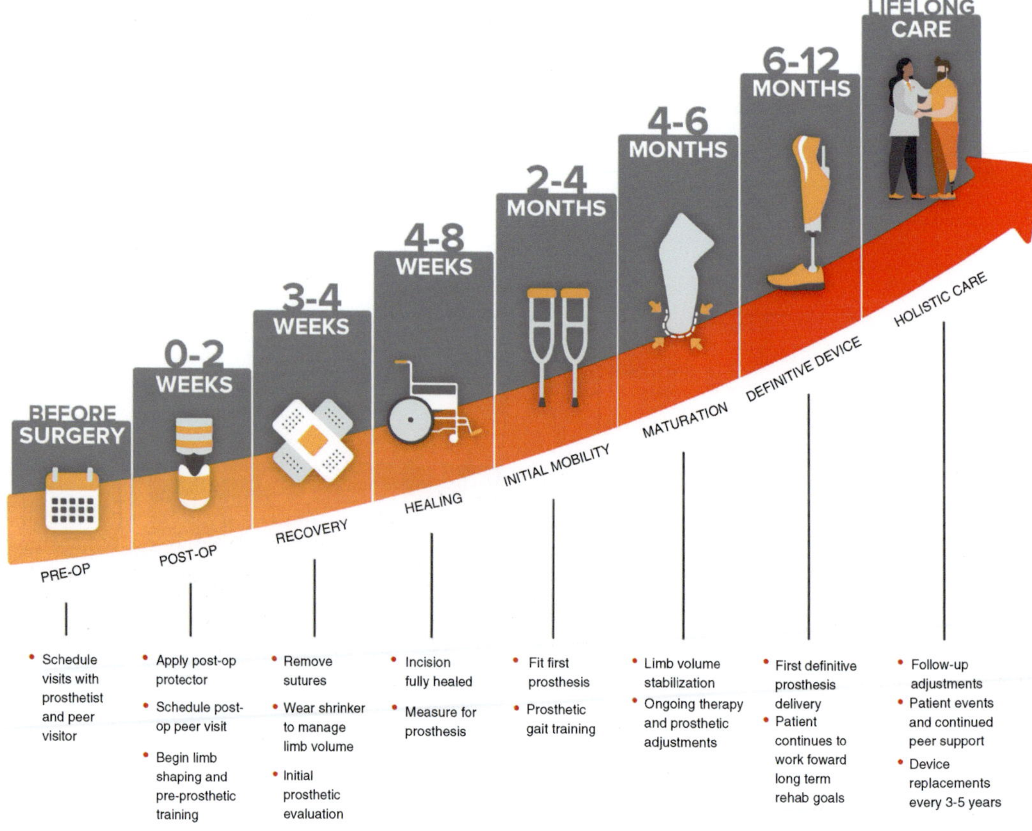

Fig. 17.2 General amputation timeline. (Courtesy of Hanger Clinic, Austin, TX)

below (Fig. 17.2). The time between milestones varies based on individual circumstances.

Upper limb amputations are most commonly observed among younger males in traumatic events [3] in contrast to lower limb amputations, which are predominantly observed among older, dysvascular individuals with comorbid health conditions. Congenital upper limb deficiencies and cancer-related amputations constitute less common causes of upper limb absence. Finger and hand amputations are ten times more common than transradial and transhumeral amputations [3]. The best available estimates from 2005 indicate that of the 1.6 million individuals living in the United States with limb loss, only 41,000 (8%) were living with major upper limb amputation [3].

Optimizing Patient Outcomes

To optimize patient outcomes, the following essential objectives should be addressed by the surgeon performing the amputation and delegated to other rehab team members, based on patients' needs and the team members' expertise: (1) reconstructive primary or revision amputation surgery with consideration of the demands of future prosthetic use including presurgical planning in collaboration with a prosthetist, (2) timely perioperative care which protects and prepares the residual limb after surgery, (3) patient education, (4) peer support and counseling, (5) physical and/or occupational therapy, (6) close collaboration with a rehabilitation team, (7) the provision of a functional prosthesis appropriate to each patient's needs and goals, (8) treatment of comorbid health conditions which may compromise function, and (9) the collection and monitoring of outcomes data on functional mobility, quality of life, and patient satisfaction.

Reconstructive Amputation Surgery

The objectives for amputation surgery are common to all patients in spite of variations in their presentations and mechanism of injury or underlying disease. A residual limb reconstructed with the following attributes will greatly enhance patients' prospects for useful prosthetic function and thus their quality of life: (1) sufficient vascular patency for healing, (2) adequate but not excessive soft tissue coverage for cushioning, (3) absence of chronic pain by effective treatment of nerves, (4) well-healed, non-adherent skin with enough mobility to withstand pressure and shear, (5) limb length which is neither too short nor too long at the level selected, (6) sufficient range of motion and muscle function in the joint proximal to amputation site without contractures created by muscle imbalances during closure, (7) limb shape which is neither too bulbous or pointed (Fig. 17.3), and (8) muscle and fascia surgically attached for soft tissue stability and power for movement. Achieving all these objectives may not always be possible. Choices and compromises are based on each patient's presentation, physical condition, other injuries requiring surgery, life needs, and goals. For example, optimal residual limb length may not be possible when there is a lack of available soft tissue coverage and skin healing. A team approach to surgical decision-making allows for consideration of different perspectives and lets patients know that the surgeon is willing to consider engaging others to achieve best possible outcome, rather than a "go-it-alone" mentality.

When multiple limb injuries are being treated in conjunction with a current or planned amputation, it is important to consider how to stage the reconstructive procedures. The amputated limb or the other injured limbs may be, at least temporarily, dependent on another limb's weight-bearing capacity. Significant weight-bearing through an amputated limb cannot commonly occur until 4 to 6 weeks postop. In these complex cases, a bent knee prosthesis may be employed for transtibial patients if weight-bearing is needed before complete surgical wound healing (Fig. 17.4) or an external fixator if the there is a fracture in a residual limb (Fig. 17.5). Rigid stabilization of other fractures to permit early weight-bearing should be considered when confronted with the patient who is likely to undergo amputation of a contralateral or distal limb. Other less critical surgical repairs, such a rotator cuff repair, can be staged until the patient regains weight-bearing capacity of the lower limbs.

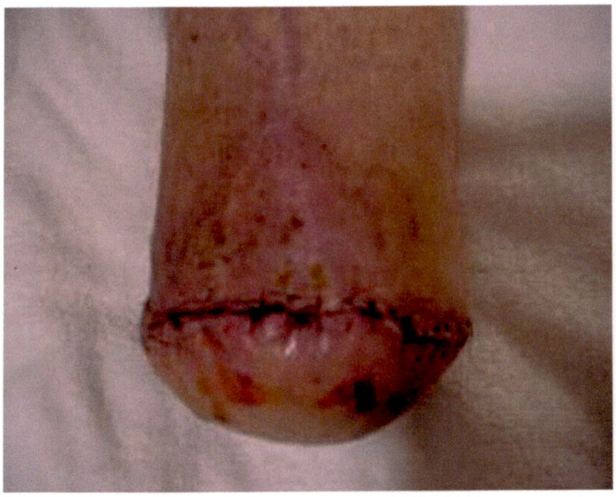
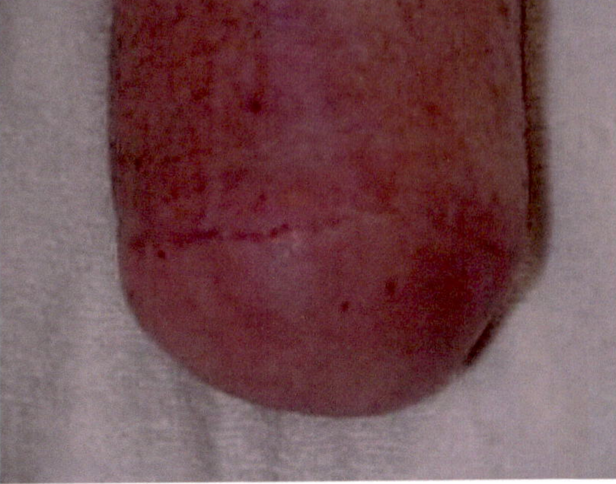

Fig. 17.3 Reconstructive amputation. (Courtesy of Dr. Lew C. Schon, Baltimore, MD)

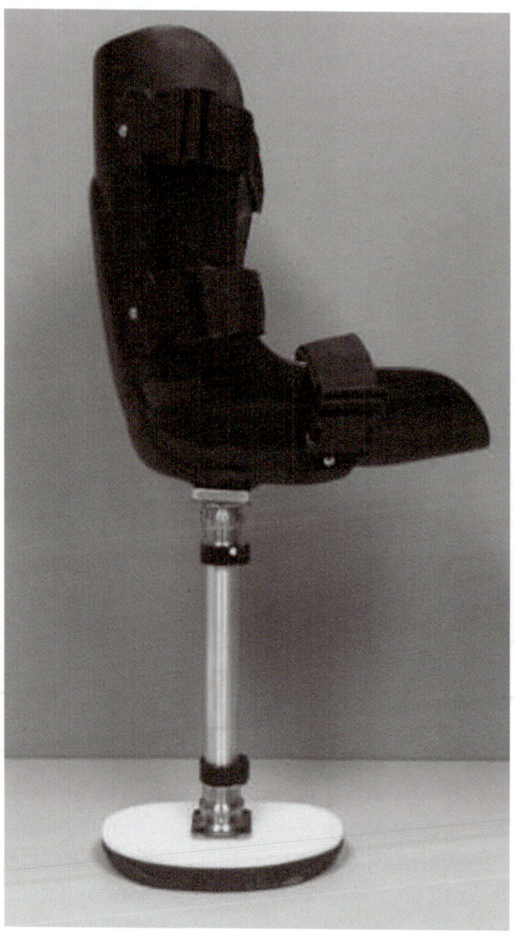

Fig. 17.4 Bent knee prosthesis. (Courtesy of Hanger Clinic, Austin, TX)

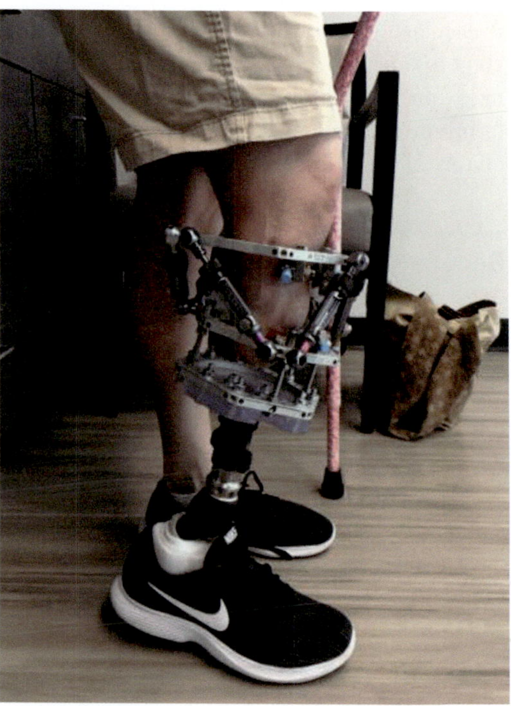

Fig. 17.5 External fixation on residual limb attached to a prosthesis. (Courtesy of Morgan Oxenrider, Hanger Clinic, Austin, TX)

Recommendations

A. *Employ surgical techniques which create an effectively reconstructed resilient residual limb.*
B. *Surgical closure should be performed with the knee in full extension and hip in full extension and adduction.*
C. *Understand the connection between surgical quality and rehab outcomes.*
D. *Encourage feedback between the rehab and surgical teams.*
E. *Whenever possible, it is beneficial for both the patient and the surgeon to have **preoperative consultations** with an experienced prosthetist.*
F. *If additional time is needed to bring surgical and rehab teams together to decide on a plan, the amputation can be **staged**, starting with a long guillotine procedure, while options for the final residual limb or hand shape are considered. Decisions regarding partial finger, partial hand, and multiple limb amputations can be especially complex and variable based on individual circumstances. Bringing surgeons and rehab specialists together also lets the patient know that this is a team effort and that the surgeon is willing to consider engaging others to achieve the best possible outcome.*

Revision Surgery

Reconstructive revision surgery should be considered when a patient is experiencing chronic pain, continual skin breakdown, or poor function, which persists in spite of multiple attempts to adjust or remake their prosthesis and/or therapy [8]. The decision to perform a revision may include many factors:

- Patient's goals, motivations, and state of mind
- Pain: degree and type
- Current function and potential for improvement
- History of prosthetic use
- Prosthetic considerations (space for components, weight, complexity, and durability)
- Cosmetic concerns
- Surgical history
- Patient's overall health and ability to tolerate surgery and anesthesia
- Healing potential
- Patient compliance with instructions
- Availability of an experienced surgeon
- Financial concerns such as insurance coverage and time away from work

Recommendations

1. *A variety of prosthetic materials and socket designs should be considered before revision surgery.*
2. *Some challenges with prosthetic wear can only be addressed by revisions to the residual limb.*

Perioperative Care

"Post-amputation management of the residual limb is an integral yet often overlooked element of surgical recovery and is instrumental in achieving optimal long-term patient outcomes." [9–11] Well-planned and vigilant postoperative care can significantly improve patients' opportunities for successful prosthetic rehabilitation. This care goes beyond healing the surgical wound by preparing the person and their residual limb to become a functioning prosthetic user. A recent set of Clinical Practice Guidelines [12] and published evidence [13] offers recommendations for three key elements of perioperative care including residual limb management, patient education, and peer mentoring.

Residual Limb Management

Postoperative, pre-prosthetic care prepares the residual limb for a more successful prosthetic fitting and earlier ambulation compared to soft dressings alone [14]. The goals of postoperative management are (1) to provide a clean wound-healing environment, (2) reduce swelling and associated pain, (3) protect the limb from external trauma, (4) reduce the incidence of knee flexion contractures, wound dehiscence, and decubitus, (5) reduce hospital length of stay, (6) decrease time before casting for initial prosthesis, (7) provide for earlier ambulation, and (8) ultimately facilitate each person's potential for their maximum rehabilitation with a faster return to activities of daily living (ADLs).

Recommendations

A. *Removable rigid dressings (RRD) (Fig. 17.6) should be used to reduce both the healing time of the residual limb and the time to prosthetic fitting following transtibial amputation.*
B. *Removable rigid dressings should be used as the preferred means of reducing postoperative edema following transtibial amputation.*
C. *Given the comparable wound infection rates observed with the two treatment options, removable rigid dressings are preferred over soft dressings for postoperative care.*
D. *Shrinker socks, tubular elastic, and silicone gel liners may be added to an RRD to aid in edema reduction and limb shaping. Appropriate padding should be in place to prevent skin breakdowns.*

Patient Education

Early education about prosthetics may also help reduce patient's anxiety about future function and the time needed for rehabilitation. An educational visit in the hospital by a board certified prosthetist is highly recommended to provide information about possible prosthetic options and the steps to prosthetic fitting. The visit should

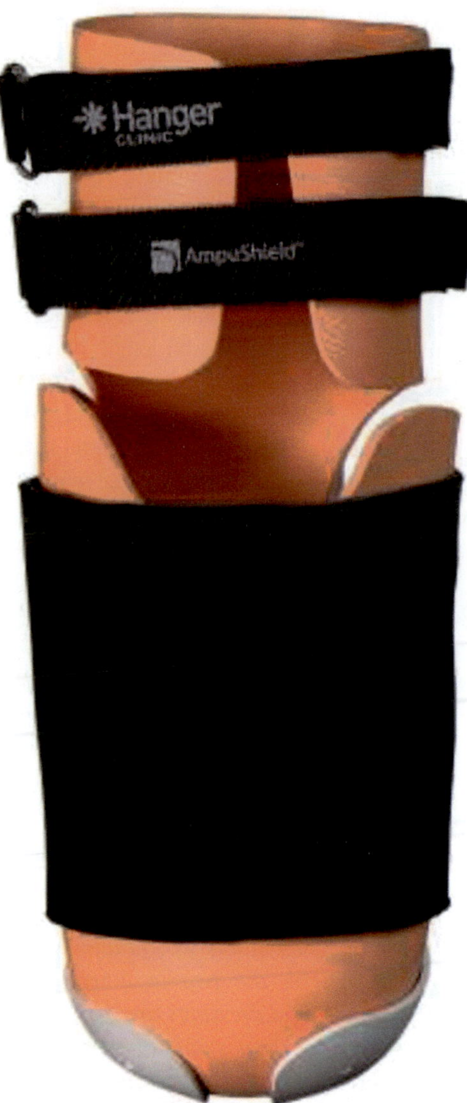

Fig. 17.6 AmpuShield postop protector RRD. (Courtesy of Hanger Clinic, Austin, TX)

stress the positive aspects of the patient's potential while setting goals and avoiding unreasonable expectations. Devastating as amputation can be, especially for a young person with so much of life still ahead of them, it is the task of the prosthetist to look beyond the tragic and terrible loss and focus on the future with the goal of restoring to each individual the capability of living their life to the fullest. Patients should also be cautioned that phantom limb sensation may lead to a

fall and injury if the missing limb is still perceived as being present and a limb protector has not been provided or is left off.

Recommendations

A. *During the perioperative period, written and/ or verbal patient education should be provided and may consist of the following topics tailored to individual conditions and needs:*

   - *Care of the residual limb*
   - *Phantom limb sensation*
   - *The rehabilitation process*
   - *Expectations and range of possible outcomes*
   - *General prosthetic information*
   - *Relevant financial information*
   - *Availability of support groups and peer mentors*

B. *Perioperative education must account for the following considerations:*

   - *Age and associated comorbidities, e.g., hearing or vision loss and cognitive or memory deficits*
   - *Current pain level and its impact on the patient's ability to absorb and retain information*
   - *Medication and its effect on a patient's ability to absorb and retain information*
   - *The current emotional state of the patient*
   - *An environment conducive to information exchange*
   - *The use of nonspecialist terms*
   - *The patient's purpose in receiving information: planning versus coping*

Peer Support and Mentoring

In addition to the many technological prosthetic solutions available, outcomes are often dramatically enhanced by the opportunity for peer visitations for the patient and their family. This provides

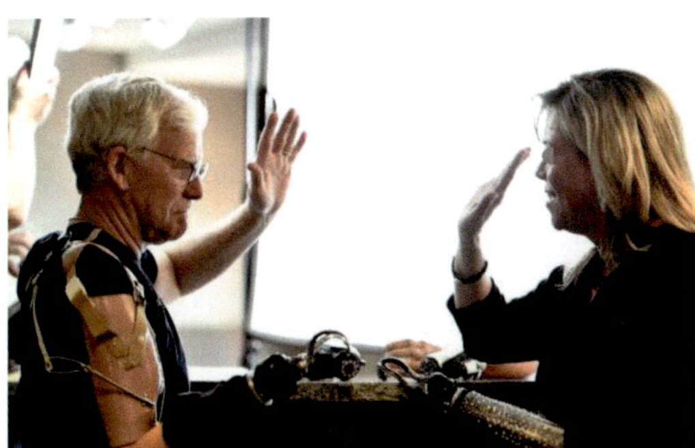

Fig. 17.7 Peer support

emotional support, motivation, and information. The amputee has likely experienced significant psychological stress from the immediate traumatic injury or the long-term struggle to save the limb [15]. A prompt initial visit by a trained peer visitor can be of immense value to the patient, and also to their family, especially in cases where the patient may have suffered brain injury or be sedated. A peer visitor, an amputee who has not only experienced firsthand the shock and adjustment to limb loss but has demonstrably succeeded as a prosthetic user, can often provide reassurance and hope. Their presence and willingness to answer questions can encourage and motivate patients for the journey that lies ahead as they heal and regain strength and mobility. Some patients also require additional help from professionals such as a psychologist or psychiatrist. Certified peer visitors can be located through AMPOWER http://www.empoweringamputees.org, the Amputee Coalition of America https://www.amputee-coalition.org, and Trauma Survivors Network www.traumasurvivorsnetwork.org. Many hospitals and rehab centers have their own support groups. If a group is not easily accessible, consider starting one with the help of one of the organizations mentioned above (Fig. 17.7).

Recommendation

A. *During the perioperative period, patients undergoing amputation should be given prompt access to appropriately trained peer mentors.*

Physical and Occupational Therapy

Physical and occupational therapists play an indispensable role in prosthetic rehabilitation. Most importantly, they help prepare patients for prosthetic use and advance their capabilities needed to effectively use their devices. The crucial objectives for therapy are scar management, range of motion, skin care, strength, balance, endurance, and prosthetic training. Therapists typically have contact with patients more frequently than other members of the rehab team and can reinforce important elements of prosthetic use such as skin care and volume management. The length of therapy and rehab may range widely depending on the patient's physical condition, cognitive abilities, and gait deviations.

In the early postoperative period, the avoidance of adherent scar tissue and flexion contractures falls largely within the purview of the therapist. Adherent scars are more susceptible to skin breakdown within a prosthesis and may also affect range of motion of the adjacent joints. The therapist will massage scar area and teach the patient self-care to keep the skin mobile to prevent it from adhering to the distal bone. This is addressed more fully in the chapter on therapy.

Preservation of range of motion and avoidance of flexion contractures should be addressed at the start of all prosthetic rehabilitation programs. Flexion contractures occur when the joint proximal to a newly amputated limb is not maintained in extension, the limb is not moved regularly, or from surgical closure in a flexed position. The restrictions that such contractures can impose may drastically limit their ambulation capabilities and thus their potential for participation in everyday, recreational, and vocational activities. As a therapist reduces a flexion contracture, the prosthetist must adjust the alignment of the prosthesis to accommodate the new joint angle. This highlights the importance of collaboration between rehab team members in providing high-quality prosthetic care for the patient. Patients should receive comprehensive physical therapy whenever new prostheses are provided and when indicated by functional deficits. This is especially important when technological improvements are made to successive designs of the prostheses.

Not every therapist is accustomed to working with prosthetic limbs, especially with a person who has suffered major traumatic injuries with one or more mangled extremities. Patients are encouraged to work with a physical therapist experienced in amputee rehabilitation to focus on balance, strength, and an efficient and symmetrical gait at a variety of walking and running speeds.

Recommendation

A. *Insure patients receive ample inpatient and outpatient physical therapy with an experienced therapist as soon as possible.*
B. *Additional physical therapy is indicated when a patient gets a new prosthesis or if they have functional deficits.*

Rehabilitation Team

The goal of restoring patients to their functional activities of daily living requires the participation of a team of skilled and experienced professionals, which includes the surgeon, prosthetist, PM&R physicians, physical and occupational therapists, and social workers. The team may also include other specialists based on each patient's unique requirements and comorbidities such as psychologists, psychiatrists, and medical specialists.

An individual's functional mobility and quality of life for many years to come may depend on the expertise of skilled providers at crucial moments in their recovery. Therefore, it is wise to carefully research and choose the most skilled and experienced prosthetists and rehabilitation specialists who can advise, support, and address a patient's specific needs, rather than settling for a convenient and readily available provider. In the case of less-frequently treated levels of amputation, such as a hip disarticulation or a hemipelvectomy, in complex injury cases, or multiple limb amputations, it is advisable to work with rehab team members who have specific experience in that area. Some patients may have to travel to receive this high level of care. Other providers and colleagues can often make referrals to recognized experts. The military is well-known for its highly knowledgeable professionals in the rehabilitation of mangled extremities and may offer guidance regarding dedicated experts in specified areas of the country.

Many victims of traumatic amputations are younger and want to go back to work. They need rehabilitation and prostheses focused on the activities specific to their vocation. The rehab team may collaborate with the local Department of Vocational Rehabilitation to help patients work around their physical challenges and provide prostheses which allow them to regain their vocation.

Recommendations

A. *A physiatrist can be extremely helpful by coordinating the efforts of the various team members.*
B. *Seek outside expertise for complex cases.*

1. **Collect and monitor outcomes**
   By collecting mobility data, the rehab team can detect changes which indicate successful treatment or the need for modifications. Recent studies highlight the relationship between mobility, quality of life, and patient satisfaction [16] (Fig. 17.8).

Recommendations

A. *Monitor patients' outcomes as they progress through rehabilitation and adjust therapy treatments and prosthetic care accordingly.*
B. *Outcomes data and clear office notes are helpful in obtaining payment for medical, therapy, and prosthetic care.*

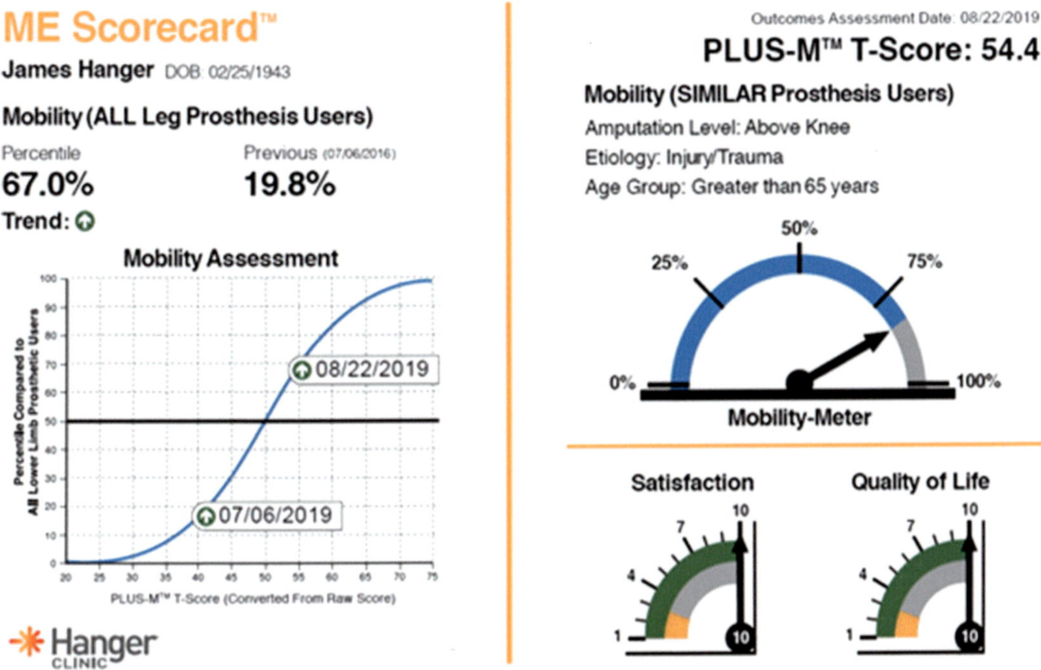

Fig. 17.8 Outcomes – mobility score card. (Courtesy of Hanger Clinic, Austin, TX)

Anticipated Outcomes for Upper and Lower Limb Prostheses

No prosthesis can fully duplicate the function and appearance of a normal human extremity. The choice of a single prosthesis or combination of prostheses is determined by the patient's physical condition, capabilities, motivation, limitations, personal preferences, and past prosthetic history as well as their requirements and goals for activities of daily living, vocation, and hobbies. Each prosthetic design has benefits and shortcomings in terms of functional capabilities, appearance, weight, environmental resilience, maintenance, and cost. These design requirements may change as patients age, progress through rehabilitation, their body and body image changes, their residual limb changes, they face different environmental conditions, their activities of daily living, and/or their goals change. Depending on their needs, different prostheses may be required for different tasks. Replacement intervals are also influenced by these factors.

There is no precise formula to predict how an individual will use prosthetic devices and which devices they will need in the future. Success is ultimately judged by the wearer and in the case of children, their parents, in terms of the utility of a prosthesis and how it meets their own individual needs and goals. Factors which may predict prosthetic use include (1) physical and cognitive capabilities and limitations, (2) motivation, (3) comorbid medical conditions, (4) psychological issues, (5) environmental factors, and (6) access to appropriate care including financial resources. Some factors may be positively influenced with interventions such as changes to prosthetic design, additional prosthetic devices, or training with a physical or occupational therapist, surgery to correct residual limb problems, and treatment of psychological or emotional issues. Other predictors such as very short limb length, poor skin quality, loss of muscle function, damaged joints, chronic pain, or traumatic brain injury are permanent and make prosthetic use more challenging, although not impossible. An individual's history of prosthetic use and the pattern of their current use are among the factors which can be used to predict their future prosthetic use.

Prosthetic Care for the Upper Extremity

Upper limb amputation presents a distinct set of challenges. Despite continued technologic advances in upper limb prosthetic rehabilitation, modern devices can only partially replicate the function, dexterity, and appearance of the lost extremity. In addition, upper limb amputation is often associated with memories of an acute traumatic event that often precipitate an unexpected and often undesirable change in vocation. Collectively, these factors and demographics may explain why up to one-third of those with upper limb amputation exhibit symptoms of clinical depression, as covered in another chapter in this text [17, 18]. As a result, individuals who have sustained an acquired amputation reported reduced life satisfaction and health-related quality of life relative to the general population [19].

Pain constitutes another core consideration in the management of upper limb amputation. The pain experienced by those with upper limb absence is more universal, frequent, and intense than that associated with lower limb amputation [16]. Some type of chronic pain is experienced by almost all individuals with upper limb loss. Painful and non-painful phantom sensations are the most prevalent sources of pain, followed by residual limb pain and pain in the sound side limb, back, or neck due to overuse injury [20]. However, while phantom limb pain is a frequent source of discomfort, for most individuals, it appears to be less disruptive to daily activity than other sources of pain [15, 18].

By contrast, overuse pain, experienced in the sound side limb, neck, and shoulder girdle, appears to be the most disruptive source of pain [18]. In fact, recent observations suggest that musculoskeletal overuse pains may have a more deleterious effect on an individual's perceived general and mental health than the absence of the limb itself [21]. Sources of overuse pain include epicondylitis, shoulder impingement, tenosynovitis, osteoarthritis, reflex sympathetic dystrophy type symptoms, and carpal tunnel syndrome [22]. Pain prevalence rates and pain locations vary with published reports with 30% to nearly 60% of queried patients reporting pain in the neck, back, and sound side limb [18–20, 23].

Anticipated Outcomes with Upper Limb Prostheses

Given the tremendous strength, dexterity, and utility of the physiologic hand, it is important for patients, family members, referring physicians, healthcare professionals, and those in case management and reimbursement to maintain and communicate to patients reasonable and accurate expectations relating to anticipated outcomes with upper limb prostheses. An international group of prosthetic users and experienced clinical specialists has attempted to define appropriate standards for success. In this effort, a number of idealistic definitions were rejected including, "the use of a prosthesis for pre-amputation job or activities," "a person's ability to perform activities to the same standards as they did before the limb loss," and "the ability to perform activities within the same time parameters as they did before." Rather, definitions of successful upper limb prosthetic rehabilitation included wearing an upper limb prosthesis for specific activities, demonstrating the ability to perform personal care and activities of daily living without help from other people, experiencing satisfaction with one's functional abilities, and performing to the best of one's ability [24].

An accurate understanding of this consensus definition is necessary to help establish and reinforce appropriate, reasonable expectations throughout the process of rehabilitation and can prevent the frustrating pursuit of unattainable goals. Individuals who have sustained upper limb loss should be made aware that successful use of a prosthesis will vary from individual to individual. While some users prefer to wear their device throughout the entire day on a daily basis, others are more measured in their use, donning their prostheses only to engage in bimanual activities and removing the device upon completion. Given the limitations of currently available prosthetic technologies compared to their missing limb, many active upper limb prosthesis users view their prosthesis as a "functional tool" rather than a restoration of the lost extremity that has been fully integrated into their body image.

The conception and pursuit of unrealistic prosthetic expectations may contribute in part to an individual's decision to abandon their upper limb prostheses. Reported definitions and rates of prosthetic abandonment within this population are extremely variable, with systematic review suggesting average abandonment rates of approximately 25% among adults with acquired limb absence [25]. Successful use of an upper limb prosthesis can be undermined by a lack of access to any of the following: appropriate prosthetic technology, an experienced upper limb prosthetist, and a knowledgeable occupational therapist. In spite of prosthesis abandonment, every person with limb loss should be given the opportunity for prosthetic use.

The provision of appropriate prostheses constitutes an important step in upper limb prosthetic rehabilitation. However, prosthetic acceptance, utilization, and integration into daily activity usually require a significant amount of work with a therapist who has experience in training individuals with upper limb prosthetics. Team rehabilitation with regular interaction between the physician, therapist, prosthetist, and end user is the ideal setting for successful integration of a prosthesis following upper limb amputation. A peer visit with a person who has a similar level of amputation, may also be helpful with a person's psychological adjustment to limb loss and motivation. A preoperative consultation with an experienced upper limb prosthetist can be helpful when deciding between amputation levels and setting patient expectations. If a visit is precluded by the traumatic nature of an upper limb amputation, an early postoperative visit is usually helpful.

Upper Limb Prosthetic Designs

The basic design elements of an upper limb prosthesis include (1) the socket in which the residual limb is placed, (2) a means of suspension, (3) one or more terminal devices which provide active or passive prehension and opposition, and (4) the mechanism of control (body or externally powered). Selections are made based on the user's needs, goals, and physical and cognitive capabilities as established from a detailed history and evaluation. For many users, restoration of a majority of pre-amputation activities and function requires more than one type of prostheses. For example, while an externally powered prosthesis with myoelectric control may serve as a primary device providing both dexterity and appropriate grip strength, such a device might be contraindicated for applications in wet or dirty environments. A more resilient, body-powered prosthesis can supplement the user's need for bimanual function in different applications and environments.

Level-Specific Considerations

Partial Finger Amputations

For decades, the prosthetic management of partial finger amputations was largely confined to high-definition silicone restorations. These prostheses provide improvements to functional dexterity by restoring finger length for opposition which is especially useful to patients when digits 1–3 are involved. They can also restore an aesthetically acceptable appearance of the fingers and protect the sensitive distal amputation site (Fig. 17.9).

Recent years have seen the development of new technologies that have expanded the range of available prosthetic solutions. Improved dexterity can be provided for finger amputations as distal as the DIP level using rigid linkage or cable mechanisms in which proximal joint movements generate movement at distal prosthetic segments (Fig. 17.10). Unfortunately, due to soft tissue compression and mechanical inefficiencies, the resultant power is comparatively weak. When grip strength and durability are the predominant objective, ratcheted manually adjustable position digit systems can facilitate a range of functional grips across various hand positions (Fig. 17.11). While these systems may provide increased function, they have a mechanical appearance which

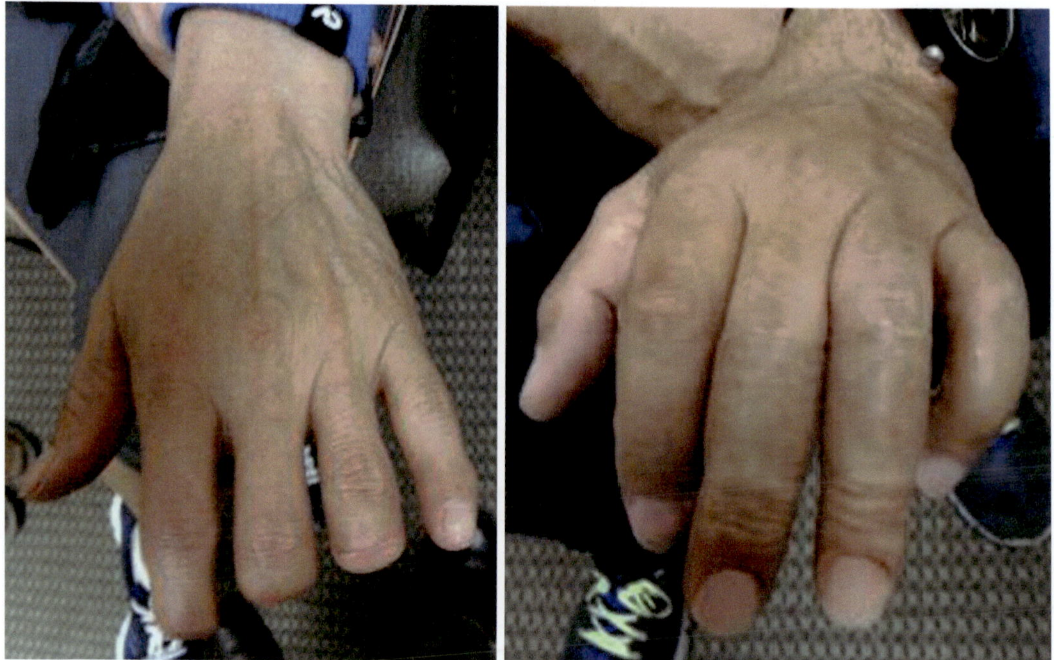

Fig. 17.9 High-definition silicone restoration of partial finger amputations. (Courtesy of Philip M. Stevens, Salt Lake City, UT)

Fig. 17.10 Partial M-finger prosthesis engineered such that MCP flexion creates flexion at a prosthetic IP joint. (Courtesy of Partial Hand Solutions, Warren, MI)

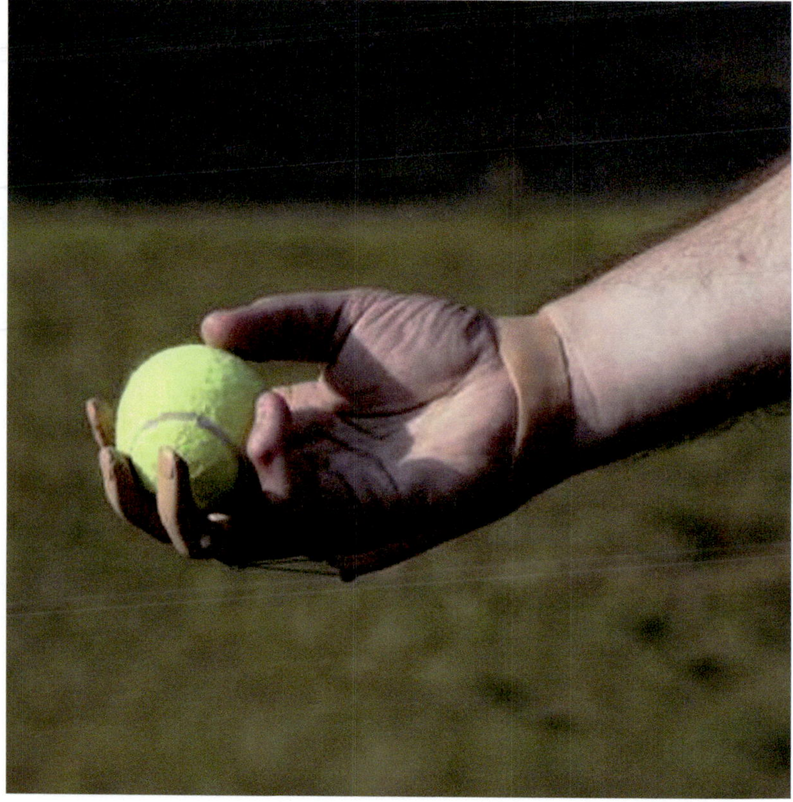

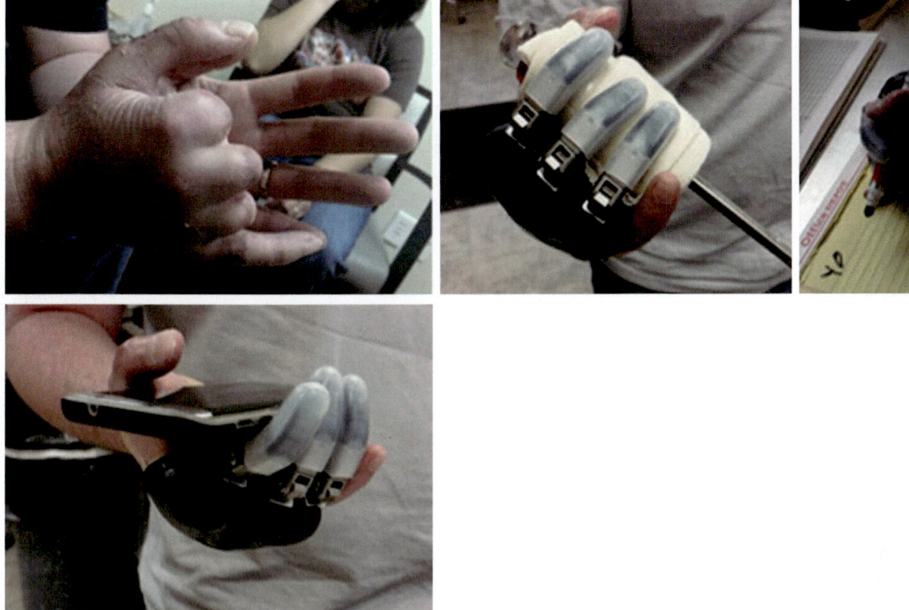

Fig. 17.11 Partial Titan Fingers that can be passively ratcheted into a desired flexion ranges. (Courtesy of Philip M. Stevens, Salt Lake City, UT), Salt Lake City, UT)

may cause patients to select the more cosmetic high-definition silicone restoration.

Partial Hand Amputations

As with partial finger solutions, partial hand solutions have historically been limited to nonadjustable opposition posts and silicone restorations (Fig. 17.12). Recent years have seen the introduction of body-powered, cable-driven digit systems for improved dexterity (Fig. 17.13) and passively adjustable digit systems for improved grip across a range of hand positions (Fig. 17.14). In addition, externally powered digit systems are available that provide light to moderate duty function, generally controlled through myoelectric inputs (Fig. 17.15). Myoelectric control in partial-hand prostheses can be enhanced by the Starfish procedure, whereby the interossei muscles for each digit are transferred to the dorsum of the hand without damaging the neurovascular pedicles. These muscles then serve as myoelectric sites for control of finger flexion by an externally powered prosthesis which allows each digit to move independently [26].

Wrist Disarticulation Amputations

Wrist disarticulation prosthetic solutions can be characterized as passive, myoelectric, body powered, or activity specific. The primary benefits are a long level arm for lifting, lower proximal trim lines, active pronation and supination, and a wide distal surface for pushing. The bulbous nature of the styloids may allow the prosthesis to be self-suspending with lower proximal trim lines for comfort. The primary limitation to prosthetic management at the wrist disarticulation level is the extended length residual limb which precludes the use of most wrist rotation components and may cause cosmetic concerns.

Transradial Amputations

Transradial amputations are the most commonly encountered major amputation level and allow patients to perform many ADLs with an appropriate prosthesis. When circumstances allow, preserving the anatomic elbow joint should be a

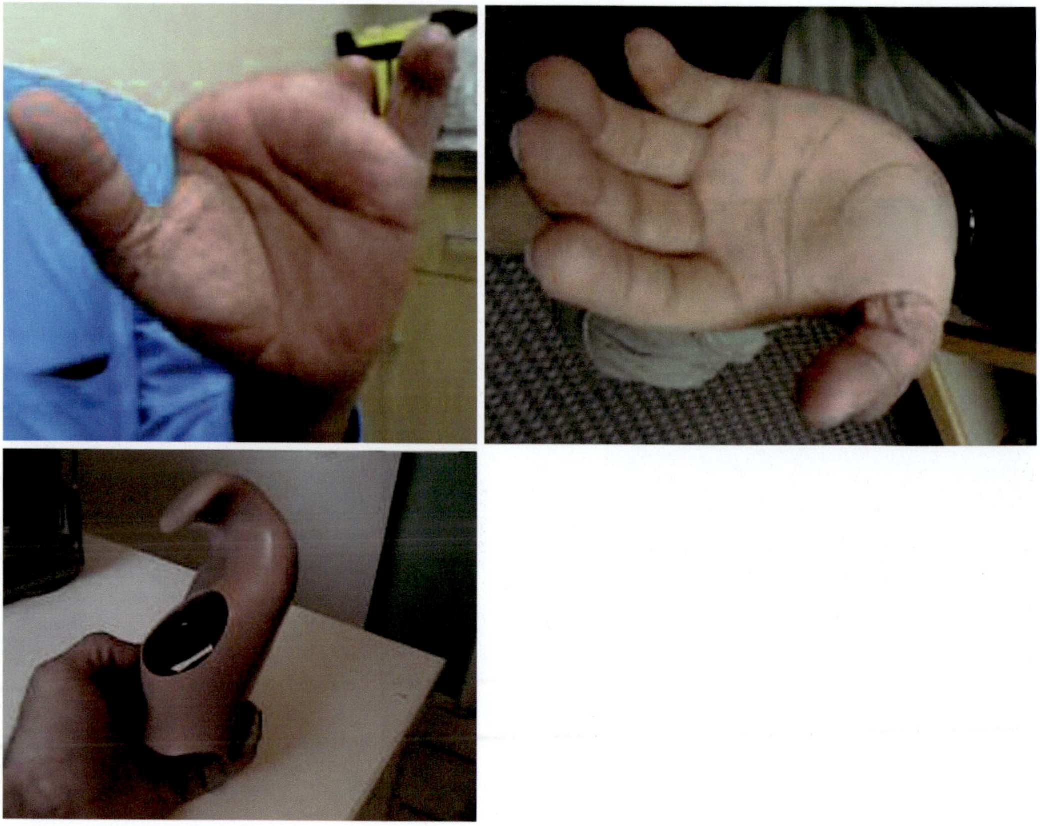

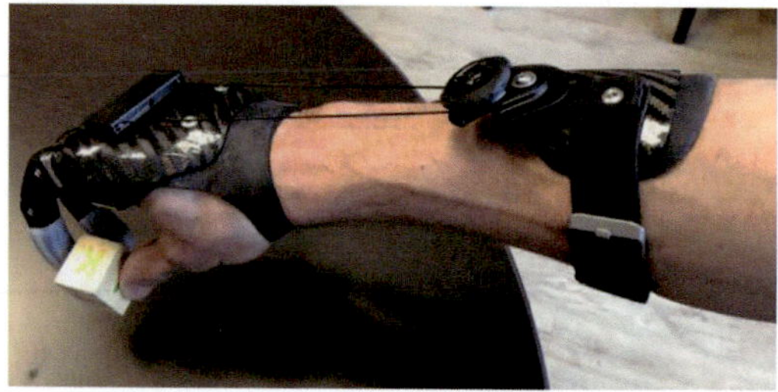

Fig. 17.12 Static opposition post and silicone restoration for partial hand amputation. (Courtesy of Philip M. Stevens, Salt Lake City, UT, and John Rheinstein, New York, NY)

Fig. 17.13 Body-powered, cable-driven M-finger prosthesis. (Courtesy of Partial Hand Solutions, Warren, MI)

priority. An amputation that retains approximately two-thirds of forearm length generally has good strength, lifting capacity, and some residual pronation/supination while still providing room for prosthetic components. Importantly, shorter transradial limbs can also be fit effectively with a prosthesis.

A range of prosthetic options are available including passive, body-powered, externally powered (usually controlled by myoelectric signals), and activity-specific prostheses. Hooks, either body powered or electric, are selected over myoelectric prostheses for their lower bulk and better visibility of objects (Fig. 17.16). Anthropomorphic terminal devices (i.e., hands) are preferred for their aesthetic benefits and broader gripping surfaces (Fig. 17.17). Recent years have seen the introduction of multi-articulate electric hand systems that provide an extensive range of grip patterns and hand gestures (Fig. 17.18). These devices are largely limited to light and moderate usage. Unfortunately, the decision between body-powered and electric systems is often determined by available insurance coverage. Myoelectric prostheses, viewed as the standard of care in many European healthcare systems, are excluded from some US healthcare plans. Externally powered terminal devices provide substantially more gripping power with less effort than their body-powered equivalents and operating motions which are closer to nor-

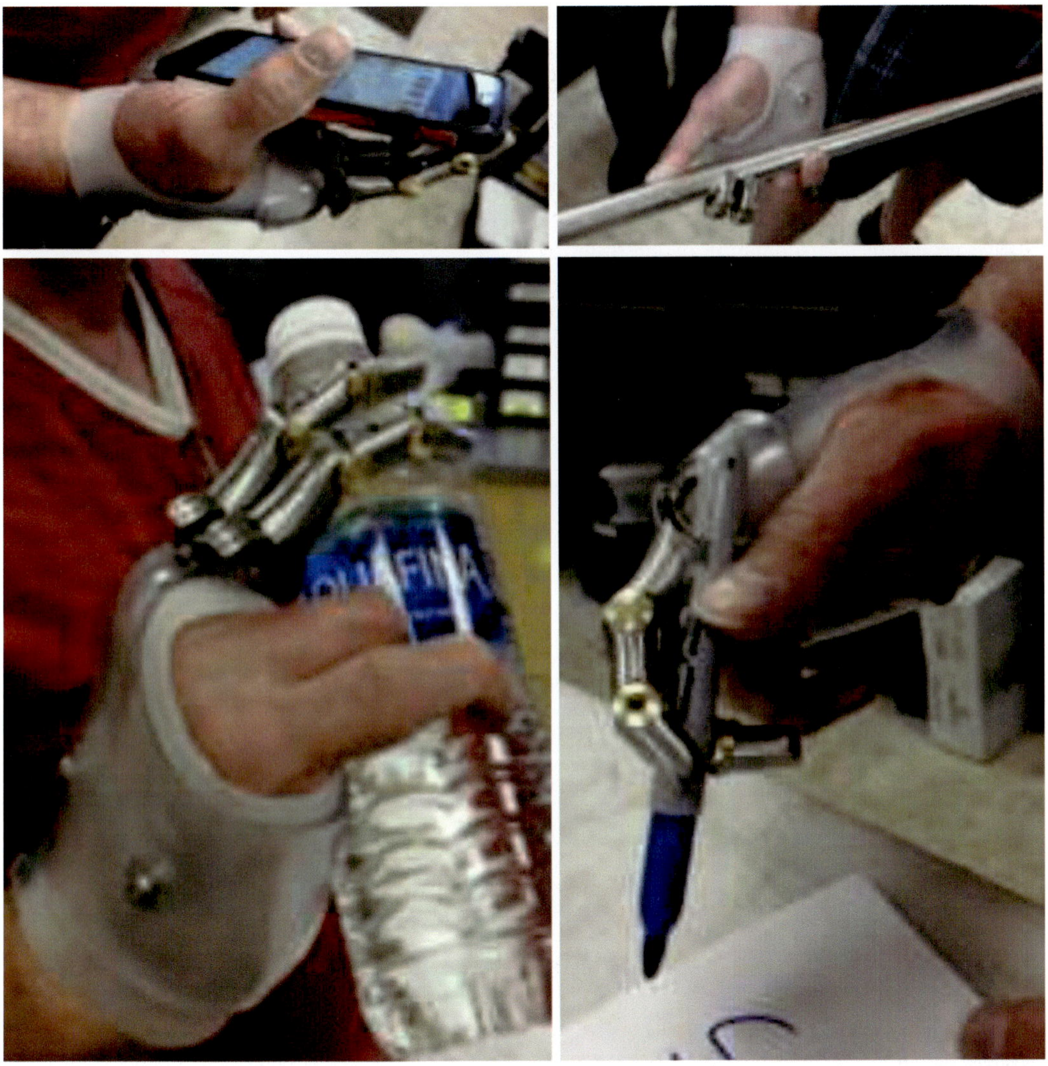

Fig. 17.14 Passively adjustable Point Design digit prosthesis demonstrating a range of grasping positions. (Courtesy of Philip M. Stevens, Salt Lake City, UT)

Fig. 17.15 Myoelectrically controlled partial hand prostheses. (Courtesy of Philip M. Stevens, Salt Lake City UT) and Ossur, Reykjavik, Iceland)

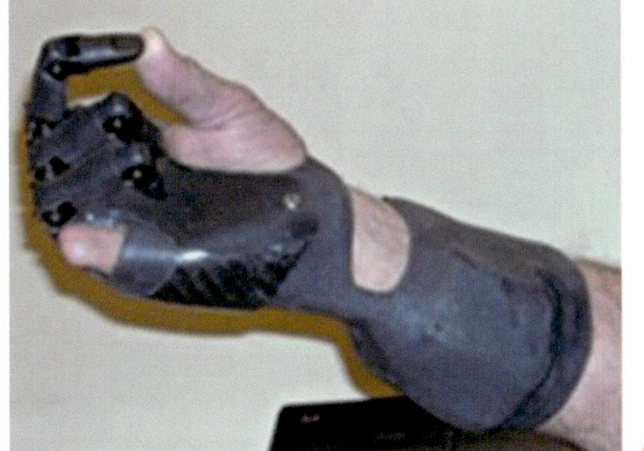
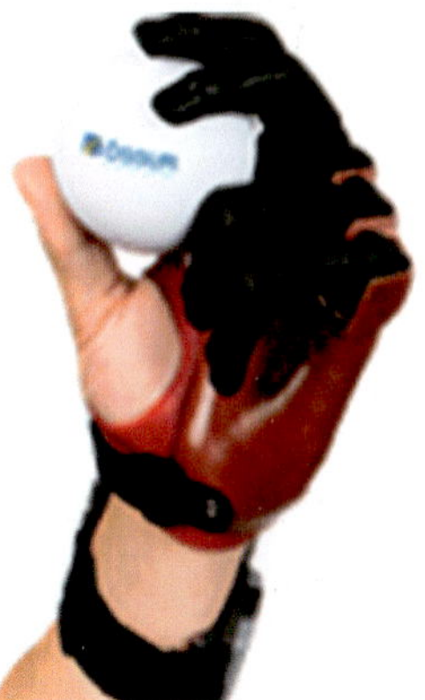

mal. Body-powered systems provide the user with proprioceptive input on the position of the hook or hand and are substantially less expensive, lighter, more resistant to environmental damage, and easier to maintain.

For myoelectric systems, electric wrist rotators can be considered, allowing active control of the relative pronation and supination of the terminal device. In traditional duel site myoelectric control, this introduces the challenge of controlling four degrees of freedom (hand open/close and wrist pronation/supination) with two myoelectric inputs (wrist flexors and wrist extensors). The timing and intensity of these signals can be used to alternate control between the wrist and hand function.

Through Elbow Amputations

Through-elbow amputations offer some advantages but have inherent limitations that make them challenging to manage with a prosthesis. The long residual limb length provides mechanical advantage for lifting and pushing activities. If the humeral condyles are preserved and redundant tissue is minimal, self-suspending sockets can be fabricated which give patients active control of internal and external humeral rotation. The length

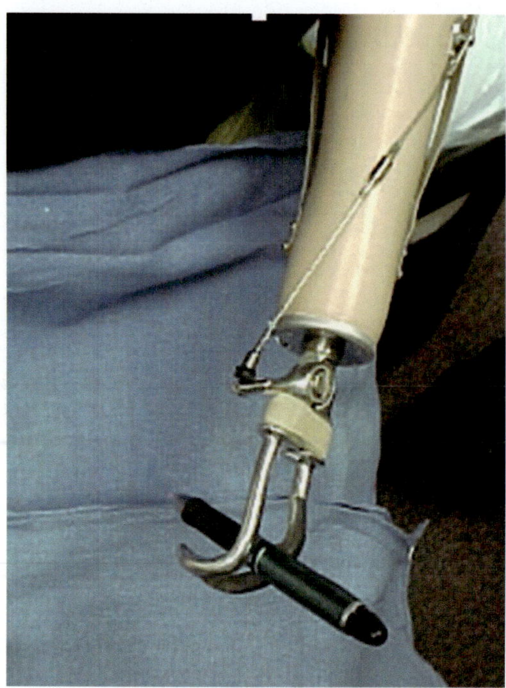

Fig. 17.16 Body-powered prosthesis with hook terminal device. (Courtesy of Philip M. Stevens, Salt Lake City, UT)

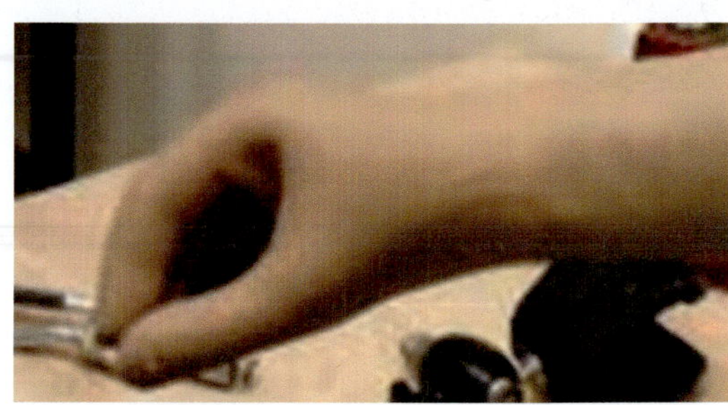

Fig. 17.17 Body-powered prosthesis with single-grip hand terminal device. (Courtesy of Philip M. Stevens, Salt Lake City, UT)

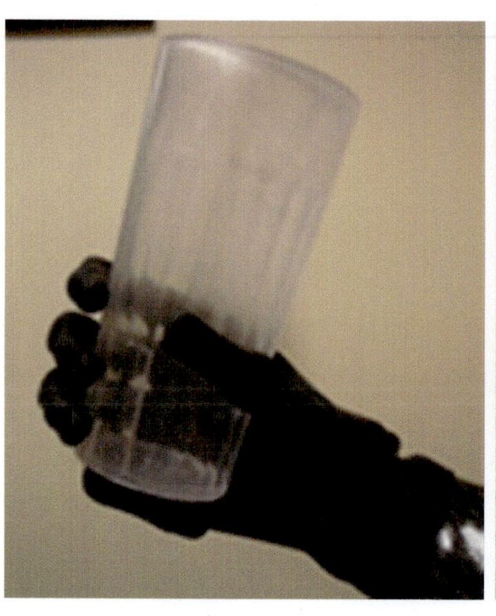
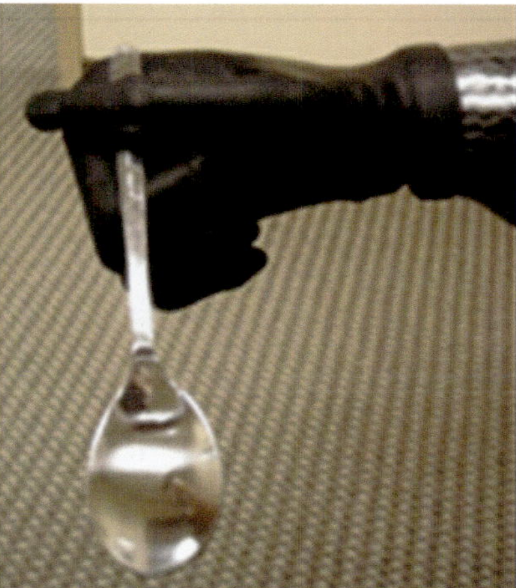
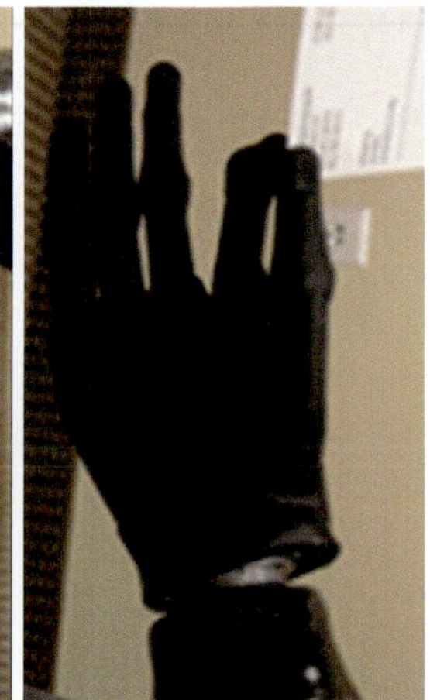

Fig. 17.18 Multi-articulate I-limb hand demonstrating a range of grip patterns. (Courtesy of Philip M. Stevens, Salt Lake City, UT)

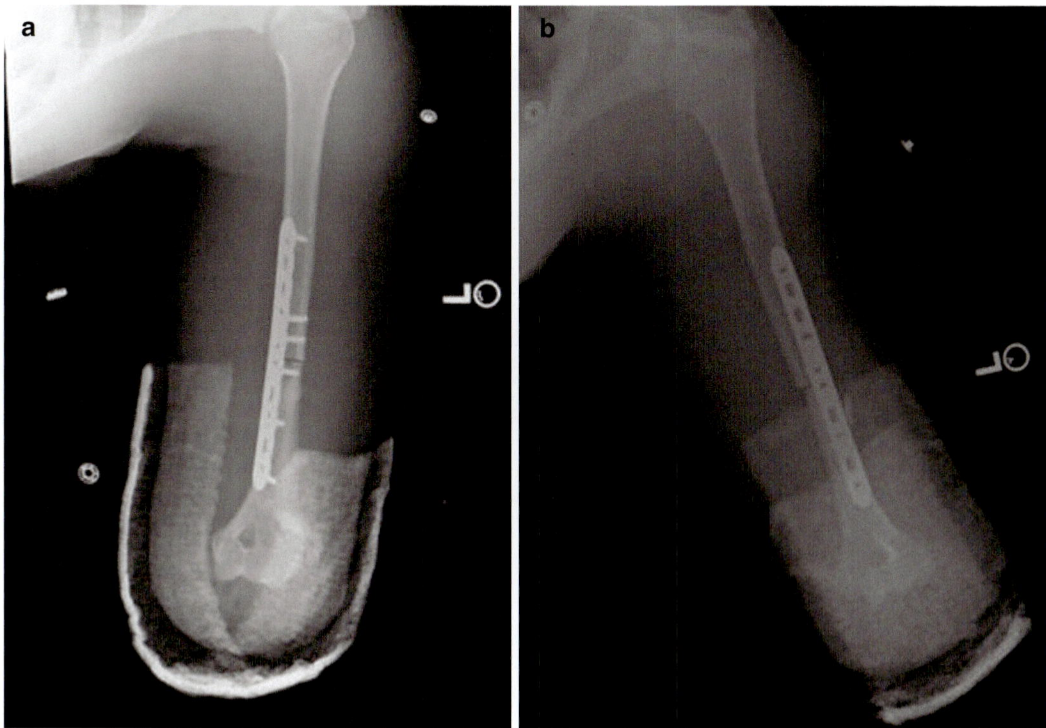

Fig. 17.19 Humeral shortening osteotomy. (Beltran, M J. Military Medicine, 175, 9:693, 2010)

of this amputation level precludes the use of self-contained prosthetic elbow joints and requires the use of outside locking elbow joints. Such joints increase the bulk of the prosthesis and are mechanically less durable than transhumeral elbow options. Prostheses at this level are generally body powered, although hybrid systems with body-powered elbow joints and electric terminal devices are an effective option. A shortening osteotomy, where a section of the humerus is removed and the condyles preserved, offers the benefits of a through-elbow amputation and allows for the use of a standard prosthetic elbow (Fig. 17.19).

Transhumeral Amputations

The standard transhumeral residual limb presents several challenges to successful prosthetic management due to the cylindrical shape of the residual humerus, the conical dimensions of the residual limb, and the lack of distal insertions of the residual muscles. These characteristics can make prosthetic suspension challenging and may allow rotation of the prosthesis about the long axis of the limb. As a result, clinicians generally attempt to stabilize the connection between the user and their prosthesis by broad proximal socket coverage as well as straps and harnesses that cross the shoulder girdle to the contralateral shoulder or chest wall, all of which limit the mobility of the affected shoulder joint. An angle osteotomy, where a piece of the distal humerus is attached at 90° to the shaft of the humerus, provides improved rotational control and suspension over a standard transhumeral amputation [27] (Fig. 17.20).

Prosthetic solutions are primarily body powered, myoelectric, or a "hybrid" combination of the two. With body-powered systems, a single shared-control cable is generally used to regulate elbow and terminal device position. A second cable locks and unlocks the elbow joint. Thus, activation of the elbow and terminal device is inherently sequential.

Myoelectric systems provide increased grip strength in the terminal device and the possibility

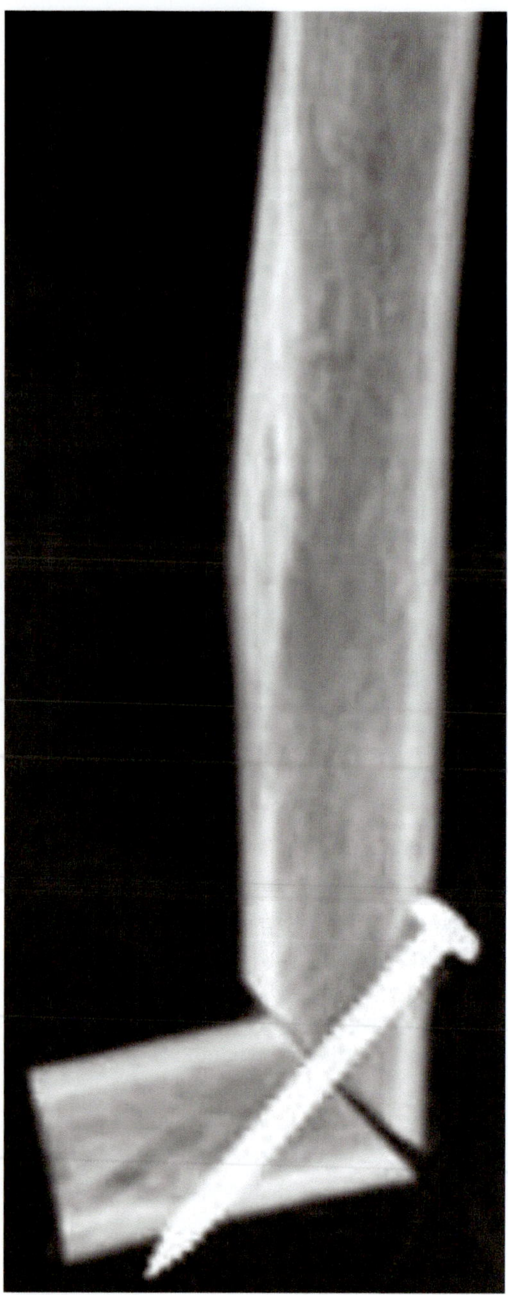

Fig. 17.20 Angle osteotomy. (Arch Orthop Trauma Surg 116, 263–265, 1997)

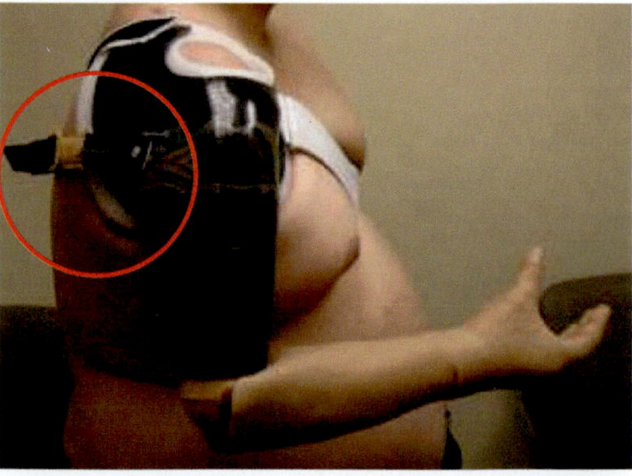

Fig. 17.21 Linear transducer incorporated in the posterior harness of a transhumeral prosthesis. (Courtesy of Philip M. Stevens, Salt Lake City, UT)

user to sequentially switch active control between the terminal device and the elbow, as well as a wrist rotator when desired. Alternately, control of the elbow position is frequently regulated by a linear transducer imbedded in the suspension harness (Fig. 17.21). Glenohumeral flexion or shoulder protraction elongates the transducer, producing elbow flexion. Glenohumeral extension or shoulder retraction permits elastic return in the transducer, signaling elbow extension. This allows myoelectric signals from the biceps and triceps to be dedicated to wrist and terminal device functions, providing the ability for simultaneous hand and elbow function.

In hybrid systems, a myoelectric terminal device is generally combined with a body-powered elbow. This reduces the weight of the prosthesis considerably by omitting the heavier electric elbow and dedicating the advanced strength and dexterity of external power to the terminal device where it is generally more beneficial to the user. Passive and activity-specific designs are less common at this level, but still available (Fig. 17.22).

of simultaneous control of the elbow and terminal device, depending upon the control strategy. When myoelectric signals are the sole means of control, the control strategy described above for transradial applications can be used to allow the

Shoulder Girdle Amputations

Shoulder-level prostheses are challenging due to the need to control multiple degrees of freedom at the terminal device, wrist, elbow, and shoulder with a limited number of control inputs

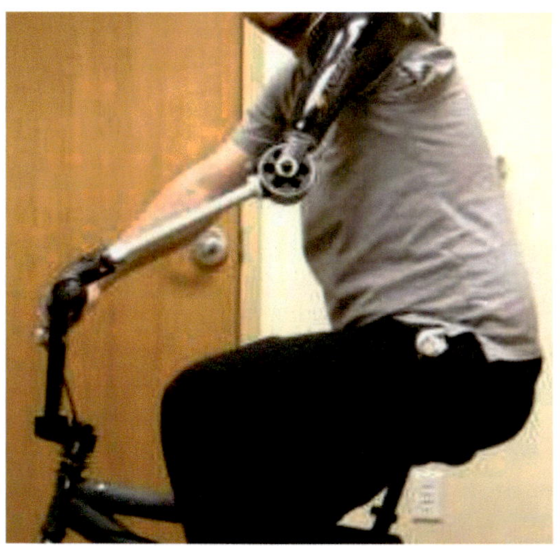

Fig. 17.22 Activity-specific cycling prosthesis for a transhumeral prosthesis user. (Courtesy of Philip M. Stevens, Salt Lake City, UT)

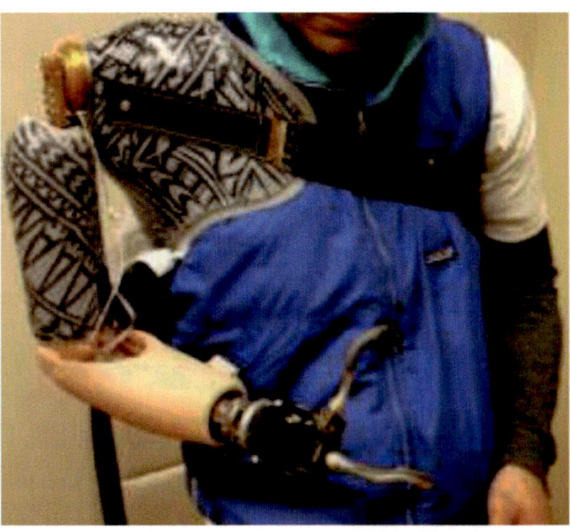

Fig. 17.23 Hybrid shoulder disarticulation prosthesis with passive shoulder, passive locking elbow, and electric hook. (Courtesy of Philip M. Stevens, Salt Lake City, UT)

and little surface area from which to suspend the prosthesis. Further, the size of the resulting device increases its weight. Purely myoelectric systems provide the highest level of dexterity and strength, but at an increased weight of the prosthesis. Purely body-powered systems are lighter and more easily tolerated by the user but provide a weaker grip force and require a series of sequential gross body motions to provide movement at the various joints throughout the system. Often there is insufficient range of motion and strength to effectively use a body-powered system at this level of amputation. Hybrid prostheses are common, in which a passively positioned shoulder joint is coupled with a passively positioned or body-powered elbow and an externally powered terminal device (Fig. 17.23). If an externally powered elbow is indicated, a linear transducer can control the elbow, while electrodes control the terminal device (Fig. 17.24).

At the shoulder level, the limited functionality and relatively high weight of available prosthetic technologies may discourage full-time daily use. Prosthetic users at this amputation level, especially unilateral users, may eventually choose to wear their devices for specific activities.

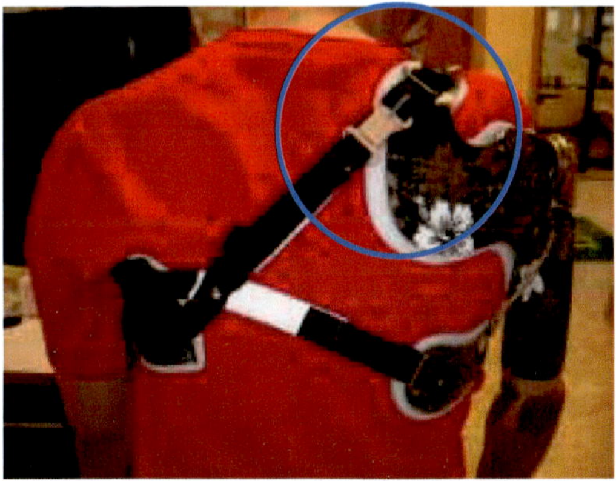

Fig. 17.24 Externally powered shoulder disarticulation prosthesis. Terminal device is controlled through two myoelectrodes on the torso. A linear transducer controls elbow position by shoulder elevation and depression. (Courtesy of Philip M. Stevens, Salt Lake City, UT)

Advancements in Upper Limb Prosthetics

There are a number of developing upper limb prosthetic advancements that are likely to have a substantial impact on future management strategies leading to improvements in functional benefits, day-to-day acceptance, and utilization rates. These include control strategies, sensory restoration, and methods of attachment.

Control Strategies

The current standard in myoelectric control is a two-site system in which two, generally antagonistic muscles on the residual limb provide input signals that directly control opposing prosthetic movements (i.e., opening and closing of a terminal device or flexion and extension of the elbow). However, even at relatively distal amputation levels, this method of control is nonnative as with wrist flexors and extensors controlling the prehension of the prosthetic hand. At more proximal amputation levels, this disparity between the muscle groups that provide input signals and the resultant prosthetic motions becomes increasingly removed, as muscles of the upper arm, shoulder girdle, and torso are called upon to signal movements of prosthetic terminal devices and wrist movements. Additionally, at increasingly proximal levels of amputation, the remaining muscle groups are often utilized to signal prosthetic motions at multiple joint segments. For example, in the management of shoulder-level amputations, muscles on the chest wall and upper back are frequently used to control movement of a prosthetic elbow, wrist, and terminal device by sequentially switching control from one joint segment to another before initiating prosthetic movement.

Targeted muscle reinnervation (TMR) represents one novel attempt to address this limitation. In this approach, proximal muscle groups are surgically divided into two or more muscle bellies, subsequently separated by a boundary of adipose tissue. Then, the residual nerves of the brachial plexus are identified, separated, and individually transferred to reinnervate these new targeted muscle bellies (Fig. 17.25). Once reinnervation has occurred, the patient can produce a greater number of independent myoelectric control signals that have a more natural association between the signaling nerve and the resultant prosthetic motions [28]. Another approach to prosthetic control is regenerative peripheral nerve interfaces (RPNIs). These free muscle grafts are used as physiological targets for peripheral nerve ingrowth providing discrete EMG implant sites. In addition both TMR and RPNI have shown efficacy for treatment of symptomatic post-amputation neuromas and phantom pain [29, 30].

A related advancement is seen in the development of myoelectric pattern recognition. In the

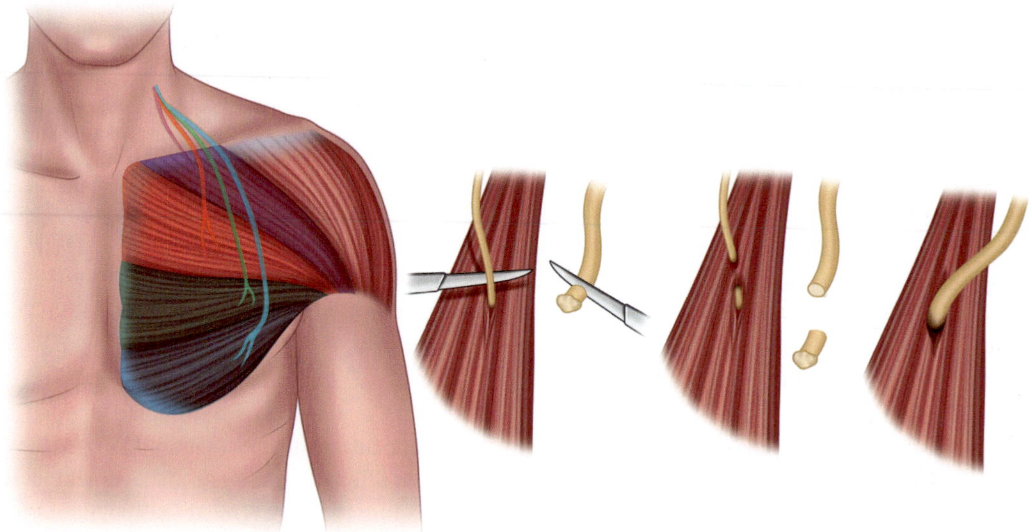

Fig. 17.25 Targeted muscle reinnervation (TMR). (Courtesy of Dr. Gregory A Dumanian, Chicago, IL)

current standard of direct myoelectric control, there is a one-to-one relationship between the signaling muscle belly and the receiving electrode. In pattern recognition, this is replaced with an array of multiple electrodes positioned around the surface of the residual limb. The patient is then asked to generate the muscle activities they associate with the desired prosthetic movements. As they do so, a processor records and later recognizes these EMG patterns, signaling the prosthesis to perform the desired motions [27]. This strategy increases the number of discrete myoelectric input signals that can be produced by the residual limb and requires less training than a two-site system since the muscle contractions are intuitive. TMR and pattern recognition have been combined to yield still further accuracy in myoelectric control [31].

Sensory Restoration

The most pronounced limitation of current upper limb prosthetic rehabilitation is the inability to relay sensory input from the prosthesis to the individual. As a result, patients may disassociate their prosthesis from themselves, viewing it merely as a tool. The ability to restore sensory input from the environment, through the prosthesis, and into the user's nervous system would likely improve both the acceptance and performance of upper limb prostheses.

Such sensory restoration has recently been described through the use of implanted cuff electrodes wrapped around peripheral nerves and connecting to the prosthesis through percutaneous electrical leads [32]. To date, the longest tenured implanted sensory electrodes have been reported at 40 months [30]. Mechanical sensors integrated into the prosthetic hand permit the realization of input signals relating to both prehensile force and hand span. These signals are then transmitted through percutaneous leads to the internal cuff electrodes, where they are experienced as sensory input. As reasonably expected, preliminary results indicate that this restoration of sensory input improves both performance and confidence with an upper limb prosthesis [30].

Attachment

An immediate connection between the residual limb and the prosthesis can be obtained through osseointegration, as the limb prosthesis is attached to a percutaneous implant that is integrated to the remaining bone or bones of the residual limb. This topic is explored in detail in the subsequent chapter.

Aggregated Advancements

Several of the advancements presented above have been creatively combined to produce an osseointegrated human-machine gateway (OHMG) [33]. Performed at the transhumeral amputation level, an osseointegrated abutment connecting the residual humerus with an external prosthesis, also houses bidirectional leads. These leads conduct motor impulses from epimysial electrodes to the prosthesis, as well as sensory impulses from the prosthesis to the sensory nerves of the limb. Myoelectric signals are processed using pattern recognition algorithms to more accurately differentiate the desired control motions of the prosthetic hand, wrist, and elbow [31]. These aggregated prosthetic advances simultaneously address the current limitations of prosthetic control, sensory restoration, and mechanical connection in a single, radically creative solution. These systems are not yet common in clinical practice.

Prosthetic Designs and Fittings for the Lower Extremity

Anticipated Outcomes with Lower Limb Prostheses

Most patients, especially young survivors of trauma who have sufficient strength, limb length, joint mobility, manageable pain, and a lack of other compounding injuries, can be expected to walk well with a lower limb prosthesis [34]. Prosthetic technology and modern materials continue to evolve at a rapid rate and now make it possible for prosthetists to design and create devices that offer the wearer greater comfort and a more natural gait than ever before. These advances give patients the function and confidence to return to active and productive lives, often in their former fields of endeavor. A few of these developments include (1) gel liners that are especially useful in cushioning and protecting unusual and challenging residual limb shapes resulting from blast, crush, and degloving injuries (some liners can also dissipate heat or perspiration), (2) adjustable sockets that allow the wearer to instantly customize the fit of their prosthesis, and (3) microprocessors and sensors which provide safety from falls, reduce energy cost, provide instant response to variations in gait and terrain, and have user selectable modes for a variety of function needs such as driving, extended standing, or playing sports. Technology is also available to assist patients who need prostheses that are custom designed or specially adapted for their vocational and recreational needs. People who work in outdoor environments, such as gardeners, fishermen, and wounded military warriors, can be provided with prosthetic devices which will function under harsh environmental conditions including the dusty and rugged conditions in conflict zones.

Honesty about expected outcomes is essential in all patient interactions; however, a positive attitude should be shared with patients to motivate them for the hard work of rehabilitation ahead.

Amputation Level-Specific Considerations

Each level of amputation presents unique considerations and challenges, especially with bilateral amputations. The higher the level of amputation, the more energy it will take to utilize the prosthesis. The basic design elements of a lower limb prosthesis include (1) a gel liner worn against the skin, (2) the socket in which the residual limb is placed, (3) suspension method, (4) prosthetics

components such as a foot, knee, and hip joint, and (5) adjustable connectors which allow for alignment changes. Crucial to the successful fitting of any prosthesis is a comfortable socket. When effectively fit, the socket connects and transfers forces from the wearer through the prosthesis to the ground and vice versa with minimal internal movement. It also distributes the pressure of weight-bearing in ways that prevent tissue breakdown. This is especially important when a mangled limb has been degloved or requires grafted skin for healing.

Patients with significant skin grafts typically become accustomed to wearing the gel coverings over their skin before they begin standing in the prosthetic device. This adjustment period can take anywhere from a few weeks to a number of months, before the wearer can be safely fitted with a weight-bearing prosthesis that will not compromise the healing skin grafts. The gel liner can be prevented from adhering to skin grafts through the use of impregnated powders which are replaced with fresh materials when they begin to lose their non-adherent properties.

Partial Foot Amputations

Partial foot amputations encompass a wide range of presentations, from missing toes to an almost complete absence of the foot with only the calcaneus remaining. Prosthetic devices for this level are similarly varied. Options range from ankle foot orthoses (AFO) with toe fillers to knee height prostheses (Fig. 17.26). Selection is based primarily on the users' need for push off at the end of stance phase, stability, and cushioning. To biomechanically substitute for the loss of the forefoot, the prosthesis must extend up to the tibial tubercle height [35].

When the entire foot has been mangled and skin grafts performed on the remaining portion of the foot, creating a prosthesis to effectively support a residual foot covered with abnormally fragile skin can present a challenge. The person's

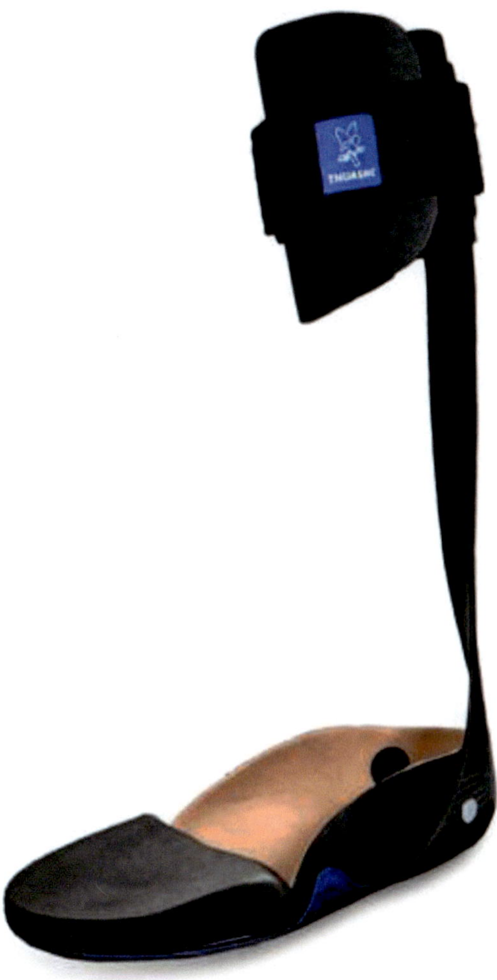

Fig. 17.26 Carbon fiber partial foot prosthesis. (Courtesy of Thuasne USA – Townsend Design, Bakersfield, CA, and Chris Toelle, LCO, Hanger Clinic, Austin, TX)

ability to ambulate comfortably on a skin-grafted foot may be limited, regardless of the prosthetic design. In such cases, the possibility of a higher level revision amputation should be raised and carefully considered. In situations where the foot is extremely painful, the patient's quality of life may be better if it is amputated so that a more successful and functional prosthesis can be fit to a healthier more resilient residual limb at the Syme's or transtibial level [34].

Syme's Amputation

An amputation at the Syme's or ankle disarticulation level can result in a very successful prosthetic outcome given the long residual limb lever arm, especially if the heel pad and plantar surface of the foot are salvaged to allow for distal end weight-bearing. The shortcomings of an amputation at this level are a somewhat bulbous prosthetic socket to accommodate the residual limb and limited space for the prosthetic foot. Patients who are especially concerned with their appearance may be unwilling to accept an unattractively shaped ankle. This cosmetic shortcoming must be explained to the patient in careful detail in advance to prevent regrets, disappointment, and potential depression following the amputation.

Transtibial (Below-Knee) Amputation

Transtibial patients with well-reconstructed residual limbs, as described above, have a high probability of successful outcomes. Prosthetic devices at the transtibial amputation level allow patients to be very active, including running and jumping unless there are complications. There are numerous design and component options which need to be individually selected for each patient.

In cases where an uninjured foot must be sacrificed due to vascular damage, the surgeon may be able to avoid a higher-level amputation by salvaging the intact tissue from the sole of the foot. Suturing that thick, strong plantar tissue into place, where the lower leg has been mangled, can create a skin graft that endows the residual limb with exceptional weight-bearing capabilities similar to those of the sole of the foot in its original position (Fig. 17.27). This procedure is best attempted by a plastic surgeon who has considerable experience and skill with skin grafting.

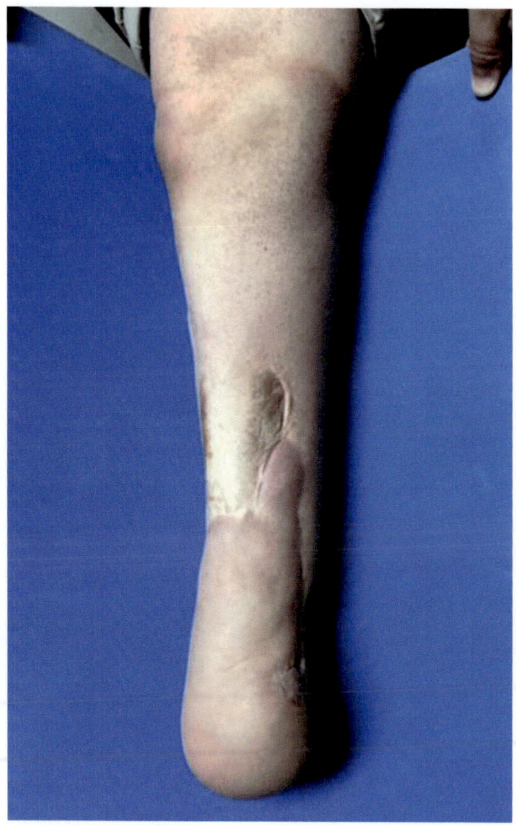

Fig. 17.27 Amputation with plantar skin of the foot transferred to distal tibia. (Courtesy of Hanger Clinic, Austin, TX)

Knee Disarticulation Amputation

A knee disarticulation is an excellent amputation choice because the patient can typically bear some or all of their weight on the end of the residual limb. The long limb length and the preservation of the thigh muscles and their insertions afford a significant mechanical advantage to patients, allowing them to walk and function with efficiency and power. Like the Syme's amputation, some patients find the appearance of the protruding femoral condyles to be unattractive. In addition, when seated, the prosthetic knee will extend outward further than the sound side. A very specific conversation needs to be scheduled with the patient to ensure that they understand what the post-amputation limb will look like, both with and without a prosthesis in place.

Transfemoral (Above-Knee) Amputation

There is good potential for prosthetic success at the transfemoral level. However, learning to walk on a device which includes a prosthetic knee is more challenging than using prosthesis designed for the more distal level amputations. The rehabilitation time is extended considerably, and the expenditure of energy to operate the prosthesis is also greater than at the more proximal levels.

Appropriately anchored musculature will enhance the chance of a successful prosthetic outcome. Myodesis, the surgical reattachment of the divided muscles to the femur, is recommended for residual limb power and stabilization. When muscles are not attached to the bone, they pull against themselves when contracted and can rotate around the femur and do not provide the strength and stability needed for optimal prosthetic control.

Ideally the patient's intact skin is used for surgical closure. However, even when skin grafts, invaginated areas, and other challenging aspects of a mangled transfemoral residual limb are present, modern flexible socket systems and new exceptional gel and silicone materials allow prosthetists to work creatively around most skin issues. User adjustable sockets provide comfort and suspension even as the wearer's residual limb changes volume throughout the day (Fig. 17.28).

Bilateral transfemoral amputation exponentially complicates and extends the rehabilitation process, as well as increasing the energy expenditure, strength, and balance needed to use prostheses. Our research and clinical experience indicate best results are achieved by starting bilateral transfemoral patients on very short prostheses and gradually increasing the length as they progress through rehab [36]. In addition, a concerted effort should be made to locate rehabilitation professionals with expertise in working with bilateral and very proximal level prosthetic patients.

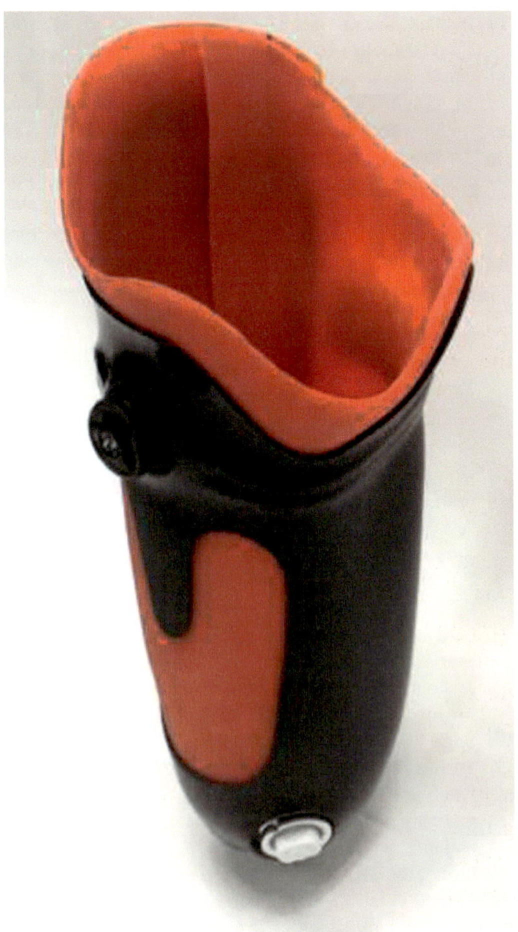

Fig. 17.28 ComfortFlex Adapt™ user adjustable transfemoral prosthetic socket. (Courtesy of Hanger Clinic, Austin, TX)

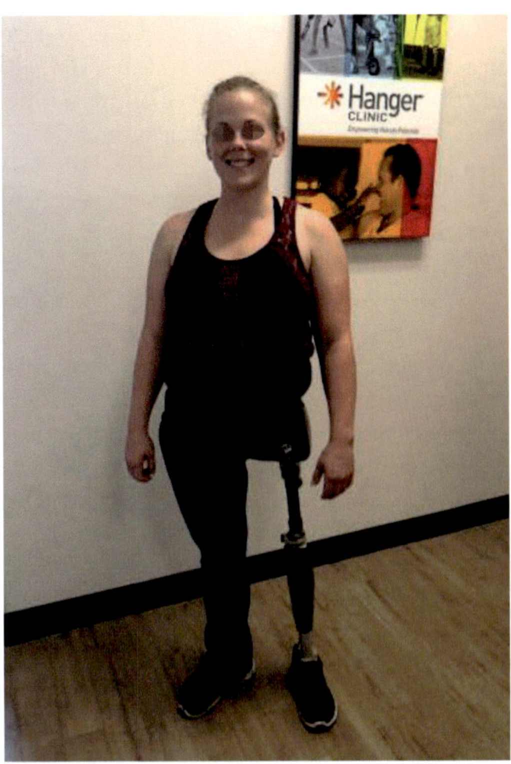

Fig. 17.29 Hip disarticulation prosthesis with flexible silicone inner socket. (Courtesy of Hanger Clinic, Austin, TX)

Hip Disarticulation and Hemipelvectomy Amputation

Injuries resulting in hip-level amputation present the most difficult challenge for a prosthetic fitting. In spite of these challenges, numerous individuals who have had crush injuries to the pelvis have successfully been rehabilitated and are walking on prostheses. Since no extrinsic muscles are available to drive the prosthesis, the patients must use their abdominals to step forward. The prosthetic hip and knee then provide stability for the stance phase of gait. Especially challenging in traumatic amputations at this level is when the skin and muscles are not available to cover the remaining bones of the pelvis. Fortunately, silicone socket technology can be configured to protect exposed bony areas while preventing the skin from chafing or breaking down. Variable durometers in different areas of the inner socket provide cushioning and firmness where needed. The natural tackiness of the silicone also prevents the prosthesis from twisting and turning (Fig. 17.29).

Advancements in Lower Limb Amputation and Prosthetics

The Ewing amputation is a recent amputation technique which prepares the limb for an agonist-antagonist myoneural interface (AMI). This system comprises a surgical construct and neural control architecture designed to serve as a bidirectional interface. It is capable of reflecting proprioceptive sensation of prosthetic joint position, speed, and torque from an advanced limb prosthesis onto the central nervous system. "The AMI offers the possibility of improved prosthetic control and restoration of muscle-tendon proprioception" [37]. Early trials of prosthetic designs include the ability to dorsiflex and plantarflex as well as invert and evert a motorized prosthetic ankle.

Advances in surgical techniques, microprocessor control, human prosthetic interfaces, and battery capacities continue to improve patients' function, comfort, and the responsiveness of their prosthetic devices. Discoveries in pain control [38, 39] and methods to help people cope with the trauma of an amputation are ongoing. We expect these innovations to continue to the benefit of prosthetic users in the future.

References

1. Doukas WC, et al. The Military Extremity Trauma Amputation/Limb Salvage (METALS) Study: Outcomes of Amputation Versus Limb Salvage Following Major Lower-Extremity Trauma. J Bone Joint Surg. 2013;95(2):138–45.
2. Staruch RMT, et al. Comparing the surgical timelines of military and civilians traumatic lower limb amputations. Ann Med Surg. 2016;6:81–6.
3. Ziegler-Graham K, MacKenzie EJ, Ephraim PL, Travison TG, Brookmeyer R. Estimating the prevalence of limb loss in the United States: 2005 to 2050. Arch Phys Med Rehabil. 2008;89:422–9.
4. Esquenazi A, Yoo SK. Lower limb amputations – epidemiology and assessment. PM&R Now website. https://now.aapmr.org/lower-limb-amputations-epidemiology-and-assessment/#references. Updated 5/03/2016.
5. Stansbury LG, et al. Amputations in U.S. Military personnel in the current conflicts in Afghanistan and Iraq. J Orthop Trauma. 2008;22:1.
6. Clasper J, Ramasamy A. Traumatic amputations. Br J Pain. 2013;7(2):67–73.
7. Wallace D. Trends in traumatic limb amputation in Allied Forces in Iraq and Afghanistan. J Mil Vet Health. 2012;20(2):31–5.
8. Honkamp N, Amendola A, Hurwitz S, Saltzman CL. Retrospective review of eighteen patients who underwent transtibial amputation for intractable pain. J Bone Joint Surg Am. 2001;83(10):1479–83.
9. Smith DG, McFarland LV, Sangeorzan BJ, Reiber GE, Czerniecki JM. Postoperative dressing and management strategies for transtibial amputations: a critical review. J Rehabil Res Dev. 2003;40(3):213–24.
10. Nawijn SE, van der Linde H, Emmelot CH, Hofstad CJ. Prosthetics Orthot Int. 2005;29(1):13–26.
11. Smith D. General principles of amputation surgery. In: Smith D, Michael J, Bowker J, editors. *Atlas of amputations and limb deficiencies: Surgical, prosthetic, and rehabilitation principles.* 3rd ed. Rosemont: American Academy of Orthopaedic Surgeons; 2004. p. 27–8.
12. Stevens P, Rheinstein J, Campbell J. Acute postoperative care of the residual limb following transtibial amputation: a clinical practice guideline. Arch Phys Med Rehabil. 2016;97(10):21.
13. Reichmann JP, Stevens PM, Rheinstein J, Kreulen CD. Removable rigid dressings for postoperative management of transtibial amputations: a review of published evidence. PM&R. 2018;10:516–23. https://doi.org/10.1016/j.pmrj.2017.10.002.
14. Churilov I, Churilov L, Murphy D. Do rigid dressings reduce the time from amputation to prosthetic fitting? A systematic review and meta-analysis. Ann Vasc Surg. 2014;28(7):1801–8.
15. Pinzur MS. The dark side of amputation rehabilitation: commentary on an article by COL (Ret) William C. Doukas, MD, et al.: "The Military Extremity Trauma Amputation/Limb Salvage (METALS) study outcomes of amputation versus limb salvage following major lower-extremity trauma". J Bone Joint Surg. 2013;95(2):e12.
16. Wurdeman SR, Stevens PM, Campbell JH. Mobility Analysis of AmpuTees (MAAT I): quality of life and satisfaction are strongly related to mobility for patients with a lower limb prosthesis. Prosthetics Orthot Int. 2018;42(5):498–503.
17. Desmond DM, MacLachlan M. Prevalence and characteristics of phantom limb pain and residual limb pain in the long term after upper limb amputation. J Rehabil Res. 2010;33:279–82.
18. Davidson JH, Khor KE, Jones LE. A cross-sectional study of post-amputation pain in upper and lower limb amputees, experience of a tertiary referral amputee clinic. Disabil Rehabil. 2010;32(22):1855–62.
19. Ostlie K, Franklin RJ, Skjeldal OH, Skrondal A, Magnus P. Musculoskeletal pain and overuse syndromes in adult acquired major upper-limb amputees. Arch Phys Med Rehabil. 2011;92:1967–73.
20. Hanley ME, Ehde DM, Jensen M, Czerniecki J, Smith DG, Robinson LR. Chronic pain associated with upper-limb loss. Am J Phys Med Rehabil. 2009;9(88):742–54.
21. Postema SG, BOngers RM, Brouwers MA, Burger H, Norling-Hermansson LM, REneman MF, Dijkstra PU, and van der Sluis CK. Musculoskeletal complaints in transverse upper limb reduction deficiency and amputation in the Netherlands: prevalence, predictors, and impact on health. Arch Phys Med Rehabil. 2016.
22. Jones LE, Davidson JH. Save that arm: a study of problems in the remaining arm of unilateral upper limb amputees. Prosthetics Orthot Int. 1999;23:55–8.
23. Datta D, Selvarajah K, Davey N. Functional outcome of patients with proximal upper limb defi-

ciency--acquired and congenital. Clin Rehabil. 2004 Mar;18(2):172–7.

24. Nimhurchadha S, Gallagher P, MacLachlan M, Wegener ST. Identifying successful outcomes and important factors to consider in upper limb amputation rehabilitation: an international web-based Delphi survey. Disabil Rehabil. 2013;35(20):1726–33.

25. Biddiss EA, Chau TT. Upper limb prosthesis use and abandonment: a survey of the last 25 years. Prosthetics Orthot Int. 2007 Sep;31(3):236–57.

26. Gaston RG, Bracey JW, Tait MA, Loeffler BJ. A novel muscle transfer for independent digital control of a myoelectric prosthesis: the starfish procedure. J Hand Surg Am. 2019;44(2):163.

27. Stevens PM, Europe's pursuit of a better transhumeral residual limb, O&P edge, May 2017. https://opedge.com/Articles/ViewArticle/2017-04-21/2017-05_02

28. Lipshutz RD. Targeted muscle Reinnervation: prosthetic management. In: Krabich JI, Pinzur MS, Potter BK, Stevens PM, editors. Atlas of amputations and limb deficiencies: surgical, prosthetic, and rehabilitation principles. 4th ed. IL, American Academy of Orthopedic Surgeons: Rosemont; 2016. p. 339–50.

29. Dumanian GA, et al. Ongers RM, Broneuroma and phantom pain in major limb. Amputees Random ClinTrial Ann Surg. 2019;270(2):238–46.

30. Woo SL, Kung TA, Brown DL, Leonard JA, Kelly BM, Cederna PSI. Regenerative peripheral nerve interfaces for the treatment of post amputation neuroma pain: A Pilot Study. Plast Reconstr Surg Glob Open. 2016;4(12):e1038.

31. Cheesborough JE, Smith LH, Kuiken TA, Dumanian GA. Targeted muscle reinnervation and advanced prosthetic arms. Semin Plast Surg. 2015;29(1):62–72.

32. Schiefer M, Tan D, Sidek SM, Tyler JD. Sensory feedback by peripheral nerve stimulation improves task performance in individuals with upper limb loss using a myoelectric prosthesis. J Neural Eng. 2016;13(1):016001.

33. Ortiz-Catalan M, Hakansson B, Branemark R. An osseointegrated human-machine gateway for long-term sensory feedback and motor control of artificial limbs. Sci Trans Med. 2014;6(257):257re6.

34. Doukas WC, et al. The Military Extremity Trauma Amputation/Limb Salvage (METALS) Study: outcomes of amputation versus limb salvage following major lower-extremity trauma. J Bone Joint Surg. 2013;95(2):138–45.

35. Berke G, Rheinstein J, Michael J, Stark G. Biomechanics of ambulation following partial foot amputation: a prosthetic perspective. J Prosthet Ortho. 2007;19(8):85–8.

36. Irolla C, Rheinstein J, Richardson R, Simpson C, Carroll K. Evaluation of a graduated length prosthetic protocol for bilateral Transfemoral amputee prosthetic rehabilitation. J Prosthet Ortho. April 2013;25(2):84–8.

37. Tyler R. The ewing amputation: the first human implementation of the agonist-antagonist myoneural interface. Plast Reconstr Surg. 2018;6(11):e1997.

38. Hunter CW, Yang A, Davis T. Selective radiofrequency stimulation of the dorsal root ganglion (DRG) as a method for predicting targets for neuromodulation in patients with post amputation pain: a case series. Neuromodulation. 2017;20(7):708–18.

39. Soin A, Shah NS, Fang ZP. High-frequency electrical nerve block for post amputation pain: a pilot study. Neuromodulation. 2015 Apr;18(3):197–205.

The Mangled Extremity: Osseointegration

Ashley B. Anderson and Jonathan A. Forsberg

Background

Civilian and military service members with trans-humeral amputations often have difficulties with currently available socket-based suspension [1, 2]. Recent advances in upper extremity prosthetics, including those with multiple degrees of freedom, improved terminal device control, and even artificial sensory feedback, have done little to improve the rate of abandonment, in part, because of the way the prosthetics interface with the upper extremity.

In conventional prosthetic usage, a range of problems encountered by amputees wearing sockets have been described including soft tissue trauma, socket discomfort, inadequate methods of suspension, excessive perspiration, and intolerance to interface materials [3–5]. Difficulties arise, in large part, due to the way

A. B. Anderson (✉)
Walter Reed National Military Medical Center, Department of Surgery Division of Orthopaedics, Bethesda, MD, USA

Uniformed Services University, Bethesda, MD, USA

J. A. Forsberg
Walter Reed National Military Medical Center, Department of Surgery Division of Orthopaedics, Bethesda, MD, USA

Uniformed Services University, Bethesda, MD, USA

Department of Orthopaedic Surgery, Johns Hopkins University, Baltimore, MD, USA
e-mail: jforsbe1@jhmi.edu

current prostheses attach to the body. Modern prostheses require a socket that transfers the force generated by a patient's environment (e.g., by the ground when walking) to the patient's skin, subcutaneous soft tissues, and muscle envelope before being transferred to the appendicular skeleton.

With traditional sockets, issues also occur with soft tissue management. For example, split thickness skin grafts are often used to preserve residual limb length but are less durable and more prone to ulceration under traditional sockets. Also, there is as much as a 60% incidence of heterotopic ossification observed in the combat-wounded population [2, 6, 7], and this high rate exacerbates socket problems by causing tissue complications, ulcerations, and local pain and increases the number of symptomatic neuromas [8, 9]. All these issues can severely restrict or curtail the amputee's ability and desire to effectively use a prosthesis, resulting in a negative impact on all aspects of function and quality of life.

Transdermal implants, conversely, allow for direct skeletal attachment of external prosthetics, therefore eliminating the need for socket-based suspension. Often called "osseointegration," the technique anchors an external prosthetic directly to the skeleton via a metallic bony implant or interface, thereby obviating the need for a socket. Bone-anchored prosthetics have the potential to facilitate an improvement in the quality of life for

© Springer Nature Switzerland AG 2021
R. A. Pensy, J. V. Ingari (eds.), *The Mangled Extremity*, https://doi.org/10.1007/978-3-319-56648-1_18

amputees who are unable to function and mobilize effectively using conventional socket prostheses [10].

Osseointegration

Osseointegration is defined as the apposition of cortical bone onto a metal implant. Professor Per-Ingvar Brånemark discovered the osseointegrative properties of bone onto titanium in the 1950s and then went on to develop a series of titanium implants for use in craniomaxillofacial reconstruction [11]. In oral surgery, the concept of direct skeletal anchorage of titanium implants is considered as state-of-the-art therapy for edentulism [4]. Since 1965 more than 600,000 edentulous patients have been treated, and a recently published meta-analysis [12] showed a long-term success rate of 92.8%. The method is also used in ENT surgery for anchorage of epistheses, for reconstruction of craniomaxillofacial defects after tumor surgery, and for anchorage of external hearing aids [13].

The surgical application of bone-anchored implants to facilitate the secure fixation of external prostheses for upper and lower extremity amputees has been the subject of increasing interest and extensive research for many years. Early experimentations both in animal and human subjects such as that described by Cutler and Blodgett [14], Mooney [15], Esslinger [16], and Hall and Rostoker [17–20] were all discontinued after relatively short periods of time. Problems encountered during the experimentation are reviewed by Ling [21].

The technique termed osseointegration developed by Professor Per-Ingvar Brånemark in the mid-1960s had become firmly established in the field of dental implant technology [11]. Professor Rickard Brånemark (Per-Ingvar's son) later applied this technique to long bones in 1990 when he introduced a pure titanium fixture into the femur of a transfemoral amputee in the first stage (Stage 1) of a two-stage surgical procedure [3, 10]. The second stage surgery (Stage 2) entailed the refashioning of the soft tissue and introduction of a titanium abutment into the internal fixture secured under tension with

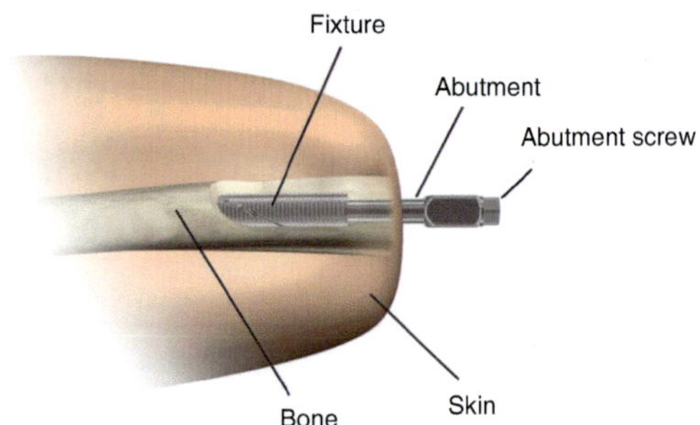

Fig. 18.1 The Osseointegrated Prostheses for the Rehabilitation of Amputees (OPRA) consists of three parts: the fixture, the abutment, and the abutment screw. Reproduced with permission and copyright © of the British Editorial Society of Bone and Joint Surgery [12]

a titanium alloy screw [10]. Now known as the Osseointegrated Prostheses for the Rehabilitation of Amputees (OPRA), the titanium abutment protruded through the skin as the point of attachment for the external prosthesis (Figs. 18.1 and 18.2) [22]. This eliminated the requirement of a prosthetic socket to transmit forces and contain the soft tissue of the residual limb during gait.

The OPRA technique is not the only method of bone-anchored prosthetic attachment. Other methods of skeletal attachment have been developed or are under development. Alternative skeletal anchorage methods include the intraosseous transcutaneous amputation prosthesis (ITAP) [23] and the method described by Aschoff et al. previously termed the endo-exo device and now termed the integral system [24]. Figure 18.2 an osseointegrated prosthesis in a transhumeral amputee (Photo courtesy of Dr. John Ingari).

Primary Aim of Prosthetic Management

Skalak and Brånemark cite several definitions of osseointegration from varying perspectives [25]. However, Esposito and coauthors summarize them nicely from the amputee's viewpoint; osseointegration can be defined as the following [12]:

> A fixture is osseointegrated if it provides a stable and apparently immobile support of a prosthesis under functional loads, without pain, inflammation, or loosening.

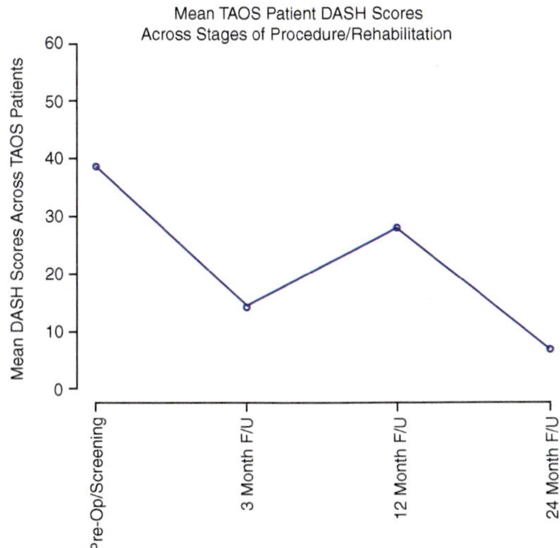

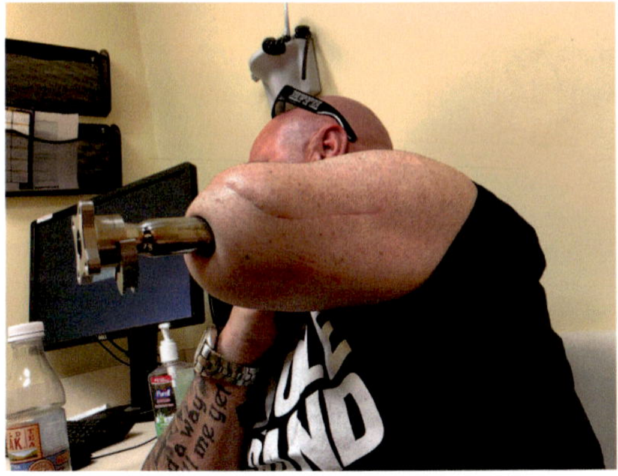

Fig. 18.2 Mean TAOS Patient DASH Scores across stages of OPRA procedure and rehabilitation where a decrease in DASH score signifies patient improvement [30, 32]. (TAOS, Transhumeral Amputee Osseointegration Study; DASH, Disabilities of the Arm, Shoulder, and Hand; OPRA, Osseointegrated Prostheses for the Rehabilitation of Amputees). Osseointegrated prosthesis for transhumeral amputee allows for multiple terminal devices

However, the biological definition is much more basic, reflecting the relationship between the bone and the internal fixation device. In this context the term is defined as:

> Osseointegration of a fixture in bone is defined as the close apposition of new and reformed bone in congruence with the fixture, including surface irregularities, so that at light microscopic level, there is no interpositioned connective or fibrous tissue and that a direct structural and functional connection is established, capable of carrying normal physiological loads without excessive deformation and without initiating rejecting mechanisms.

With this in mind, the primary objective in the early postoperative stage following osseointegration surgery is to promote this close apposition between new and reformed bone and the internal fixture [26]. Failure to achieve this objective through the premature application of excessive torsional or axial forces to the system will jeopardize the integrity of the fixture within the bone [12]. This may result in the formation of interposing fibrous tissue between the implant and bone, therefore forming what is effectively a pseudarthrosis. Failure to achieve proper osseointegration will likely necessitate implant removal.

For this reason, OPRA has been developed as both a surgical technique and a rehab agenda focused on ensuring that osseointegration occurs, which will maintain the prosthesis over time and protect the long-term integrity of the internal fixture and associated components. As such, prosthetic components should not be considered or prescribed in isolation. The sum of the prosthetic components including the implant, abutment, retaining bolt failsafe mechanism, and the external prosthetic components must be viewed as a system working in harmony to preserve the intraosseous implant as well as facilitate optimal mobility and function for the amputee (Fig. 18.1) [22].

Previous Research

Although prior research in transdermal amputation osseointegration surgery focused primarily on the lower extremity, many principles apply to the upper extremity. For example, in transfemoral amputees, 51 patients treated with OPRA were followed for a minimum of 2 years [10]. Before and after assessments demonstrated statistically significant improvements in prosthetic use, mobility, and functional status. In addition, there were fewer interface issues when compared to their previous socket-based prosthesis [10]. Importantly, safety outcomes demonstrated 92% implant survival rate at 2 years, despite a relatively high rate of superficial infections [10]. Although infections occurred 41 times in 28 patients (54.9%), most were treated effectively with oral antibiotics [10]. Overall, four implants required removal, three for aseptic loosening, and one for infection [10].

One of the most interesting findings resulting from this cohort with skeletally anchored prostheses was their increased ability for distinguishing between different types of contact stimuli to the prosthetic foot. This phenomenon is called "osseoperception" and is particularly important for osseointegrated implants of the upper extremity [27]. It is also important to note that the forces generated by the upper extremity are far lower than those generated by the process of weight-bearing ambulation. In addition, the soft tissue envelope is typically more stable in the arm when compared to the thigh, which may result in a decreased rate of superficial infection. Therefore, osseointegrated implants for the upper extremity are theorized to be less problematic than those used for the lower extremity.

Tsikandylakis et al. reported on 18 transhumeral amputees that underwent osseointegration using the OPRA [22]. The 2- and 5-year implant survival was 85% and 82%, respectively. Like the lower extremity, superficial infections were the most common adverse events, and the 2- and 5-year incidence was 18% (3 of 16) and 35% (5 of 14), respectively [22]. However, infections in the upper extremity were much less frequent than in the lower extremity. Their treatment included local mechanical cleaning of the transdermal interface, local or oral antibiotics and restriction of soft tissue mobility by using a silicone liner, and surgical revision of the prosthesis in two of the five cases. Only one implant required removal due to deep infection that occurred 3.5 years after the Stage 2 procedure. Importantly, all but one patient was able to continue using their prosthesis during the infection treatment process [22].

Lower Extremity Application

Like the upper extremity, multiple lower extremity percutaneous implant systems exist for clinical use [28]. Each system balances the goal to generate a stable bone-implant interface while avoiding complications such as infection and loosening. Patients with lower extremity amputations often experi-

ence problems related to the use of socket-suspended prostheses. The clinical development of osseointegrated percutaneous prostheses for patients with a transfemoral amputation started in 1990 [10]. Today, there are numerous osseointegrated implants under development for patients with lower extremity amputation. The five most commonly available systems are the following: OPRA, the compress transcutaneous implant (CTI), the integral leg prosthesis (ILP), the osseointegrated prosthetic limb (OPL), and the percutaneous osseointegrated prosthesis (POP) [28]. However, the only implant that is currently FDA approved is the OPRA system [28]. Like the upper extremity, the clinical indications include the following key patient characteristics: complications with a conventional socket prosthesis, skeletal maturity, adequate bone stock in the residual limb, compliance with a rehabilitation protocol, and good overall health [10, 24, 26, 28–32].

Where We Are Today

The Department of Defense is conducting a clinical safety trial called the Transhumeral Amputee Osseointegration Study (TAOS) with OPRA device for transhumeral amputee during the stages of procedure through the course of rehabilitation [33]. So far, in the six-patient cohort, Disabilities of the Arm, Shoulder, and Hand (DASH) scores as well as Patient-Reported Outcomes Measurement Information System (PROMIS) both show trends toward improvement at 24-month follow-up when compared to preoperative screening (Figs. 18.2 and 18.3) [34, 35]. Importantly, at a median follow-up of 1 year, none of the study participants demonstrated any implant-related complications or adverse events related to osseointegration surgery. However, as more patients enroll, we are continuing to establish and verify the safety and the performance of the transhumeral OPRA and compare functional status to transhumeral amputees with their socket-based prostheses. A similar study, the Transfemoral Amputee Osseointegration Study (TFAOS), is also underway with the Department of Defense.

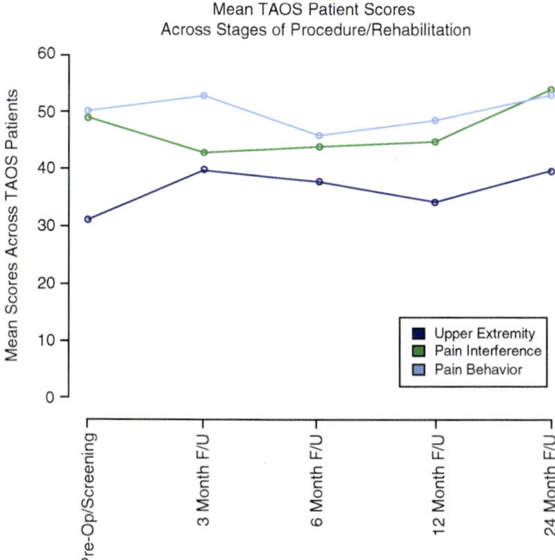

Fig. 18.3 Mean TAOS Patient PROMIS Scores across stages of OPRA procedure and rehabilitation where an increase in PROMIS score signifies patient improvement [31, 32]. (TAOS, Transhumeral Amputee Osseointegration Study; PROMIS, Patient-Reported Outcomes Measurement Information System; OPRA, Osseointegrated Prosthesis for the Rehabilitation of Amputees)

In conclusion, bone- anchored, or "osseointegrated," prosthetics continue to have the potential to facilitate an improvement in the quality of life for amputees who are unable to function and mobilize effectively using conventional socket prostheses [10, 22]. With continued research, these prosthetics are promising rehabilitation and functional alternatives for patients with transhumeral amputations when compared to traditional socket prostheses. However, comparative studies are still needed to support its potential utility for a broader patient population and demonstrate possible superiority as a prosthetic system.

References

1. Wright TW, Hagen AD, Wood MB. Prosthetic usage in major upper extremity amputations. J Hand Surg. 1995;20(4):619–22. https://doi.org/10.1016/s0363-5023(05)80278-3.
2. Alfieri KA, Forsberg JA, Potter BK. Blast injuries and heterotopic ossification. Bone Jt Res. 2012;1(8):174–9. https://doi.org/10.1302/2046-3758.18.2000102.
3. Krajbich JI, Pinzur MS, Potter BK, Stevens PM. Atlas of amputations and limb deficiencies: surgical, prosthetic and rehabilitation principles. 4th ed. 2004.
4. Adell R, Eriksson B, Lekholm U, Brånemark PI, Jemt T. Long-term follow-up study of osseointegrated implants in the treatment of totally edentulous jaws. Int J Oral Maxillofac Implant. 1990;5(4):347–59.
5. Aschoff H-H, Clausen A, Tsoumpris K, Hoffmeister T. Implantation der Endo-Exo-Femurprothese zur Verbesserung der Mobilität amputierter Patienten. Oper Orthop Traumatol. 2011;23(5):462–72. https://doi.org/10.1007/s00064-011-0054-6.
6. Potter BK, Burns TC, Lacap AP, Granville RR, Gajewski DA. Heterotopic ossification following traumatic and combat-related amputations. J Bone Jt Surg. 2007;89(3):476–86. https://doi.org/10.2106/jbjs.f.00412.
7. Potter MBK, Forsberg LJA, Davis TA, et al. Heterotopic ossification following combat-related trauma. J Bone Jt Surg. 2010;92:74–89. https://doi.org/10.2106/jbjs.j.00776.
8. Tintle LSM, Baechler LMF, Nanos CGP, Forsberg LJA, Potter MBK. Traumatic and trauma-related amputations. J Bone Jt Surg. 2010;92(18):2934–45. https://doi.org/10.2106/jbjs.j.00258.
9. Tintle LSM, Baechler LMF, Nanos CGP, Forsberg LJA, Potter MBK. Reoperations following combat-related upper-extremity amputations. J Bone Jt Surg. 2012;94(16):e119. https://doi.org/10.2106/jbjs.k.00197.
10. Brånemark R, Berlin O, Hagberg K, Bergh P, Gunterberg B, Rydevik B. A novel osseointegrated percutaneous prosthetic system for the treatment of patients with transfemoral amputation: a prospective study of 51 patients. Bone Jt J. 2014;96-B(1):106–13. https://doi.org/10.1302/0301-620x.96b1.31905.
11. Brånemark PI, Hansson BO, Adell R, et al. Osseointegrated implants in the treatment of the edentulous jaw. Experience from a 10-year period. Scand J Plastic Reconstr Surg Suppl. 1977;16:1–132.
12. Esposito M, Hirsch J, Lekholm U, Thomsen P. Biological factors contributing to failures of osseointegrated oral implants, (I). Success criteria and epidemiology. Eur J Oral Sci. 1998;106(1):527–51. https://doi.org/10.1046/j.0909-8836..t01-2-.x.
13. Håkansson B, Carlsson P. Skull simulator for direct bone conduction hearing devices. Scand Audiol. 1989;18(2):91–8. https://doi.org/10.3109/01050398909070728.
14. Murphy EF. History and philosophy of attachment of prostheses to the musculoskeletal system and of passage through the skin with inert materials. J Biomed Mater Res. 1973;7(3):275–95. https://doi.org/10.1002/jbm.820070319.
15. Mooney V, Predecki PK, Renning J, Gray J. Skeletal extension of limb prosthetic attachments–problems in tissue reaction. J Biomed Mater Res. 1971;5(6):143–59. https://doi.org/10.1002/jbm.820050612.

16. Esslinger JO. A basic study in semi-buried implants and osseous attachments for application to amputation prosthetic fitting. Bull Prosthet Res. 1970;10(13):219–25.
17. Hall CW. Developing a permanently attached artificial limb. Bull Prosthetic Res. 1974;22:144–57.
18. Hall CW, Cox PA, Mallow WA. Sketeal exension development: criteria for future designs. Bull Prosthetic Res. 1976;10:69–94.
19. Hall CW. A future prosthetic limb device. J Rehabilitation Res Dev. 1985;22(3):99. https://doi.org/10.1682/jrrd.1985.07.0099.
20. Andersson GB, Gaechter A, Galante JO, Rostoker W. Segmental replacement of long bones in baboons using a fiber titanium implant. J Bone Jt Surg Am. 1978;60(1):31–40. https://doi.org/10.2106/00004623-197860010-00005.
21. Ling RSM. Observations on the Fixation of Implants to the Bony Skeleton. Clin Orthop Relat R. 1986;210(NA):80–96. https://doi.org/10.1097/00003086-198609000-00012.
22. Tsikandylakis G, Berlin Ö, Brånemark R. Implant survival, adverse events, and bone remodeling of Osseointegrated percutaneous implants for Transhumeral amputees. Clin Orthop Relat Res. 2014;472(10):2947–56. https://doi.org/10.1007/s11999-014-3695-6.
23. Kang NV, Pendegrass C, Marks L, Blunn G. Osseocutaneous integration of an intraosseous transcutaneous amputation prosthesis implant used for reconstruction of a transhumeral amputee: case report. J Hand Surg. 2010;35(7):1130–4. https://doi.org/10.1016/j.jhsa.2010.03.037.
24. Aschoff HH, Kennon RE, Keggi JM, Rubin LE. Transcutaneous, distal femoral, intramedullary attachment for above-the-knee prostheses. J Bone Jt Surg. 2010;92(Supplement & lowbar;2):180–6. https://doi.org/10.2106/jbjs.j.00806.
25. Skalak R. Biomechanical considerations in osseointegrated prostheses. J Prosthet Dent. 1983;49(6):843–8. https://doi.org/10.1016/0022-3913(83)90361-x.
26. Hagberg K, Brånemark R. One hundred patients treated with osseointegrated transfemoral amputation prostheses–rehabilitation perspective. J Rehabil Res Dev. 2009;46(3):331–44. https://doi.org/10.1682/jrrd.2008.06.0080.
27. Hagberg K, Häggström E, Jönsson S, Rydevik B, Brånemark R. Psychoprosthetics. London: Springer-Verlag London Limited; 2008. p. 131–40. https://doi.org/10.1007/978-1-84628-980-4_10.
28. Zaid MB, O'Donnell RJ, Potter BK, Forsberg JA. Orthopaedic osseointegration. J Am Acad Orthop Surg. 2019;27:e977–85. https://doi.org/10.5435/jaaos-d-19-00016.
29. Sullivan J, Uden M, Robinson KP, Sooriakumaran S. Rehabilitation of the trans-femoral amputee with an osseointegrated prosthesis: the United Kingdom experience. Prosthetics Orthot Int. 2003;27(2):114–20. https://doi.org/10.1080/03093640308726667.
30. Tillander J, Hagberg K, Hagberg L, Brånemark R. Osseointegrated titanium implants for limb prostheses attachments: infectious complications. Clin Orthop Relat Res. 2010;468(10):2781–8. https://doi.org/10.1007/s11999-010-1370-0.
31. Hagberg K, Brånemark R, Gunterberg B, Rydevik B. Osseointegrated trans-femoral amputation prostheses: prospective results of general and condition-specific quality of life in 18 patients at 2-year follow-up. Prosthetics Orthot Int. 2008;32(1):29–41. https://doi.org/10.1080/03093640701553922.
32. Muderis MA, Khemka A, Lord SJ, de Meent HV, Frölke JPM. Safety of osseointegrated implants for transfemoral amputees. J Bone Jt Surg. 2016;98(11):900–9. https://doi.org/10.2106/jbjs.15.00808.
33. Forsberg, JA. Transhumeral Amputee Osseointegration Study (TAOS) FDA Early Feasibility Study IDE#G150155.
34. Hudak PL, Amadio PC, Bombardier C, et al. Development of an upper extremity outcome measure: the DASH (disabilities of the arm, shoulder, and head). Am J Ind Med. 1996;29(6):602–8. https://doi.org/10.1002/(sici)1097-0274(199606)29:6<602::aid-ajim4>3.0.co;2-l.
35. Cella D, Yount S, Rothrock N, et al. The patient-reported outcomes measurement information system (PROMIS). Med Care. 2007;45(5):S3–S11. https://doi.org/10.1097/01.mlr.0000258615.42478.55\.

Index

© Springer Nature Switzerland AG 2021
R. A. Pensy, J. V. Ingari (eds.), *The Mangled Extremity*, https://doi.org/10.1007/978-3-319-56648-1

Printed by Printforce, the Netherlands